NEW DEVELOPMENTS IN MEDICAL RESEARCH

OREGANO

PROPERTIES, USES AND HEALTH BENEFITS

New Developments in Medical Research

Additional books in this series can be found on Nova's website
under the Series tab.

Plant Science Research and Practices

Additional e-books in this series can be found on Nova's website
under the e-book tab.

NEW DEVELOPMENTS IN MEDICAL RESEARCH

OREGANO

PROPERTIES, USES AND HEALTH BENEFITS

GEMA NIETO
EDITOR

nova
Medicine & Health
New York

Library of Congress Cataloging-in-Publication Data
ISBN: 978-1-53616-284-4
Library of Congress Control Number:2019950425

Published by Nova Science Publishers, Inc. † New York

CONTENTS

PREFACE

Humans have employed medicinal plants for thousands of years in traditional medicine. Oregano has been cultivated mainly for centuries in the Mediterranean area, although it now can be found on most continents. Oregano is one of the most popular plants in Spanish traditional remedies and its leaves have been used in traditional medicines in order to treat illness such as aching muscle, skin sores, asthma, digestion disorders, infections, inflammation or maintaining general health. In addition, oregano has been used since ancient times as an ingredient in Mediterranean diet. In this sense, there are several species of oregano, being Spanish thyme or Origanum vulgare, the spice variety sold most in the United States and Europe.

Nowadays the use of oregano is not exclusive for culinary proposes, because the consumers' concerns about the use of synthetic additives into foods have led the food industry to the search for green strategies.

In this sense, oregano extracts, essential oils and individual compounds from this herb have demonstrated antioxidant, anti-inflammatory, anticancer, and antimicrobial actions, which may contribute to the capacity to avoid human infections or to protect the cardiovascular and nervous systems by blood glucose and lipid modulation.

Therefore, based on the current scientific literature, oregano essential oil can be considered as a rich source of bioactive compounds and its addition to food matrices transmit these benefits; this approach can be used as a tool to generate functional foods.

This book reviews and discusses oregano containing several potent antimicrobial, antioxidant compounds that may contribute to benefit the nervous and cardiovascular systems. In addition, the opportunity of using Origanum vulgare as potential platform for producing polyphenols, biogas and energy under biorefinery approach has been discussed. Moreover, the possibility to be added into foods as natural additives and a strategy in order to improve human health was also discussed. In this sense, the inclusion of oregano into meat products, yogurt, juices and others could be an interesting strategy to produce functional foods.

The oregano extract and essential oil represents a good strategy in order to substitute synthetic antioxidants and to produce functional foods with an extended shelf life.

Several industries are now looking for sources of new, natural and safe agents. Essential oil from Origanum spp. has shown efficacy retarding lipid oxidation in food matrices. Oregano essential oil possesses strong antimicrobial activity against food pathogen bacteria highlighting its potential as a tool to achieve food safety. Oregano essential oil has shown efficacy in reducing microbial growth of deteriorative microorganisms (bacteria, yeast, molds), representing the potential to increase shelf-life of food. Oregano essential oil can be considered as a rich source of bioactive compounds and its addition to food matrices transmit these benefits; this approach can be used as a tool to generate functional foods. Results obtained from numerous studies can help to exploit the use of the Origanum EOs studied as the functional food and pharmacological ingredients for promoting health.

Chapter 1 - Oregano is a widely used spice in the food industry. It is mainly used for its aromatic properties with a primary role to enhance the taste and aroma of food. Oregano has been shown to exhibit antioxidative and antimicrobial activity due to the high content of oleanolic, ursolic, caffeic, rosemarinic, lithospermic acids, flavonoids, hydroquinones, tannins, and phenolic glycosides. Oregano, one kind of labiate *Origanum* plant that has been known for a long time as a popular remedy, is a very versatile plant. It was reported that *Origanum compactum* Benth., *Origanum minutiflorum* O. Schwarz and P.H. Davis, and *Origanum majorana* L. exhibit antifungal activity, antibacterial activity, and antimicrobial activity, respectively. In addition, it has been used widely in China as a kind of feed additive because it has a broad spectrum of action against bacteria, a rapid effect, and little residue, and now its antibacterial effect has been researched *in vitro* and *in vivo* all over the world. The oregano also exhibited antimicrobial properties against Gram-positive and Gram-negative bacterial strains including clinical isolates, against microscopic filamentous fungi and yeasts. The mechanism of antimicrobial activity is based on its principal components, i.e., thymol and carvacrol, which have antimicrobial properties. Plants which are rich in antioxidant compounds are presented in food industry. There are evident requirements for increasing application of natural antioxidants obtained from plant material. The use of synthetic antioxidants for prevention of free radical damage can involve questionable nutritional value and toxic side effects while natural antioxidants which occur in many plants reduce oxidative damage and help in preventing mutagenesis, carcinogenesis, and aging due to their radical scavenging activities. A number of studies focused on antioxidant activities of essential oils from various aromatic plants reported that the oregano essential oil has a considerable antioxidant effect on the the fat oxidation process. Many publications showed antioxidative activities of oregano. Nowadays there is an increasing interest for alternative and efficient compounds for food preservation, having the goal to replace antimicrobial chemical additives.

Chapter 2 - Along the years, cosmetics, fragrances and health care industry have been the basis for developing huge research on aromatic plants as a fundamental raw material for natural products. The demand for these products as well as the possibility to enhance the growing of strategic crops in isolated rural areas is very well connected with the idea of exploiting industrially all valuable compounds in the aromatic plants resulting in new profitable feedstocks. Colombia has been characterized as a potential natural products producer due to its large biodiversity. So many aromatic plants are cultivated in this country (e.g., basil, cilantro, laurel, oregano, rosemary, sage, calendula, etc.) being European oregano (Origanum vulgare) and American oregano (Lippia graveolens) two of the most commercialized oregano types. However, the bioactive compounds (carvacrol and thymol in case of oregano) are not totally used despite their renowned application in natural care and health industry as antioxidants, fungicidal and bactericidal compounds. The main industrial use of oregano is for culinary purposes, but technological extraction of polyphenols and antioxidants from leaves and flowers represent a great opportunity. Besides, the stem of the plant is obtained as a residue and it can be used as lignocellulosic substrate for anaerobic digestion in order to produce biogas, electricity and steam as integral products. This chapter states an opportunity of using Origanum vulgare as potential platform for producing polyphenols, biogas and energy under biorefinery approach. A techno-economic assessment will be carried out in order to compare the feasibility of stand-alone and biorefinery processes. Biorefinery approach enhances the economic performance at high scales and the stand-alone process is profitable at low scales, the environmental impact using all residues generated by the oregano processing is comparable with other biorefineries.

Chapter 3 - Oregano (*Origanum vulgare L.*) is an herbaceous plant native to the Mediterranean regions that has been used for medicinal purposes, owing to its antimicrobial, antioxidant and antifungal properties. In particular, the essential oil (EO) of this plant is extracted with the aim of being used mainly in pharmaceutical, cosmetic and food industry. Many of these EOs are safe compounds classified as GRAS (generally recognized as safe). The primary components of the oregano EO are:carvacrol and thymol. These main components are phenolic substances, responsible for the antimicrobial properties. The objective of this work was to evaluate the effect of the carvacrol addition (0.10% or 0.5% w/w) on the antimicrobial, mechanical and physical properties of self-supporting edible films based on native cassava starch (2.67% w/w) and hydroxypropyl methylcellulose (HPMC, 0.67% w/w), plasticized with glycerol (1.70% w/w) and additionally added with potassium sorbate (0.30% w/w). Moreover, the effect of different emulsification speeds (6500 rpm or 21500 rpm) on the film properties was analyzed. It was observed that the films were structurally amorphous and prone to yellow color. A high shear rate generated a higher solubility and tensile strength than the film obtained at a lower speed, while the deformation showed no significant differences between studied films. To evaluate the antimicrobial action, films were formulated with 0.50% w/w of carvacrol and the agar diffusion assay was carried out. The spoilage microorganisms of foods such as *Z. bailii, L. plantarum,* and *P. fluorescens* were tested, observing a complete inhibition of the microbial growth in the contact zone of the film with the agar. For this formulation, the physical properties were evaluated and compared with films containing only sorbate. It was evidenced that Elastic Modulus, rupture stress and deformation decreased with respect to those films that did not contain the component of the oregano EO. On the other hand, films did not show differences in color, water solubility and water vapor permeability. The results obtained provide essential information on the carvacrol performance as edible films component to increase the shelf life of food products and improve their quality, helping to optimize their production and behavior and to satisfy consumer demand for more natural and safe products, benign with the environment.

Chapter 4 - Oregano is one of the main seasonings used worldwide in the preparation of dishes at both household and industrial level because of its unique sensory properties. Moreover, the composition of oregano leaves has been associated with a preservative effect in food matrixes. The investigation of oregano composition revealed that products of secondary metabolism in plant tissues, mainly essential oils (e.g., terpenes) and phenolic compounds are the main classes of compounds to exert such an effect in food. Consequently, several studies explored the impact of oregano components in food. Some approaches have been developed in order to prevent food quality loss such as addition of oregano as an ingredient in the product formulation, soaking food matrix into a solution with oregano active compounds, production of nanoparticles, inclusion into films and into food package material. It is worth mentioning that the antimicrobial potential of oregano has been reported in meat, meat products, fish, fish products, vegetables, bread, oils, salad dressing and fruits. This chapter discusses the use of oregano extracts in food matrixes, which also includes technologies, antimicrobial mechanisms, and the relation between food matrix characteristics and enhancement of shelf life.

Chapter 5 - Oregano (*Origanum vulgare*) is a perennial herb used as condiment, that mainly grows in the Mediterranean region. However, different varieties of oregano also grow around Europe, Asia and Latinoamerica, each one with distinctive compounds that has been tested in order to know their possible health benefits. This aromatic spice is rich in antioxidant compounds such as monoterpens as carvacol, flavonoids as epicatechine, epigallocatechine, catequin, rutin, kaempferol, and luteonin, and phenolic acids as rosmarinic. Due to its molecular structure, its regular consumption has reported several beneficial effects such as antioxidant, anti-inflammatory, anticancer, and antimicrobial. For these reasons, the use of oregano extract is a good strategy to use in meat products to replace synthetics additives. Additionally, this extract has a pleasant odour and flavour, so it could be used in order to improve the organoleptic quality of the meat products when it is added as ingredient. The present review exposes the health benefits provided by oregano consumption and the latest research about its use on meat, together new trends about its application as ingredient in functional meat products will be exposed.

Chapter 6 - Oregano (*Origanum vulgare* L.) is a popular aromatic herb that belongs to the mint family (Lamiaceae). This plant is originally from warm to temperate regions of Eurasia and the Mediterranean regions and has been naturalized in parts of America. This popular medicinal plant is well known for its flavorful dried leaves and flowering tops. Oregano is a culinary herb and is widely used in kitchens all over the world, extensively through the Mediterranean cuisine. Furthermore, the oregano medicinal values were acknowledged by Greeks from ancient times. The Oregano's essential oil has been largely studied and reported to have several biological properties, including, antioxidant, antimicrobial, and antimutagenic activities. It also has been found to have great potential in the food industry as a food additive. More specifically, oregano's essential oil contains carvacrol, thymol, ρ-cymene, thymoquinone, and γ-terpinene. Currently, studying properties of this plant's extracts are attracting more interest due to the growing interest for the research of alternatives for potential treatment and prevention of certain diseases like cancer. Therefore, there is much interest in investigating Oregano properties for medical purposes. In this chapter, the focus is laid on the chemical composition, pharmacological and biological properties of Oregano and its health benefits.

Chapter 7 - Oregano is one of the most famous culinary herbs used all over the world. The genus *Origanum* L. is represented by several species. The most important is *Origanum vulgare* which predominate in occurrence. Oregano has been used in traditional medicine since ancient times. Greek and Roman used oregano for diarrhea, asthma and to maintain general health. Oregano contains many bioactive compounds such as essential oil. Oregano essential oils present a characteristic odor due to the main compounds carvacrol and thymol. Oregano essential oils have been largely investigated for their potential as antimicrobial and antioxidant agents. In addition, they are used in food products and cosmetic. However oregano use and benefit is not limited to human but is also related to animal. Natural products are gaining interest. They are considered as an alternative to synthetic ones. Moreover, the use of natural additives is considered more safety and will assure a better quality to food products. In the last recent years, products containing essential oil have been used as growth promoters and feed additives in animal nutrition. This chapter discusses actual and potential uses of oregano as an alternative food and feed additive.

Chapter 8 - Infections with the ectoparasitic protozoans *Ichthyobodo salmonis* and *Trichodina truttae* cause severe mortalities among juvenile chum salmon *Oncorhynchus keta* reared in hatcheries for the salmon stock enhancement program in Japan. This chapter first focused on dietary supplementation with oregano essential oil as a preventive against *I. salmonis* and *T. truttae* infections in juvenile chum salmon, then discussed the mechanism of control shown by the preventive measure, and finally characterized the susceptibility of various pathogens known to infect chum salmon to oregano essential oil as compared with other essential oils. Feeding juvenile chum salmon a diet supplemented with 0.02% oregano oil for at least 7 successive days prior to parasite exposure effectively controlled *I. salmonis* and *T. truttae* infection outbreaks. Among juvenile chum salmon reared in hatchery ponds, this method practically suppressed *I. salmonis* and *T. truttae* infections, and substantially reduced juvenile mortalities caused by the two protozoans. Dietary supplementation with carvacrol, the principal component of oregano essential oil, prevented *I. salmonis* and *T. truttae* infections. Carvacrol exterminated both of the protozoans from the body surface of juvenile salmon already infected with *I. salmonis* or *T. truttae*, and was detected in the skin of juveniles given feed supplemented with oregano oil. Of seven herb essential oils tested, only oregano oil intensively prevented infections of *I. salmonis* and *T. truttae* as well as the growth of other bacterial and fungal pathogens known to infect chum salmon. Together, these results demonstrate the feasibility of dietary supplementation with oregano essential oil as a preventive measure against ectoparasitic protozoan diseases in juvenile chum salmon; implicate the antiparasitic action of carvacrol as a possible mechanism of the prevention; and indicate the potential use of oregano oil as an antimicrobial against bacterial and fungal diseases in juvenile chum salmon.

Chapter 9 - In recent years, aromatic plants and the products derived from them have gained attention as phytogenic feed additives in animal nutrition, more so as in January 2006, the European Union banned the use of antibiotic growth promoters in animal feeds. Oregano (*Origanum vulgare L.),* sovarv in Romanian, is a perennial aromatic herb from the Lamiaceae family, which displays important antibacterial and antioxidant properties (particularly due to is phenolic compounds carvacrol and thymol) and a high content of trace elements (for example: Cu, Fe, Mn, Zn). The data on the chemical composition of *Origanum vulgare L.*, even the data on the same subspecies, are rather varied, being closely related to the climacteric conditions and the geographical areas of growth. Some authors studied the antimicrobial activity of the oils obtained from several oregano varieties and noticed that their efficacy depends on the location from where the plants have been harvested. Numerous studies show that oregano helps digestion and nutrient absorption, displays antibacterial properties and prevents imbalances in animal gut. These effects are more so important when young animals are reared under heat stress conditions, which bear upon the balance of the intestinal microflora. Due to these properties, oregano has been studied as phytoadditive in the diet formulations for broiler reared under heat stress (32°C). This chapter presents a review of findings regarding the chemical characterisation of oregano (as powder and essential oil) harvested from a culture (located at Livezeni, Mures County, latitude 46.55°N, longitude 24.63°E) of a Romanian producer of aromatic plants, with special emphasis on their impact on the microflora of the broiler reared under heat stress conditions.

Chapter 10 - The aim of this study was to study the antioxidant activity and the antimicrobial activity against Salmonella, of the essential oil of oregano (EOs) and the posterior addition at doses of 0.05% (O_1) and 0.4% (O_2) in pork patties. For that 3 batches of pork burgers (minced to 5 mm and 2% salt) were prepared: the control group C, Level1 (0.05% EOs), and Level2 (0.4% EOs). The burgers were packed with modified atmosphere

(70% O_2: 20% CO_2: 10% N_2) and stored for a maximum of 6 days at 4°C in natural lighting conditions. The total Salmonella counts was determined using Brilliant green agar medium (BGA), 37°C, 48h. A validated PCR identification protocol from the EU ''Food PCR'' for Salmonella, was used both for the confirmation of presumptive colonies and for determining presence or absence of the pathogen. In addition, the antioxidant activity of the essential oil in a model system (Fenton reaction), and in burgers with ESR (electron spin resonance) evaluated by free radical formation during heating at 55°C and its binding to PBN (α-fenil-N-tert-butilnitrona) on days 0, 3 and 6 of storage was studied. The results showed that O showed antimicrobial effect and prooxidat effect at phenol concentration ≥ 12 mg GAE/L. In patties O1, the radical formation after 3 hours of heating at 55°C was significantly lower ($P < 0.05\%$) than in control samples (C) and O_2 throughout the storage. In general, all patties inoculated and stored in modified atmosphere, the results showed that Salmonella spp. survived after 9 days of storage. However, in treated patties with 0.4% of O the growth of Salmonella was significantly lower ($P < 0.05\%$) than control meat from day 3 of storage. The results indicate that the use of 0.05% essential oil of oregano, as a natural antioxidant in pork burgers, being a good strategy of conservation.

In: Oregano: Properties, Uses and Health Benefits
Editor: Gema Nieto Martínez
ISBN: 978-1-53616-284-4

Chapter 1

ANTIMICROBIAL AND ANTIOXIDANT ACTIVITY OF OREGANO (*ORIGANUM SP.*)

Miroslava Kačániová[1,2,*], PhD and Eva Ivanišová[3], PhD
[1]Slovak University of Agriculture, Nitra, Slovakia
[2]Department of Bioenergy Technology and Food Analysis, Rzeszow University, Rzeszow, Poland
[3]Department of Plant Storage and Processing, Slovak University of Agriculture, Nitra, Slovakia

ABSTRACT

Oregano is a widely used spice in the food industry. It is mainly used for its aromatic properties with a primary role to enhance the taste and aroma of food. Oregano has been shown to exhibit antioxidative and antimicrobial activity due to the high content of oleanolic, ursolic, caffeic, rosemarinic, lithospermic acids, flavonoids, hydroquinones, tannins, and phenolic glycosides. Oregano, one kind of labiate *Origanum* plant that has been known for a long time as a popular remedy, is a very versatile plant. It was reported that *Origanum compactum* Benth., *Origanum minutiflorum* O. Schwarz and P.H. Davis, and *Origanum majorana* L. exhibit antifungal activity, antibacterial activity, and antimicrobial activity, respectively. In addition, it has been used widely in China as a kind of feed additive because it has a broad spectrum of action against bacteria, a rapid effect, and little residue, and now its antibacterial effect has been researched *in vitro* and *in vivo* all over the world. The oregano also exhibited antimicrobial properties against Gram-positive and Gram-negative bacterial strains including clinical isolates, against microscopic filamentous fungi and yeasts. The mechanism of antimicrobial activity is based on its principal components, i.e., thymol and carvacrol, which have antimicrobial properties. Plants which are rich in antioxidant compounds are presented in food industry. There are evident requirements for increasing application of natural antioxidants obtained

[*] Corresponding Author's E-mail: miroslava.kacaniova@gmail.com.

from plant material. The use of synthetic antioxidants for prevention of free radical damage can involve questionable nutritional value and toxic side effects while natural antioxidants which occur in many plants reduce oxidative damage and help in preventing mutagenesis, carcinogenesis, and aging due to their radical scavenging activities. A number of studies focused on antioxidant activities of essential oils from various aromatic plants reported that the oregano essential oil has a considerable antioxidant effect on the the fat oxidation process. Many publications showed antioxidative activities of oregano. Nowadays there is an increasing interest for alternative and efficient compounds for food preservation, having the goal to replace antimicrobial chemical additives.

Keywords: herbals, antimicrobial activity, antioxidants, food, human body, essential oils

INTRODUCTION

Antioxidants are the compounds produced by the body to neutralize the effect of free radicals, but the effect is limited to specific antioxidants. Oxidants and anti-oxidate ratio is maintained in human body, an alteration in these oxidants and antioxidats cause accumulation of reactive oxygen species within the body, this process is sign as oxidative stress. Oxidative stress has an important role in tissue damage and leads to pathological conditions such as inflammation, DNA damages regarding different types of cancer (Topdag et al. 2005, 269; Kuttappagari et al. 2015, 71). Oxidants and antioxidants may play a role in the last stages of cancer development. At this stage the levels of antioxidants play a very important role in prevention and progression of carcinogenesis.

Antioxidants are substances that delay or inhibit the oxidation of food, and therefore they are of great interest to food scientists. These biological active substances are naturally present in food, but sometimes at very low levels. Therefore, an additional quantity is added to control oxidation, increases shelf life, and improve overall quality. The mechanism by which this occurs is termed free radical termination, and is accomplished through the donation of an electron or hydrogen atom. Antioxidants can also protect food by the deactivation of metal ions and singlet oxygen. The most extensively used synthetic antioxidants in food are butylated hydroxyanisole (BHA – usually added to meat and milk products, vegetable oil, chewing gums), butylated hydroxytoluene (BHT – usually added to meat and milk products, potato chips), propyl gallate (PG – usually added to meat and milk products, vegetable oils, spices), and tertiary butylhydroquinone (TBHQ - usually added to meat, fish and milk products) (Haworth 2003, 95-96).

Metal ions like magnesium, iron and copper, chelators are also used extensively in the food industry due to the prooxidant effects of transition. Chelators such as citric acid (natural), ethylenediamintetraacetic acid (EDTA) and polyphosphates or their derivatives are used to chelate metal ions. For many years there has been strong debate and concern regarding the safety of certain synthetic antioxidants as potential carcinogens. BHA, BHT, PG and TBHQ still remain on the generally recognized as safe list, although limitations to their use have been implemented in the USA and EU, while BHT, PG and TBHQ still lack approval in many countries. Therefore, there is growing interest by consumers and the food industry in replacing currently used synthetic compounds with natural alternatives that are perceived to be safer and have wider consumer acceptance (Haworth 2003, 95-96; Kumar 2011, 129-130).

Nowadays, consumer interest and demand for natural and organic products has increased in the world. As a result, use of synthetic additives has declined while additives are considered to be natural have grown, largely because the latter are perceived as safer. The natural trend, coupled with the growing market for premium food products, has driven the use of natural antioxidants like tocopherols (vitamin E), natural herbal flavourings, and ascorbic acid (vitamin C). Many herbal extracts have antioxidant properties, and therefore they are used as food antioxidants (Haworth 2003, 95-96; Carocho and Ferreira 2013, 15-16. The antioxidant function can be generally linked to the presence of phenolic compounds such as phenolic acids, flavonoids and essential oils. The herbal extract most commonly used in cosmetic and pharmaceutical industry and also as a food antioxidant is oregano (*Origanum* sp.) (Leyva-López et al. 2017, 1-2).

ANTIOXIDANT ACTIVITY OF *ORIGANUM VULGARE* (L.)

The genus *Origanum* (*Lamiaceae*), with about 40 known species, is native to Mediterranean, Euro-Siberian and Irano-Siberian regions (Vazirian et al. 2015, 41). Now it is cultivated all over the world, including the USA, South America, Asia, Europe to central Asia, Mediterranean region, Middle East, and Crete (Charles 2013, 449) (Figure 1).

Dried leaves in whole or ground form (with light to dark green color) and essential oil are used from *Origanum vulgare* (Figure 2). Dark green leaves are available whole or in chopped or minced form. The dried light green leaves are available whole, in flaked form or ground. Essential oil is obtained by stem distillation of the dried flowering herb. The oil is a yellow to dark-brown mobile liquid with yield 1-2%. Flavour and aroma of *Origanum vulgare* is strongly aromatic, camphoraceous, slightly bitter and pungent flavour. The pungent flavour has some green, musty, hay, and minty notes. It imparts a slightly astringent mouth feel (Charles 2013, 450).

According to Kikuzaki and Nakatani (1989, 520) and Charles (2013, 452) the main active compounds of *Origanum vulgare* are carvacrol, thymol, *p*-cymene, γ-terpinene, sabinene, linalool, borneol, β-caryophyllene which are the major compounds found in the essential oil. *Origanum vulgare* also contains proteins, vitamins, acids, tannins, sterols, flavonoids, and bitter principle. These authors also reported presence of five antioxidant phenolic compounds, rosmarinic acid derivate, caffeic acid, protocatechuic acid, phenyl glucoside and 2-caffeyloxy-3-[2-(4-hydroxybenzyl)-4, 5-dihydroxy]-phenyl propionic acid. Koukoulitsa et al. (2006, 1655) and Charles (2013, 452) also published presence of the polar constituents – apigenin, luteoin, chrysoeriol, diosmetin, quercetin, eriodictyol, cosmocide, vicenin-2, caffeic acid, rosmarinic acid, *p*-menth-3-ene-1,2-diol 1-*O*-*β*-glucopyranoside, thymoquinol 2,5-*O*-*β*-glucopyranoside, thymolquinol 2,5-*O*-*β*-diglucopyranoside, 12-hydroxyjasmonic acid and its *β*-glucopyranoside, lithospermic acid B, epi-lithospermic acid B and 10-epi-lithospermic acid. There are some selected nutritional constituents and antioxidant activity of dried oregano presented in Table 1.

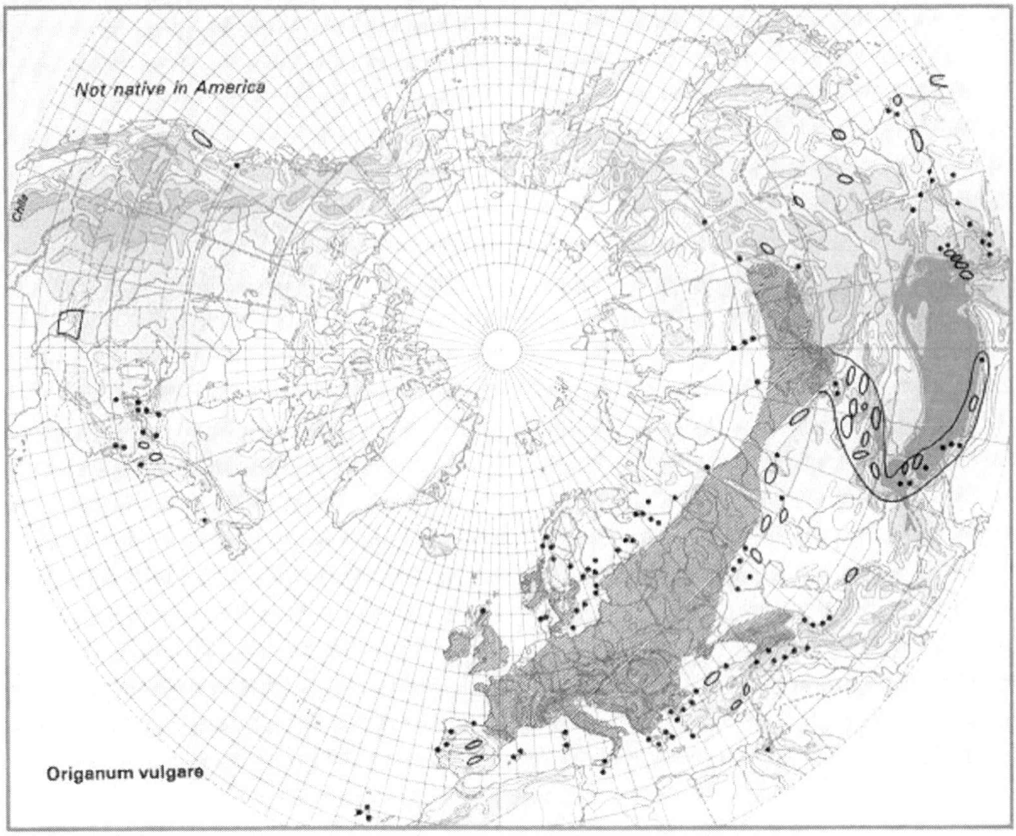

Figure 1. Distribution of *Origanum vulgare* L. in world (Botanical photogalery, 2018).

Oregano had a strong dose-dependent protective effect on the copper-induced low-density lipoproteins oxidation (Kulisić et al. 2007, 87). In study of Baricevic and Bartol (2002, 177-180) oregano has been used as stabilizers of edible oils (0.1% concentration) or of finished meat products (0.25% concentration). The supplements from oregano protected chickens against stress-induced increases in tiobarbituric acid reactive substances, in different muscles (Young et al. 2003, 1343). Oregano showed nitric oxide supressing activity because of the inhibition of inducible nitric oxide synthase expression (Tsai et al. 2007, 440). Treatment with oregano oil (200 mg oregano oil per kg) significantly retarded lipid oxidation in breast and thigh meat patties of turkey storage times compared with controls (Govaris et al. 2004, 115-117). Five polar constituents from oregano were found to inhibit aldose reductase, the first enzyme of the polyol pathway implicated in the secondary complications of diabetes (Koukoulitsa et al. 2006, 1653).

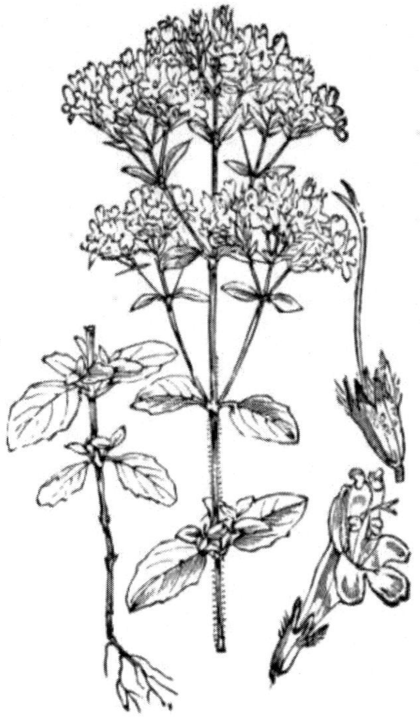

Figure 2. *Origanum vulgare* L. (Botany online, 2018).

In study of Botsoglou et al. (2004, 210) there was indirectly provided evidence that antioxidant components present in oregano essential oils were absorbed by the rabbit and increased the antioxidant capacity of tissues. A significant increase in the oxidative stability of fried chips, measured as the rate of peroxide formation during storage at 63 °C, was achieved by addition of ground oregano (10 g of oregano powder per kg) or its petroleum ether extracts (Lolos et al. 1999, 1526-1526). Oregano extract enriched with rosmarinic acid yielded higher than expected amylase inhibition than purified rosmarinic acid, suggesting the involvement of other phenolic compounds or phenolic synergies (McCue and Shetty 2004, 101). Carvacrol from oregano essential oil protected the liver against defects caused by ischemia and reperfusion, and carvacrol was not hepatoxic (Canbek et al. 2008, 447). The aqueous-methanolic extract of oregano showed antiurolithic activity, and this was possibly mediated through inhibition of calcium oxalate crystallization, antioxidant, renal epithelial cell protective and antispasmodic activities (Khan et al. 2011, 125). Srihari et al. (2008, 787) found out that oregano supplementation to have a modulatory role on tissue lipid peroxidation and antioxidant profile in colon cancer-bearing rats, and this suggests a possible anticancer activity of oregano. Carvacrol was shown to afford a significant hepatoprotective and antioxidant effect against d-GalN-induced rats (d-galactosamine) (Aristatile et al. 2009, 15). The protective effect of dietary oregano on the alleviation of carbon tetrachloride-induced oxidative stress in rats was studied in the study of Botsoglou et al. (2008, 209), and they found that oregano effectively improved the impaired antioxidant status in tetrachloride-induced toxicity in rats. The use of 1% oregano oil in broiler diets improved feed conversion ratio and feed utilisation in Alagawany et al. (2018, 463) study. Moreover, oregano can induce a marked improvement on the intestinal microbiota and ileal villus height of broilers when it is combined with attapulgite by ratio 15 mg/kg of oregano. A positive effect on digestible nutrient intake of fifteen 7-month old male goats which were fed on diets with 0, 10 and 50 g/kg of dried oregano was obtained with both oregano concentrations (Williams et al. 2018, 19). Cooking hamburgers with spice mixture containing rosmarinic acid (19 mg/250 g) from oregano decreased statistically the malondialdehyde suggesting potential health benefits for atherogenesis and carcinogenesis (Li et al. 2010, 1180-1182). Oregano has also shown the activity as an effective quencher of oxidative attackers with antimelanogenesis properties (Chou et al. 2010, 742). There were analyzed hot and cold ethanol 50% extracts of *Origanum vulgare* in terms of qualitative and quantitative chemical composition, and their antioxidant and antimicrobial potential in study of Bubueanu et al. (2015, 157). The obtained results showed no significant differences in terms of chemical composition and bioactivity, between the extracts. Thus, in industry sector these results can be used for reducing cost production. Morshedloo et al. (2017) analyzed different plant parts and phenological growth stages of oregano. The highest levels of carvacrol were identified in the essential oils from flowers (79.2%), roots (70%), and the early vegetative growth (67.34%).

Table 1. The nutrient compounds and antioxidant activity of dried oregano (Charles 2013, 452)

Nutrient	Units
Water	9.93 g/100 g
Energy	265 kcal
Protein	9.00 g/100 g
Total lipid	4.28 g/100 g
Total dietary fiber	42.5 g/100 g
Total sugars	4.09 g/100 g
Calcium	1.60 mg/100 g
Vitamin C	2.3 mg/100 g
Vitamin B_6	1.04 mg/100 g
Vitamin E	18.26 mg/100 g
Fatty acid, total saturated	1.55 g/100 g
Fatty acid, total monosaturated	0.72 g/100 g
Fatty acid, total polyunsaturated	1.37 g/100 g
ORAC (antioxidant activity)	175.30 μmol TE/100 g
Total polyphenols	3.79 mg GAE/100 g

TE – trolox equivalent; GAE – gallic acid equivalent.

All the essential oils exhibited high radical-scavenging properties are shown in the DPPH* assay. The essential oils from flowers, however, exhibited in their study the highest antioxidant activity and could be used as a preservative agent on an industrial scale. Oregano and compounds isolated from it have been found to have antioxidant activity.

ANTIOXIDANT ACTIVITY OF *ORIGANUM COMPACTUM* (BENTH.)

Origanum compactum (Figure 3) is an endemic species which grow in the north of Morocco. It is traditionally used for culinary and medical preparations (Sbayou et al. 2014, 3562). It is mainly used as a culinary condiment and largely employed in popular medicine for the treatment of ailments such as dysentery, colitis, bronco-pulmonary, gastric acidity, and gastro-intestinal diseases. *Origanum compactum* is also used as preservative for the melted butter (Bouyahya et al. 2016, 2). There are dried leaves in whole or ground form and essential oil used from *Origanum compactum*. Essential oil is obtained by stem distillation of the dried flowering herb. The oil has strong, hot and spicy odour, it is colourless to very slightly yellow mobile liquid with yield 1-2,5%. Flavour and aroma of *Origanum compactum* is strongly aromatic, slightly bitter and pungent flavour. Only a few studies aimed to investigate the chemical composition of *Origanum compactum*; the main constitutes are polyphenols, which are grouped in three major chemical classes – phenolic acids, tannins and flavonoids. Extraction of dried and powered aerial parts of oregano yielded thymohydroquinone, betulinic acid, β-amyrin, betulin, oleanolic acid, ursolic acid, aromadendrin, 21 α-hydroxyuleanolic acid, and 21 α-hydroxyursolic acid (Amakran et al. 2014, 2111; Bouyahya et al. 2016, 2). The total amount of flavonoids in oregano ethyl acetate extract, was the highest one (54.7 ±1.8 g QE/kg; QE – quercetin equivalent), while the petroleum ether extract was the richest in polyphenols (707.8 ±13.4 g GAE/kg; GAE – gallic acid equivalent) according to El Babili et al. (2011, 512). The anthocyanins (5.63 ±0.19 mg CE/kg; CE – cyanidin equivalent) were presented in higher amounts in the petroleum ether extract. Tannins were found in all extracts with an amount between 12.4 (ethanol extract) to 510.3 (petroleum ether extract) as catechin equivalent in g/kg. The main compounds of *Origanum compactum* essential oils are carvacrol, thymol, *p*-mecyne, and γ-terpenine (Bouyahya et al. 2016, 2-3).

Several studies demonstrate the antioxidant activities of organic extracts and essential oil of *Origanum compactum*. Bouhdid et al. (2008, 1558) evaluated the antioxidant activity of oregano essential oils by reducing power, DPPH assay and β-carotene-linoleic acid assay. The results of this study revealed evidence that the essential oil (250 mg/L) of *Origanum compactum* possesses a strong antioxidant effect by these methods. The antioxidant capacity in their study depended on the oil concentration and was attributed to the phenolic compounds present in the oil. El Babili et al. (2011, 512) evaluated the antioxidant activity of oregano essential oil, ethyl acetate, petroleum ether, ethanol extract and decoction using ABTS (acid 2,2'-azino-bis(3-éthylbenz-thiazoline-6-sulfonique) radical-scavenging assay and DPPH (1,1-diphényl-2-picrylhydrazyl) free radical scavenging. The results showed that the essential oil showed a higher antioxidant activity with an IC50 (2 ±0.1 mg/L). The aqueous extract (50 g of oregano powder per 0.5 mL of water) had the highest antioxidant activity with an IC50 (4.8 ±0.2 mg/L) by DPPH assay among the extracts.

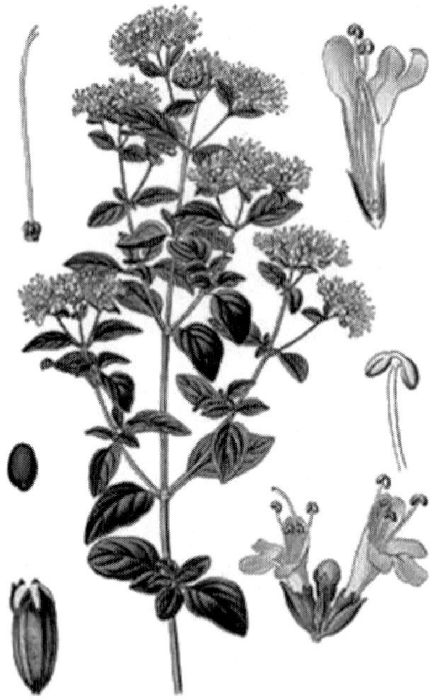

Figure 3. *Origanum compactum* Benth. (Pinterest, 2018).

ANTIOXIDANT ACTIVITY OF *ORIGANUM MINUTIFLORUM* (O. SCHWARZ AND P. H. DAVIS)

Origanum minutiflorum (Figure 4) is an endemic plant which occurs in the mountains of southern Turkey. It is used as a spice for seasoning, as the herbal tea, and also as a medicinal herb for curing stomach-aches and respiratory colds (Elmastas et al. 2018, 374). *Origanum* essential oil, mainly rich in carvacrol, is used as a painkiller in rheumatism by rubbing externally on painful limbs. The aromatic oregano water, rich in carvacrol, is consumed to check gastrointestinal disorders, reduce blood cholesterol and glucose level and also for tumor suppressive activities (Goze et al. 2010, 2156). Dried leaves in whole or ground form and essential oil are used from *Origanum minutiflorum* Essential oil is obtained by stem distillation of the dried flowering herb. The oil has strong, hot and spicy odour, it is colourless to very slightly yellow mobile liquid with yield 0.35 – 4.4%

(Altundag and Aslim 2011, 37). Flavour and aroma of *Origanum minutiflorum* is strongly aromatic.

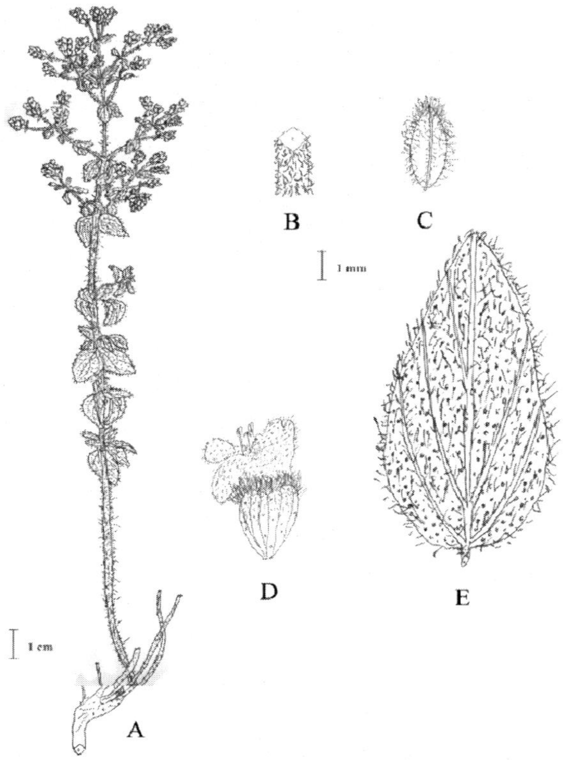

Figure 4. *Origanum minutiflorum* O. Schwarz and P.H. Davis (A-general view; B-stems; C-bracts; D-flower; E-leaves) (Sadikoglu and Ozhatay 2015, 89).

Only few studies aimed to investigate the chemical composition of *Origanum minutiflorum*; the main constitutes of essential oil are: *α*-pinene (1.04-1.28%), *α*-thujene (0.03%), camphene (0.03-0.62%), *β*-pinene (0.14-0.16%), sabinene (0.02-0.06%), *δ*-3-carene (0.05-0.06%), myrcene (0.18-0.19%), *α*-terpinene (0.55-0.59%), limonene (0.18-0.24%), 1,8-cineole (0.27-0.58), 2-hexanol (0.01-0.04%), *γ*-terpinene (0.03-2.28%), (E)-*β*-ocimene (0-0.02%), *p*-cymene (3,39-9.38%), terpinolene (0.09-0.11%), (Z)-3-hexanol (0.01-0.02%), 3-octanol (0.04%), 1-octen-3-ol (0.22-1.00%), *α*-cubebene (trace-0.02%), *cis*-sabinene hydrate (0.26-0.38%), linalool (0.06-0.07%), terpinen-4-ol (0.7-0.84%), *β*-caryophyllene (0.74-1.56%), allo-aromadendrene (0.04-0.09%), limonene oxide (0.03-0.05%), *α*-terpineol (0.02-0.05%), isoborneol (1.27-2.16%), (Z)- *β*-farnesene (0.09-0.12%), *cis*-piperitol (0.02-0.03%), (E)-isoeugenol (0.01-0.91%), methyl salicylate (0.02-0.04%), cuminaldehyde (0.02%), caryophyllene oxide (0.26-0.45%), eugenol (0.24-0.51%), thymol (0.22-0.28%) and carvacrol (75.40-82.00%) (Baser et al. 1991, 445-446). In study of Elmastas et al. (2018, 374) isolation of bioactive compounds from *Origanum minutiflorum* was executed on n-butanol extract to yield the compounds responsible for the activities. Tricosan-1-ol, (8*E*,16*E*)-tetracosa-8,16-diene-1,24-diol, azepan-2-one, 3,4-dihydroxybenzoic acid, apigenin, eriodictyol, globoidnan-A, luteolin, rosmarinic acid, apigenin-7-*O*-glucuronide, and vicenin-2 were isolated by chromatographic methods (column chromatography and semi-preparative high performance liquid chromatography (HPLC) and structures were elucidated on the basis of spectroscopic techniques including 1D/2D nuclear magnetic resonance (NMR) and liquid chromatography/time-of-flight/mass spectrometry (LC-TOF/MS). The isolated compounds and extracts in their study were applied for antioxidant assays including 1,1-diphenyl-2-picrylhydrazyl ($DPPH^{\bullet}$) scavenging, 2,2'-azino-bis (3-ethylbenzothiazoline-6-sulphonic acid) ($ABTS^{\bullet+}$) scavenging, reducing power, and cuprac techniques. 3,4-Dihydroxy benzoic acid, eriodictyol, luteolin, and rosmarinic acid revealed the considerable antioxidant activities. Their results confirmed that *Origanum minutiflorum* has a potency to be a promising medicinal plant for food and pharmaceutical industries on account of including significant bioactive compounds. There was suggested that feeding rainbow trouts with feeds containing essential oils or lyophilized extract of *Origanum minutiflorum* at the concentrations of 500 and 1000 mg/kg for 8 weeks could increase nonspecific immune system parameters and antioxidant activity in a study of Sari and Ustuner (2018, 1013). In study of Kilicgun and Kilicgün and Korkmaz (2014, 260) there were found posibble antidiabetic (150 mg of dry oregano powder per kg of body weight) and hepatoprotective activities (150 mg of dry oregano powder per kg of body weight) of four infusions of *Origanum minutiflorum*.

Antioxidant Activity of *Origanum majorana* (L.)

Origanum majorana L. (Figure 6) is a tender perennial herb of *Origanum* genus. It is commonly known as sweet marjoram and native to Cyperus, Antolia (Turkey) and it is naturalised in parts of Mediterranean region especially Egypt. It is cultivated all over the world (Figure 5) in different parts of India, France, Hungry and the United States for its flavour and fragrance. It is a well-liked home remedy for chest infection, cough, sore throat, rheumatic pain, nervous disorders, cardiovascular diseases, epilepsy, insomnia, skin care, flatulence and stomach disorders (Goel and Vasudeva 2015, 261-263). The fresh leaves are used whole or in chopped form. They are used as garnish and also in salads. The dried leaves are used whole, in cut or ground form. The aromatic seeds are employed in French comfitures and confectionery *Origanum majorana* has pleasant, aromatic, and spicy aroma. It has fresh, spicy, bitter and slightly pungent, camphor-like notes. It has delicate, sweet aroma of sweet basil and thyme and has fragrant, spicy, minty-sweet sharp, with bitter and camphoraceous undertones (Charles 2013, 394).

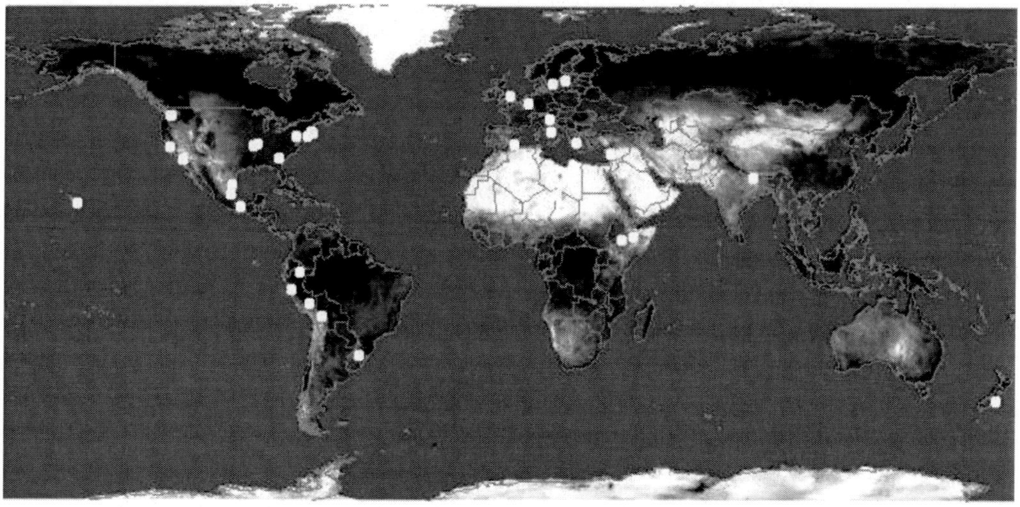

Figure 5. Distribution of *Origanum majorana* (L.) in world (Discover life, 2018).

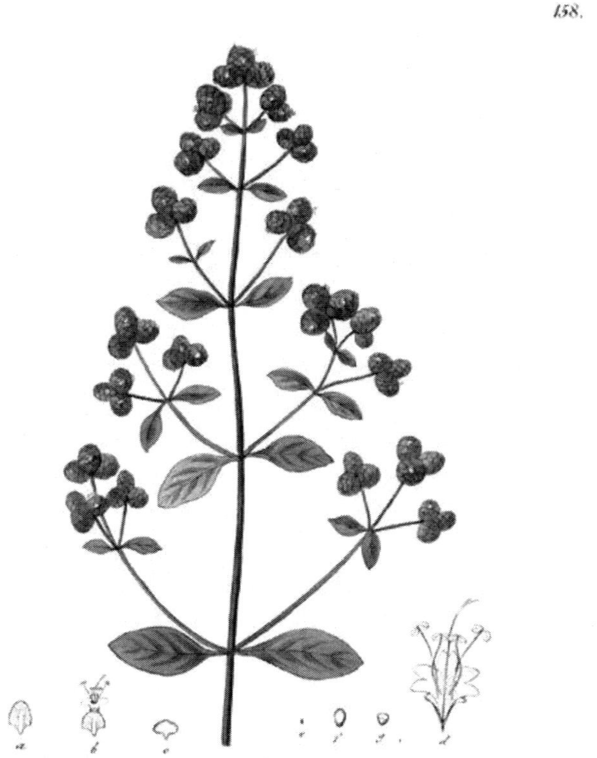

Figure 6. *Origanum majorana* (L.) (Pinterest, 2018).

The main bioactive compounds include flavonoid glycosides, tannins, steroids and vitamins (especially A and C). The major constituents of essential oil are terpin-4-ol (20%), sabinene hydrate (12-15%), α-terpineol, sabinene, and linalool. The major phenolic acids are sinapic, ferulic, coumaric, caffeic, syringic, vanillic, and 4-hydroxybenzoic acid (Petr et al. 2008, 3940; Charles 2013, 394). The plant is rich in polyphenols such as arbutin, 6-O-4-hydroxybenzoyl arbutin, and 2-hydroxy-3-(3,4-dihydroxyphenyl) propionic acid, isolated as moderate antioxidants. Catechin, rutin (quercetin 3-o-rhamnose glycoside), quercetin and eriodictyol are the flavonoids reported in different extracts of water, 60% methanol, 60% acetone and ethyl acetate. Amentoflavone is a flavonoid which has been determined by reversed phase HPLC in two different varieties of *O. majorana* L. Luteolin-7-diglucoside, apigenin-7-glucoside, and diosmetin-7-glucuronide, 6-hydroxyluteolin and 6-hydroxyapigenin glycosides, arbutin, methylarbutin are present as flavonoid glycosides in marjoram. Aqueous and methanol extracts from sweet marjoram contain multiple compounds e.g., phenolic derivatives (phenolic acids, flavonoids as apigenin, luteolin, quercitin and their glycosides as rutin or isovitexin. β-sitosterol is reported in the aerial parts of the plant. Linolenic, linoleic and oleic acid are the fatty acids present in its leaves. Vitamin A and C are reported in the leaves and floral parts of marjoram herb. Caffeic acid, carnosic acid, carnosol, labiatic acid and rosmarinic acid are various types of tannins found in aerial parts of the herb (Goel and Vasudeva 2015, 263). The nutritional compounds and antioxidant activity of *Origanum majorana* are given in Table 2.

Table 2. The nutrient compounds and antioxidant activity of dried *Origanum majorana* (Charles 2013, 451)

Nutrient	Units
Water	7.64 g/100 g
Energy	271 kcal
Protein	12.66 g/100 g
Total lipid	7.04 g/100 g
Total dietary fiber	40.3 g/100 g
Total sugars	4.09 g/100 g
Calcium	1.99 mg/100 g
Vitamin C	51.4 mg/100 g
Vitamin B_6	1.19 mg/100 g
Vitamin E	1.69 mg/100 g
Fatty acid, total saturated	0.529 g/100 g
Fatty acid, total monosaturated	0.940 g/100 g
Fatty acid, total polyunsaturated	4.405 g/100 g
ORAC (antioxidant activity)	27.297 μmol TE/100 g fresh matter
Total polyphenols	964 mg GAE/100 g fresh matter

TE – trolox equivalent; GAE – gallic acid equivalent.

Origanum majorana – marjoram is known to possess various positive properties to human body including antioxidant activity. Saito et al. (1976, 505) reported strong antioxidant activity at 0.02% against lard than tocopherol. The antioxidant activity of marjoram was found to be much stronger than α-tocopherol and comparable with butylated hydroxytoluene (BHT) in the egg yolk assay (Charles 2013, 451. The ethanol extract of the leaves of marjoram (25 g/150 mL) showed an antioxidant and free radical-scavenging activity using colorimetric assays. The extract exhibited a marked inhibitory effect in 1,1-diphenyl-2-picrylhydrazyl (DPPH) scavenging assay. The ethanol extracts (0.008; 0.018; 0.028 and 0.04%) of both stem and root have shown *in vitro* antioxidant activity, respectively using spectrophotometric method by DPPH, H_2O_2 free radical scavenging, metal chelating and ferric reducing power assay. Both the extracts have showed potent antioxidant activity in all models. The IC50 values were found comparable with ascorbic acid and the reducing ability of root ethanol extract was found to be high compared to stem ethanol extract (Goel and Vasudeva 2015, 264). The ethyl-alcohol, n-hexane and aqueous extracts obtained from leaves and flowering tops of two marjoram herbs from Hungary and Egypt showed antioxidant activity *in vitro* by spectrophotometric and chemiluminometric methods using DPPH and Rancimat method. The Egyptian herb and its aqueous extract (0.04%) was better antioxidant than Hungarian one (Vagi et al. 2005, 17). Saxena et al. (2016, 321) reported the effect of marjoram and thyme on the quality of semi fried mullet fish fillets during cold storage. Oxidation of fat is very common problem in food industry. Microbial analysis, may report that both essential oils of thyme and marjoram have antimicrobial properties too. Marjoram and thyme oils are also rich in phenolic compound being particularly active in both antioxidants and antimicrobials. Amarowicz et al. (2009, 1111) investigated the free radical scavenging and antiacetyl cholinesterase activities of marjoram (25 g/250 mL), thyme and oregano extracts. They observed antioxidant activities of extracts were higher in marjoram than in thyme and oregano. Nakatani (2000, 263) studied the compounds from various herbs and spices for their antioxidant activity and isolated 26 active compounds from marjoram, rosemary, thyme and oregano. The aqueous extract from marjoram was shown to have a remarkable capacity in retarding lipid oxidation, and these extracts were found to be a rich in bond forms of phenolic compounds such as hydroxycinnamic acids and flavonoids (Triantaphyllou et al. 2001, 313). Marjoram extract was shown to alleviate the kidney and liver antioxidant activities and lower the lipid peroxidation levels that were disrupted by cadmium in albino rats. Marjoram (1 g/kg) showed both protective and curative effects on cadmium-induced hepatoxicity and nephrotoxicity (Shati 2011, 797). In study of Heo et al. (2002, 5-7) was found ursolic acid (0.1-10 iM) from marjoram to reduce the micromolar Abeta-induced oxidative cell death. Ursolic acid activity was assessed by MTT ((3-[4,5-dimethylthiazol-2-yl]-2,5 diphenyl tetrazolium bromide)), lactate dehydrogenase, and trypan blue assay. *Origanum majorana* extract (250-500 mg/kg) was found to significantly decrease the incidence of ulcers, basal gastric secretion and acid output, and the concentration of malondialdehyde (Al-Howiriny et al. 2009, 531). In studies of El-Ashmawy et al. (2005, 238) were concluded that marjoram plays an important role in ameliorating liver and kidney functions and genotoxicity induced by lead toxicity. They found the essential oil, alcoholic, and aqueous extract of marjoram (0.5%) to significantly reduce the serum activities of alanine and aspartate transaminases, alkaline phosphatise urea, and creatine and improved the kidney and liver histology in comparison with lead acetate treated group. The essential oil of marjoram was able to reduce that damaging effects of ethanol toxicity on male fertility, liver, and brain tissues. The effect of polyphenolic compounds of commercial culinary herbs including marjoram on fructose-mediated protein glycation was study by Dearlove et al. (2008, 275). They found that these extracts can to be potent inhibitors of protein glycation and this is an example of the antidiabetic potential of these culinary herbs and spices.

ANTIMICROBIAL ACTIVITY OF OREGANO SPP.

The problems regarding application of conventional antibiotics, including antimicrobial resistance, environmental problems, cancerogenity, side effects and high costs, have reinforced a tendency to replace synthetic antimicrobials with natural alternative agents (Gortzi et al. 2007, 934). Plant based products are among the alternative agents examined in order to replace conventional antibiotics. Accordingly, extensive research has been carried out in order to evaluate the antimicrobial effect of the essential oils and extracts which showed the ability to inhibit the growth of various pathogenic microorganisms (Burt 2004, 231).

It has been demonstrated in previous studies, that the content of essential oil and extracts of medicinal plants like *Origanum* species containing antimicrobial, antioxidant and other biological activities may change. It is based on the differences in cultivation, origin, vegetative stage and growing seasons of the plants (Deans et al. 1992, 230; Kustrak et al. 1996, 8; Leung and Foster 1996, 316; Milos et al. 2000, 80; Muller-Riebau et al. 1995, 2263). *Origanum vulgare* ssp. *vulgare* is one of the most widely distributed subspecies growing in the Eastern Anatolia region of Turkey. However, there have been no attempts to study the chemical composition and biological activities of essential oils and extracts from *O. vulgare* ssp. *vulgare* plants collected from the Eastern Anatolia region of Turkey up to now. In recent years, multiple drug/chemical resistance in both human and plant pathogenic microorganisms have been developed due to indiscriminate use of commercial antimicrobial drugs/chemical commonly used in the treatment of infectious diseases (Davis 1994, 375; Loper et al. 1991, 287). On the other hand, foodborne diseases are still a major problem in the world, even in well developed countries, like the USA (Mead et al. 1999, 607). Food spoilage caused by a variety of microorganisms has often been recognized as an inconvenient and one of the most important concerns for food industry. Many bacteria (*Escherichia coli*, *Enterobacter* spp., *Bacillus* spp., *Salmonella* spp., *Staphylococcus aureus*, *Klebsiella pneumoniae*, *Listeria monocytogenes* and *Campylobacter jejuni*), yeast and fungi (*Candida* spp., *Zygosaccharomyces* spp., *Fusarium* spp., *Aspergillus* spp., *Rhizopus* spp., and *Penicillium* spp.) species has been reported as the causal agents of foodborne diseases and/or food spoilage so far (Betts et al. 1999, 29;

Deak and Beuchat 1996, 65; Pitt and Hocking 1997; Walker 1988, 91). The contamination of raw and/or processed food with microflora can take place at various stages from the production to the sale and distribution (Deak and Beuchat 1996, 212). Thus, food industry at present uses chemical preservatives to prevent the growth of food spoiling microbes (Sagdıc and Ozcan 2003, 141). Due to the economical impacts of spoiled food and the consumer's concerns over the safety of food containing synthetic chemicals, a lot of attention has been paid to naturally derived compounds or natural products (Alzoreky and Nakahara 2003, 224; Hsieh et al. 2001, 38). Recently, there has been considerable interest in extracts and essential oils from aromatic plants with antimicrobial activities for controlling pathogens and/or toxin producing microorganisms in food (Alzoreky and Nakahara 2003, 224; Soliman and Badeaa 2002, 1970; Valero and Salmeron 2003, 74; Sahin et al. 2004, 550).

The traditional use of plants as medicine provides the basis for suggesting that essential oils and plant extracts may be useful for specific medical conditions. The antimicrobial activity of natural compounds is well documented, including a few reports focused on the effects of essential oils against *H. pylori* (Ohno et al. 2003, 207-210; Imai et al. 2001, 32; Kalpoutzakis et al. 2001, 881).

The herbs of two aromatic species *O. vulgare* L. and *O. basilicum* L. (Lamiaceae) are used as spices in everyday life, as well as medicine for treating different conditions, including respiratory and digestive disorders (Zhang et al. 2014, 300). *O. basilicum* was used as mild sedative, antihelmintic, and also against flatulence or urinary infections, while *O. vulgare* has a long tradition in the treatment of respiratory infections, gastrointestinal diseases (particularly diarrhoea) and against inflammation of skin and mucous membranes in Serbian traditional medicine, except for culinary use. The chemistry of essential oil of *O. vulgare* and *O. basilicum* and its antimicrobial activity is well studied (De Falco et al. 2013, 14948; Stefanakis et al. 2013, 539), as well as the chemistry and activity of different herb extracts. Phenolic compounds, phenolic acids and flavonoids are major compounds of oregano and basil herb according to the literature (Zhang et al. 2014, 300; Esen et al. 2007, 371; Faleiro et al. 2005, 8162; Karakaya et al. 2011, 645; Zaidi et al. 2009, 286; Kiferle et al. 2011, 946). Recent reports have shown a very good antimicrobial activity of the essential oils of *O. vulgare* subsp. *glandulosum* rich in carvacrol, while some phenolics isolated from *O. vulgare* possessed weak to moderate antiviral activity (Zhang et al. 2014, 300; Lu et al. 2014, 262). Several reports presented the results of weak or moderate antiH.pylori activity of the essential oil or different extracts of *Oregano* species (Ohno et al. 2003, 207-208; Karakaya et al. 2011, 645; Stamatis et al., 2003, 175). Some reports also suggested synergistic effects against *H. pylori in vitro* of phenolics from oregano and cranberry water soluble extracts (0.1 mg of phenolics/disc) through urease inhibition and disruption of the energy production by inhibition of proline dehydrogenase at the plasma membrane (Lin et al. 2005, 8558).

Table 3. Antimicrobial activity of *Origanum* sp. against Gram positive bacteria (García-Beltrán and Esteban 2015)

Origanum species	Bacteria	References
O. syriacum	*Staphylococcus aureus*	[El Gendy et al. 2015, 201-207]
	Enterococcus faecalis	[El Gendy et al. 2015, 201-207; Hakki et al. 2010, 1725-1729]
	Bacillus brevis	[Hakki et al. 2010, 1725-1729]
	Bacillus megaterium	[Hakki et al. 2010, 1725-1729]
	Bacillus subtilis	[Hakki et al. 2010, 1725-1729]
	Micrococcus luteus	[Hakki et al. 2010, 1725-1729]
	Mycobacterium smegmatis	[Hakki et al. 2010, 1725-1729]
	Listeria innocua	[Viuda-Martos et al. 2010, 436-443]
O. vulgare	*Staphylococcus epidermidis*	[Martins et al. 2014, 73-80]
	Staphylococcus aureus	[Martins et al. 2014, 73-80]
	Staphylococcus saprophyticus	[Saeed and Tariq 2009, 421-424]
	Micrococcus sp	[Saeed and Tariq 2009, 421-424]
	Bacillus sp	[Saeed and Tariq 2009, 421-424]
	Bacillus cereus	[Abdullah et al. 2011, 943-952]
	Bacillus subtilis	[Abdullah et al. 2011, 943-952]
	Bacillus pumilis	[Abdullah et al. 2011, 943-952]
	Enterococcus faecalis	[Melo et al. 2015, 285-289]
	Listeria innocua	[Teixeira et al. 2013, 2707-2714]
	Listeria monocytogenes	[Teixeira et al. 2013, 2707-2714; Dimitrijevic et al. 2007, 774-782]
	Bochothrix thermosphacta	
	Micrococcus luteus	[Hernández-Hernández et al. 2014]
O. dictamnus	*Staphylococcus aureus*	[Mitropoulou et al. 2015; Marrelli et al. 2016, 735-739]
	Staphylococcus epidermidis	[Mitropoulou et al. 2015; Marrelli et al. 2016, 735-739]
	Listeria monocytogenes	[Mitropoulou et al. 2015]
	Bacillus cereus	[Marrelli et al. 2016, 735-739]
	Bacillus subtilis	[Marrelli et al. 2016, 735-739]
	Streptococcus faecalis	[Marrelli et al. 2016, 735-739]
	Staphylococcus hominis	[Economakis et al. 1999, 189-191; Economakis et al. 2002, 6276-6280]
	Streptococcus mutans	[Liolios et al. 2009, 77-83]
	Streptococcus viridans	[Liolios et al. 2009, 77-83]
O. michrophyllum	*Bacillus cereus*	[Marrelli et al. 2016, 735-739]
	Bacillus subtilis	[Marrelli et al. 2016, 735-739]
	Staphylococcus aureus	[Marrelli et al. 2016, 735-739]
	Staphylococcus epidermidis	[Marrelli et al. 2016, 735-739]
O. libanoticum	*Bacillus cereus*	[Marrelli et al. 2016, 735-739]
	Bacillus subtilis	[Marrelli et al. 2016, 735-739]
	Staphylococcus epidermidis	[Marrelli et al. 2016, 735-739]
O. majorana	*Bacillus cereus*	[Abdullah et al. 2011, 943-952]
	Bacillus subtilis	[Abdullah et al. 2011, 943-952]
	Bacillus pumilis	[Abdullah et al. 2011, 943-952]
	Staphylococcus aureus	[Abdullah et al. 2011, 943-952]
O. acutidens	*Bacillus macerans*	[Sökmen et al. 2004, 3309-3312]
	Bacillus megaterium	[Sökmen et al. 2004, 3309-3312]
	Bacillus subtilis	[Sökmen et al. 2004, 3309-3312]
	Clavibacter michiganense	[Sökmen et al. 2004, 3309-3312]
	Enterococcus faecalis	[Sökmen et al. 2004, 3309-3312]
	Staphylococcus aureus	[Sökmen et al. 2004, 3309-3312]
	Staphylococcus epidermis	[Sökmen et al. 2004, 3309-3312]
O. glandulosum	*Enterococcus hirae*	[Mechergui et al. 2015, 102-108]
	Staphylococcus aureus	[Mechergui et al. 2015, 102-108]
O. minutiflorum	*Listeria monocytogenes*	[Dadalioglu and Evrendilek 2004, 8255-8260]
	Staphylococcus aureus	[Dadalioglu and Evrendilek 2004, 8255-8260]

Table 4. Antimicrobial activity of *Origanum* sp. against Gram negative bacteria (García-Beltrán and Esteban, 2015)

Origanum species	Bacteria	Reference
O. syriacum	*Pseudomonas aeruginosa*	[El Gendy et al., 2015; Hakki et al. 2010, 1725- 1729]
	Escherichia coli	[El Gendy et al. 2015, 201-207]
	Klebsiella oxytoca	[Hakki et al. 2010, 1725-1729]
	Yersinia enterocolitica	[Hakki et al., 2010 1725-1729]
	Klebsiella pneumoniae	[Hakki et al. 2010, 1725-1729]
	Escherichia coli O157:H7	[Al-Mariri and Safi 2014, 36-43]
	Proteus spp.	[Al-Mariri and Safi 2014, 36-43]
	Yersinia enterocolitica O9	[Al-Mariri and Safi 2014, 36-43]
	Brucella melitensis	[Al-Mariri and Safi 2013, 44-50]
O. vulgare	*Enterobacter aerogenes*	[Martins et al. 2014, 73-80]
	Enterobacter sakazakii	[Martins et al. 2014, 73-80]
	Proteus vulgaris	[Martins et al. 2014, 73-80]
	Escherichia coli	[Martins et al., 2014, Melo et al. 2015, 285-289]
	Pseudomonas aeruginosa	[Martins et al. 2014, 73-80]
	Salmonella poona	[Abdullah et al. 2011, 943-952]
	Salmonella Enteritidis	[Melo et al. 2015, 285-289]
	Salmonella Typhimurium	[Melo et al. 2015, 285-289]
	Pseudomonas fragi	[Hernández-Hernández et al. 2014]
	Salmonella spp.	[Hernández-Hernández et al. 2014]
	Aeromonas hydrophila	[Chaudry et al. 2007, 609-613]
	Citrobacter spp.	[Chaudry et al. 2007, 609-613]
	Enterobacter aerogenes	[Chaudry et al. 2007, 609-613]
	Flavobacterium spp.	[Chaudry et al. 2007, 609-613]
	Klebsiella ozaenae	[Chaudry et al. 2007, 609-613]
	Klebsiella pneumoniae	[Chaudry et al. 2007, 609-613]
	Proteus mirabilis	[Chaudry et al. 2007, 609-613]
	Salmonella typhi	[Chaudry et al. 2007, 609-613]
	Salmonella paratyphi	[Chaudry et al. 2007, 609-613]
	Serratia marcescens	[Chaudry et al. 2007, 609-613]
	Shigella dysenteriae	[Chaudry et al. 2007, 609-613]
	Helicobacter pylori	[Chaudry et al. 2007, 609-613]
O. dictamnus	*Salmonella* Enteritidis	[Mitropoulou et al. 2015]
	Salmonella Typhimurium	[Mitropoulou et al. 2015]
	Escherichia coli	[Mitropoulou et al. 2015;
	Enterobacter cloacae	Marrelli et al. 2016, 735-739]
	Klebsiella pneumoniae	[Liolios et al. 2009, 77-83]
	Pseudomonas aeruginosa	[Liolios et al. 2009, 77-83]
	Helicobacter pylori	[Liolios et al. 2009, 77-83]
	Acinetobacter hemolyticus	[Liolios et al. 2009, 77-83]
	Empedobacter brevis	[Liolios et al. 2009, 77-83]
	Erwinia carotovora	[Liolios et al. 2009, 77-83]
	Clavibacter michiganensis	[Liolios et al. 2009, 77-83]
O. michrophyllum	*Escherichia coli*	[Marrelli et al. 2016, 735-739]
O. majorana	*Escherichia coli*	[Abdullah et al. 2011, 943-952]
	Pseudomonas aeruginosa	[Abdullah et al. 2011, 943-952]
	Salmonella poona	[Abdullah et al. 2011, 943-952]
	Helicobacter pylori	[Stamatis et al. 2004, 175]
O. acutidens	*Acinetobacter baumanii*	[Sökmen et al. 2004, 3309-3312]
	Acinetobacter lwoffi	[Sökmen et al. 2004, 3309-3312]
	Brucella abortus	[Sökmen et al. 2004, 3309-3312]
	Cedecea davisae	[Sökmen et al. 2004, 3309-3312]
	Enterobacter cloacae	[Sökmen et al. 2004, 3309-3312]
	Escherichia coli	[Sökmen et al. 2004, 3309-3312]
	Klebsiella pneumoniae	[Sökmen et al. 2004, 3309-3312]
	Morgonella morganii	[Sökmen et al. 2004, 3309-3312]
	Proteus vulgaris	[Sökmen et al. 2004, 3309-3312]
	Pseudomonas aeruginosa	[Sökmen et al. 2004, 3309-3312]
	Pseudomonas pseudoalkaligenes	[Sökmen et al. 2004, 3309-3312]
	Salmonella cholerasuis arizonae	[Sökmen et al. 2004, 3309-3312]
	Salmonella enteritidis	[Sökmen et al. 2004, 3309-3312]

Table 4. (Continued)

Origanum species	Bacteria	Reference
	Serratia plymuthica	[Sökmen et al. 2004, 3309-3312]
	Shigella sonnei	[Sökmen et al. 2004, 3309-3312]
	Xanthomonas campestris	[Sökmen et al. 2004, 3309-3312]
O. glandulosum	*Escherichia coli*	[Mechergui et al. 2015, 102-108]
	Klebsiella pneumoniae	[Mechergui et al. 2015, 102-108]
	Pseudomonas aeruginosa	[Mechergui et al. 2015, 102-108]
O. minutiflorum	*Escherichia coli O157:H7*	[Dadalioglu and Evrendilek 2004, 8255-8260]
	Salmonella typhimurium	[Dadalioglu and Evrendilek 2004, 8255-8260]

Table 5. Antimicrobial activity of *Origanum* sp. against microscopic filamentous fungi (García-Beltrán and Esteban, 2015)

Origanum species	Fungi	Reference
O. syriacum	*Aspergillus fumigatus*	[El Gendy et al. 2015, 201-207]
	Aspergillus flavus	[El Gendy et al. 2015, 201-207]
	Aspergillus niger	
	Saccharomyces cerevisiae	[Hakki et al. 2010, 1725- 1729]
O. dictamnus	*Candida albicans*	[Liolios et al. 2010, 229-241]
	Candida tropicalis	[Liolios et al. 2010, 229-241]
	Candida glabrata	[Liolios et al. 2010, 229-241]
	Botrytis cinerea	[Liolios et al. 2010, 229-241]
	Fusarium sp.	[Liolios et al. 2010, 229-241]
	Aspergillus niger	[Mitropoulou et al. 2015]
	Saccharomyces cerevisiae	[Mitropoulou et al. 2015]
	Penicillium digitatum	[Daferera et al. 2000, 2576-2581]
	Yarrowia lipolytica	[Karanika et al., 2001, 175-181]
O. acutidens	*Candida albicans*	[Sökmen et al. 2004, 3309-3312]
	Alternaria solani	[Sökmen et al. 2004, 3309-3312]
	Aspergillus flavus	[Sökmen et al. 2004, 3309-3312]
	Aspergillus niger	[Sökmen et al. 2004, 3309-3312]
	Aspergillus variecolor	[Sökmen et al. 2004, 3309-3312]
	Fusarium oxysporum	[Sökmen et al. 2004, 3309-3312]
	Fusarium solani	[Sökmen et al. 2004, 3309-3312]
	Microsporum canis	[Sökmen et al. 2004, 3309-3312]
	Moniliania fructicola	[Sökmen et al. 2004, 3309-3312]
	Mortieraula alpina	[Sökmen et al. 2004, 3309-3312]
	Penicillum spp.	[Sökmen et al. 2004, 3309-3312]
	Rhizopus spp.	[Sökmen et al. 2004, 3309-3312]
	Rhizoctonia solani	[Sökmen et al. 2004, 3309-3312]
	Trichophyton rubrum	[Sökmen et al. 2004, 3309-3312]
O. glandulosum	*Candida albicans*	[Mechergui et al. 2015, 102-108]
	Candida tropicalis	[Mechergui et al. 2015, 102-108]
O. majorana	*Candida rugosa*	[Kunicka-Styczyńska 2011, 326-328]
	Debaryomyces hansenii	[Kunicka-Styczyńska 2011, 326-328]
	Kluyveromyces marxianus	[Kunicka-Styczyńska 2011, 326-328]
	Rhodotorula glutinis	[Kunicka-Styczyńska 2011, 326-328]
	Rhodotorula minuta	[Kunicka-Styczyńska 2011, 326-328]
	Saccharomyces cerevisiae	[Kunicka-Styczyńska 2011, 326-328]
	Trichosporon cutaneum	[Kunicka-Styczyńska 2011, 326-328]
	Yarrowia lipolytica	[Kunicka-Styczyńska 2011, 326-328]
	Zygosaccharomyces rouxii	[Kunicka-Styczyńska 2011, 326-328]
O. vulgare	*Candida glabatra*	[Soares et al. 2015, 213]
	Microsporum canis	[Nardoni et al. 2005, 1473-1478]
	Microsporum gypseum	[Nardoni et al. 2005, 1473-1478]
	Trichophyton mentagrophytes	[Nardoni et al. 2005, 1473-1478]
	Trichophyton erinacei	[Nardoni et al. 2005, 1473-1478]
	Trichophyton terrestre	[Nardoni et al. 2005, 1473-1478]

O. basilicum is also an aromatic plant which is rich in essential oil and phenolic compounds (flavonoids, phenolic acids) with known antimicrobial activity. Nakhaei et al. (2006, 2887) studied antiH. pylori activity of *O. basilicum* extracts using the agar-diffusion method, while Castillo-Juárez et al. (2009, 403) obtained significant minimal inhibitory concentrations (MICs) of *O. basilicum* extracts of different polarity.

Antimicrobial activity of *Origanum* sp. is summarized in Table 3-5.

ANTIMICROBIAL ACTIVITY OF *ORIGANUM VULGARE*

The ability of some herbs and seaweeds to inhibit the activity of bacterial fish pathogens is of great interest (Direkbusarakom 2014, 7-14; Muniruzzaman and Chowdhury 2009, 75-82; Zilberg et al. 2010, 361-369; Borisutpeth et al. 2005; Dubber and Harder 2008, 196-200). However, our knowledge about the bactericidal activity of oregano as a natural treatment for fish bacterial pathogens is limited. Therefore, another objective of the present study was to study the effects of *O. vulgare* extracts against three opportunistic pathogenic bacteria, *V. harveyi, V. anguillarum* and *P. damselae* (formerly *V. damselae*) (Amar et al. 2017, 153; Frans et al. 2011, 643), which were selected because of their responsibility for infections that affect a variety of marine animals, including fish, crustaceans, molluscs and cetaceans, and also humans. Furthermore, *Vibrionaceae* represents the major cause of mortality in farmed marine species (Rivas et al. 2013, 283; Nguyen and Jacq 2014, 382). In this respect, past results demonstrate that Gram-positive marine bacteria are generally more susceptible to herbal extracts than Gram-negative marine *Vibrionaceae* (Dubber and Harder 2008, 196-200). Nevertheless, some herbals act as inhibitors of the quorum-sensing pathways in *Vibrio* sp. (Citarasu 2010, 403-404). It is important to underline that in the present study, both extracts showed bactericidal activity against the three fish pathogen tested in a dose-dependent manner. Our results demonstrated that ethanolic extracts showed higher bactericidal activity than aqueous extracts. Low-medium and high concentrations of ethanolic extracts showed bactericidal activity against the three pathogens tested, while only the highest concentration of the aqueous extract showed activity against *P. damselae*. The present results are in conformity with other studies that demonstrated that ethanolic extracts have stronger bactericidal activity than aqueous ones (Teixeira et al. 2013, 2709; Coccimiglio et al. 2016, 6; Karaboduk et al. 2014, 1289; Klūga et al. 2017, 79). The different bactericidal activity between aqueous and ethanolic extracts observed in this study may be the consequence of the different components extracted in each case. Among the most abundant components present in oregano leaves, flavonoids, phenolic acids and specially terpenoids present bactericidal activity and are much more abundant in ethanolic than in aqueous extracts (García-Beltrán and Esteban 2016; Teixeira et al. 2013, 2707).

The aqueous extracts of *V. harveyi*, did not show a bactericidal activity against this bacterium, and the number of viable bacteria increased in a dose-dependent manner. Previous studies indicated that aqueous extracts of oregano had no (Teixeira et al. 2013, 2711; Karaboduk et al. 2014, 1289) or just low (Martins et al. 2014, 73-80; Teixeira et al. 2013, 2711; Ashraf et al. 2011, 257; Akrayi et al. 2015, 35; Masood et al. 2007, 609) bactericidal activity against different human bacteria. Furthermore, the available results indicate that the temperature is also important for the composition of the obtained extracts and can be a very significant factor in terms of bactericidal activity. In this sense, an aqueous decoction was prepared by boiling oregano leaves in sterile distilled water for 15 min and the obtained extract did not have bactericidal activity (Masood et al. 2007, 609; Saeed and Tariq 2009, 421-424). However, when an aqueous infusion was prepared by soaking the oregano leaves in sterile distilled water for two days with occasional shaking, the obtained infusion had bactericidal activity against many bacteria (including *E. coli, P. aeruginosa, P. mirabilis, A. hydrophila, E. aerogenes, S. marcescens, S. dysenteriae, Staphylococcus* sp., *Klebsiella* sp., *Micrococcus* sp., *Bacillus* sp., *Salmonella* sp., *Citrobacter* sp. and *Flavobacterium* sp.) (Martins et al. 2014, 73-80; Masood et al. 2007, 609; Saeed and Tariq 2009, 421-424).

The antimicrobial activity of the EOs was initially tested by measuring the inhibition zone diameter observed, using a well diffusion method (Sarikurkcu et al. 2015, 178). It is obvious that the EOs showed significant activity against the tested microorganisms with inhibition zones ranging from 8.33-34.67mm. However, the EOs differs significantly in their activity against test microorganisms. *O. vulgare* subsp. *vulgare* was the most active against *S. lutea, S. aureus, C. albicans, E. faecalis* and *B. cereus* 34.67, 26.67, 24.67, 22.33 and 20.33mm, respectively. *O. vulgare* subsp. *hirtum* showed promising antifungal activity against *C. albicans* with inhibition zone 32.33mm. In general, most of the tested gram-positive bacteria and *C. albicans* were sensitive to the EOs. However, *S. typhimurium, E. coli* and *P. aeroginosa* were the most resistant bacteria. The EOs of *O. vulgare* was analyzed by several authors. De Falco et al. (2013, 14948) reported OVV under different growth conditions showed antimicrobial action, mainly against Gram-positive pathogens and particularly *B. cereus* and *B. subtilis*. On the other hand, Khosravi et al. (2011, 95) evaluated the EOs exhibited the broad spectrum of antifungal activity against *C. glabrata* isolates with mean inhibition zone of 27.1mm. The antimicrobial activity of the EOs was examined by microdilution susceptibility assay against 7 bacterial and 1 yeast strains selected on the basis of their relevance as human pathogens. The experiments revealed that the EOs exhibited variable MICs and significant antimicrobial activity, depending on the microbial strains. The MIC values of OVV and OVH ranged from 85.3 to 426.7g/ml and 85.3 to >512, respectively. *O. vulgare* subsp. *vulgare* showed very strong activity against *S. lutea* with the best MIC (85.3g/ml). The lowest MIC for *E. coli* was 213.3g/ml, whereas the highest MIC was 426.7g/ml for *S. typhimurium*. Many previous researchers (De Falco et al. 2014, 243; Stefanakis et al. 2013, 539-546) reported the antimicrobial activity of

Origanum species but their findings were different from those of present study. According to Ozkalp et al. (2010, 273) the antimicrobial activities of EO from oregano were found effective in inhibiting the growth of *M. luteus* and *B. cereus* with MICs values 16 and 32g/ml, respectively. In another study (De Martino et al. 2009, 2735) the EO of *O. vulgare* was found active mainly against the Gram-positive pathogens, among which *S. epidermidis* was the most affected (MIC 25g/ml). In the present study, MIC values for *C. albicans* were 128 and 85.3g/ml for OVV and OVH, respectively. Cleff et al. (2010, 116) demonstrated the antifungal effect of *O. vulgare* EO against *Candida* spp. suggest its administration may represent an alternative treatment for candidiasis. Also, *O. vulgare* EO was exhibited antifungal activity against three *Monilinia* species (Mancini et al. 2014, 639-642). In another study conducted by Esen et al. (2007, 371-376) the EOs of wild-growing *O. vulgare* subsp. *hirtum* from the Marmara region of Turkey found effective in inhibiting the growth of Gram-positive and Gram-negative bacteria with MICs values between 62.5 and 500g/ml. It is thought that the observed dissimilar results may be attributed to differences in methods and composition of the EOs and the variable sensitivity of different microorganisms to EOs relates to different resistance levels between the strains used in each particular study. The data in relation to the composition of the oils, it appears evident that the antimicrobial activity was mainly linked to the presence of significant proportion of carvacrol, and thymol as phenolic constituents that their mechanism of action would therefore be similar to other phenolics (Lambert et al. 2001, 453-462; Burt, 2004, 226). p-ymene (in this study its rate was % 13.45 for EO of OVV) is not an effective antibacterial when used alone, but when combined with carvacrol synergism has been observed against microorganisms (Burt, 2004, 235). According to our results, EO of OVH having linalool as a major component was showed better antifungal activity than EO of OVV against *C. albicans*. The importance of the antifungal activity of linalool has been previously reported (Hristova et al. 2013, 39-42). Their data suggest that although linalool differs slightly from the other monoterpene alcohols because it is acyclic, this component showed significant inhibitory activity chiefly against *C. albicans*.

The results of *in vitro* antimicrobial activity of five extracts from *O. vulgare* against 29 strains of bacteria and fungi, was determined by microdilution method (Ličina et al. 2013, 498-500). The intensity of antimicrobial activity varied depending on the species of microorganisms and on the type of plant extract. The water extract showed the greatest inhibitory effects against tested bacteria among tested extracts. The extracts were more effective against Gram-positive than Gram-negative bacteria. The significant effect was exhibited against species from genus *Bacillus*, especially against *Bacillus pumilis* NCTC824 with MIC<0.3mg/ml. Moreover, the extracts demonstrated strong antibacterial effect on *Sarcina lutea*. The most effective was diethyl ether extract. Further, all strains of *S. aureus* showed high sensitivity to all oregano extracts. Water extract indicated the best antibacterial effect. *S. aureus* PMFKGB12, the strain isolated from food, was the most sensitive among tested strains. Human pathogenic bacteria, *Escherichia coli, Pseudomonas aeruginosa, Klebsiella pneumoniae, Enterococcus faecalis*, showed low sensitivity to tested oregano extracts. Weerakkody et al. (2010, 1408) tested antimicrobial activity of water, ethanol and hexane extract and they also noticed low sensitivity of *E. coli* (MIC>5mg/ml). The methanol extracts of aerial parts of oregano did not show antimicrobial activity (Sahin et al. 2004, 549) while Chaudry et al. (2007, 609) demonstrated significant antimicrobial activity of aqueous infusion. Water extract showed good antibacterial activity in this study. The water extract was rich in total phenols and it could explain its activity. Kursat et al. (2011, 413) confirmed the effects of flavonoids on Gram positive bacteria and fungi (*Trichophyton* sp. (15.4±0.2mm), *Candida albicans* (9.2±0.3mm) and *Candida glabrata* (9.1±0.1mm)). The yeasts were more sensitive than molds in the study of Ličina et al. (2013, 498). Ethanol, acetone, ethyl acetate and diethyl ether extract inhibit the growth of *C. albicans* and *Rhodotorula* sp. at concentrations between 2.5mg/ml and 10mg/ml. Water extract was the least active against the yeasts. Antifungal activity of oregano essential oils was more investigated than activity of plant extracts according to literature review. Manohar et al. (2001, 111) have demonstrated that oregano oil effectively inhibits *in vitro* and *in vivo* growth of *C. albicans*. The experiment with mice indicated administration of oregano oil in the prevention and treatment of candidiasis. Moreover, Rosato et al. (2009, 972) have demonstrated synergistic effect between *O. vulgare* oil and nystatin. Also, essential oil of oregano was found to inhibit the growth of *Aspergillus niger* (Rahbar et al. 2012, 2681). *Aspergillus restrictus* and *Penicillium chrysogenum* were the most sensitive in study, among the tested molds. In relation to these molds, acetone, ethyl acetate and diethyl ether extract showed interesting results with MICs at 2.5 and 5mg/ml.

ANTIMICROBIAL ACTIVITY OF *OREGANO MAJORANA*

In Tunisia, *O. majorana* is commonly known by the name of "khezama" or marjoram and is frequently used for culinary and medicinal purpose (Veres et al. 2007, 1155). This plants exhibits rather high diversity of both taxonomic and chemical aspects (Hazzit et al. 2006, 6314). It is cultivated for its aromatic leaves, which have commonly been used in fresh and dried forms as a spice or condiment in various cuisines. Marjoram leaves also contain EO that has been widely used in folk medicines. Marjoram oil has been reported to be non-toxic, non-irritant and non-sensitizing, but to be avoided during pregnancy. Marjoram oil has also been used in perfumes, soaps, and detergents for its spicy herbaceous notes and as stomachic, antiseptic, expectorant, and sedative, for the treatment of insomnia, rheumatism, migraines, dysmenorrhoea and diarrhoea. In Tunisia, the plant has been widely employed to add flavor to the cooking liquid used in preparing carrots, peas, spinach and zucchini and salad dressing. *O. majorana* has also been widely prepared in an infusion form and applied as a stimulant, sudorific, emmenagogue and galactagogue for the treatment of several health diseases and disturbances, including heart and blood diseases, fevers, leucoderma, inflammations, asthma, hysteria, and paralysis (European Pharmacopoeia, 1975).

The antimicrobial activities of *O. majorana* EO were evaluated using the agar diffusion and the microtiter broth methods against 25 test microorganisms, including 12 bacteria (six Gram-positive and six Gram-negative) and 13 fungi (nine yeast and four dermatophytic strains). Their potency was assessed quantitatively by IZ, MIC, MFC, MBC/MIC, MFC/MIC and IC50 values. The results obtained were almost the same observed for antibiotic gentamicin and Amphotericin B used as a positive probe. The EO was noted to be active against all microbial strains but in different degrees. The data indicated that the IZ from 8±0mm to 18.33±0.57mm with MIC from 0.097 mg/ml to 3.125 mg/ml for bacterial strains, and from 11±0mm to 28±0mm with MIC from 0.058mg/ml to 0.468 mg/ml for fungal strains. *M. luteus* NCIMB 8166 (18.33±0.57mm) and *Candida albicans* ATCC 90028 (28±0mm) were the most sensitive bacteria and fungus, respectively. *P. aeruginosa* ATCC 27853 (IZ¼ 8±0 mm and MIC¼ 3.125mg/ml) seems to be the most tolerant strain. The results of antifungal activity assays showed that the oil moderately reduced the growth of all strains, expect for Candida albicans ATCC 90028, which was strongly inhibited by the EO with an IZ value of 28±0 mm and a MIC value of 0.058 mg/ml. MBC or MFC are defined as the lowest concentration of EO or antibiotic at which inoculated bacteria or fungi are completely killed. The evaluation MBCs and MFCs values showed variability of inhibition among all strains, with values ranging from 0.39mg/mL to 6.25mg/mL for bacteria and from 0.234mg/mL to 1.875mg/ml for fungi. *M. luteus* NCIMB 8166, *Candida albicans* ATCC 90028 and *Candida parapsilosis* ATCC 22019 seems to be the most sensible towards EO effect because these strains showed the weaker values of MBC. The MBC/MIC and MFC/MIC ratio was used to determine the antimicrobial powers of EO (Hajlaoui et al. 2016, 92). According to the classification of Soro et al. (2010, 307), when this ratio is greater than 4, the oil is considered bacteriostatic or fungistatic whereas it is bactericidal or fungicidal when it is lower or equal to 4. This ratio has shown a bacteriostatic effect of the oil to the half of the strains tested and a fungicidal effect for the majority of the fungal strains. These results highlight the potential utilization of marjoram oil in dermatomycoses, which are common infections caused by filamentous fungi and by some yeasts that can be severe in immuno-compromised patients. Antifungal actions are quite similar to those described for bacteria. However, two additional phenomena inhibiting the action of yeast are worth mentioning: the establishment of a pH gradient across the cytoplasmic membrane and the blocking of energy production of yeasts which involve the disruption of the bacterial membrane (Abdelouaheb and Amadou 2012, 170).

The antimicrobial properties of EO have purportedly been associated with the high proportion of oxygenated monoterpenes and especially to their major constituents, such as terpin-4-ol (Tabanca et al., 2001, 4300), a-terpinol (Cosentino et al. 1999, 131), a-pinene, and p-cymene. Other compounds such as g-terpinene, b-caryophyllene, and sabinene are also known to have efficient antimicrobial properties (Andrews et al. 1980, 302; Cimanga et al. 2002, 214; Burt 2004, 224; Nada et al. 2005, 1427). These compounds increase fungal cell permeability and membrane fluidity and inhibit medium acidification. Moreover, terpenes are thought to be inducing alterations in cell permeability by entering between the fatty acyl chains that make up the membrane lipid bilayers, thus disrupting lipid packing and causing changes to membrane properties and functions (Sikkema et al. 1995, 212). However, and since EO consist of various major to minor constituents, the synergistic effects of some compounds should be taken into consideration as for as antibacterial activity is concerned. The results obtained in the present study showed that gram-positive bacteria were more sensitive than gram-negative bacteria, which is in agreement with some previous reports in the literature (Harpaz et al. 2003, 415; Hajlaoui et al. 2009, 2227-2229). Among the tested microorganisms, bacteria, including Gram-positive and Gram-negative strains, were less sensitive to the oil than yeasts. However, they were not as active as gentamicin. These results are in disagreement with several previous works reporting that *Origanum basilicum* EO displayed greater activity against bacterial than antifungal strains (Karaman et al. 2003, 231).

The differences in the susceptibility of the test organisms to EO could be attributed to variation in the rate of EO constituents penetrating through the cell wall and cell membrane structures. As shown, the obtained data showed that Gram-positive bacteria were more sensitive than Gram-negative ones. These differences could be due to the differences in the cell membrane of those bacterial groups with the presence of the lipopolysaccharides in the outer membrane for Gram-negative bacteria, which makes them inherently resistant to external agents, such as hydrophilic dyes, antibiotics, detergents, and lipophilic compounds (Djenane et al. 2011, 1046; Gupta et al. 2011, 102). Without this barrier, the membrane in Gram-positive bacteria can be permeated more easily and disrupt the proton motive force, electron flow, active transport, and coagulation of the cell contents (Ennajar et al. 2009, 364).

Antimicrobial Activity of *Origanum compactum*

The antibacterial properties of *O. compactum* essential oils and extracts against pathogenic bacteria were reported in many studies and obtained results are promising (Bellakhdar et al. 1988, 94), indicated antibacterial effect of *Oregano* flowers, leaves and stems essential oil against five of pathogenic bacteria of salmonella sp isolated from food borne.

Essential oil of *O. compactum* was tested against six Gram positive (*Staphylococcus aureus, Listeria monocytogenes* serovar 4b, *Listeria innocua* and *Enterococcus faecium*) and 4 Gram negative bacteria (*Escherichia coli* K12, *Escherichia coli* serovar O157:H7, *Proteus mirabilis, Pseudomonas aeruginosa, Pseudomonas fluorescens* and *Bacillus subtilis*), and inhibited the growth of all tested bacteria MICs range from 0.0078 for *S. aureus* (MBLA) to over >1ml/ml for *P. aeruginosa* (Bouhdid et al., 2008, 1567).

Different modes of action are involved in the antimicrobial activity of essential oils and extracts. Because of the variability of quantity and chemical profiles of the essential oil and extract components, it is likely that their antimicrobial activity is not due to a single mechanism. It is considered that these components have several sites of action at the cellular level. Generally, there are six possible mechanisms of antimicrobial action, which include: (1) disintegration of cytoplasmic membrane, (2) interaction with membrane proteins (ATPases and others), (3) disturbance of the outer membrane of gram negative bacteria with the release of lipopolysaccharides, (4) destabilization of the proton motive force with leakage of ions, (5) coagulation of the cell content, and (6) inhibition of enzymes synthesis (Nazzaro et al. 2013, 1457).

The mechanism of antibacterial action seems to have a relationship with a great number of complex constituents in Eos and extracts instead of just specific bioactive metabolites, which may result in different action modes and difficult identification from molecular point of view (Burt, 2004, 239; Carson et al. 2002, 1918).

Carvacrol (main coumpound of Origano oil) has been demonstrated able to destabilize the cytoplasmic membrane and acts as a proton exchanger, thereby reducing the pH gradient across the cytoplasmic membrane. The resulting collapse of the proton motive force and depletion of the ATP pool eventually lead to cell death (Ultee et al. 2002, 1563).

O. compactum essential oil showed a strong antibacterial activity against *Staphylococcus aureus* and *Pseudomonas aeruginosa*. This activity may be associated with the presence of carvacrol and thymol, which is the major component of the oil. The mechanism of action is related with the capacity of *O. compactum* essential oil to induce leakage of intracellular K+ from cells, induce alterations of membrane potential and induce alterations in the bacterial membrane. These alterations led to the loss of membrane-selective permeability and thus the inhibition of respiratory activity, and also the loss of other essential enzymatic activities, all these changes led to cell death (Bouhdid et al. 2009, 1568).

The compounds of phenolic structures, such as carvacrol and thymol presented as the main compounds (chemotypes) of *O. compactum* essential oil are highly active against several pathogenic bacteria. These compounds have been reported to be bacteriostatic or bactericidal agents, depending on the concentration used (Pelczar et al. 1988, 325). These compounds are highly active despite their relatively low capacity to dissolve in water (Hili et al. 1997, 270; Lis-Balchin and Deans 1997, 760; Sivropoulou et al. 1996, 1203; Suresh et al. 1992, 255). In general, the EO having the most important antibacterial properties contain a high percentage of phenolic compounds such as carvacrol (Periago et al. 2006, 18) and thymol (Cosentino et al. 1999, 131; Juliano et al. 2000, 516; Lambert et al. 2001, 453).

Their mechanism of action is related to the capacity of these compounds in the disruption of the cell membrane, movement of protons, the flow of electrons, active transportation and the coagulation of the cell content (Davidson 1997; Sikkema et al. 1995, 218).

Furthermore, carvacrol destabilizes the cytoplasmic membrane and also acts as a proton exchange, thereby reducing the pH gradient across the cytoplasmic membrane. The collapse of the force protons movement and resulting depletion of ATP pool lead to cell death (Ultee et al. 1999, 4608).

The importance of the presence of the hydroxyl group in the phenolic compounds such as carvacrol and thymol was confirmed (Dorman and Deans 2000, 310; Ultee et al. 2002, 1563). The relative position of the hydroxyl group on the phenol ring does not appear to strongly influence the level of antibacterial activity. Indeed, the action of thymol against *Bacillus cereus, Staphylococcus aureus* and *Pseudomonas aeruginosa* appears to be comparable to that of carvacrol (Lambert et al. 2001, 453-462; Ultee et al. 2002, 1562). However, in a study on the effects of carvacrol and thymol, it was shown that they act differently against Gram-positive and Gram-negative species (Dorman and Deans 2000, 310).

Carvacrol and thymol are able to disintegrate the outer membrane of Gram negative bacteria, releasing lipopolysaccharides (LPS) and inducing the increase in the permeability of the cytoplasmic membrane toward ATP (Lambert et al. 2001, 455).

On other hand, studies of *B. cereus* showed that carvacrol interacts with the cell mebrane, which it dissolves in the phospholipid bilayer and fit between the fatty acid chains (Ultee et al. 2002, 1564). This distortion of the physical structure lead to the expansion and destabilization of the membrane, increased membrane fluidity which and consequently increase the passive permeability (Ultee et al. 2002, 1564).

The management of fungal infections possesses many problems, including a limited number of antifungal drugs, toxicity, and resistance to commonly used antifungal drugs, relapse of infections and the high costs. For that, it is very important and necessary to discover new antifungal agents to combat the strains expressing resistance to the available antifungal drugs. One of natural products used as therapeutic agent against fungi is *Oregano*, e.g., its essential oils and extracts. Considerable Oregano petroleum ether, hexane, chloroform and methanol extract activity were estimated by Fadel et al. (2013, 11019) against *Penicillium digitatum.*

The petroleum ether extracts of *O. compactum* were highly active against the mycelial growth of *P. digitatum*, The effectiveness of petroleum ether extract might be due to its high levels of carvacrol, p-cymène, thymol and terpinene (Bouchra et al. 2003, 165), the antifungal activity of carvacrol, the main compound of lamiaceae essential oil has been the subject of several studies (Daferera et al., 2000, 2576-2581).

The methanol 80% extracts of *O. compactum* aerial parts were also highly effective against *P. digitatum* mycelial growth. It was demonstrated that the mechanism of toxicity of total phenols against the fungi is based on the inactivation of the fungal enzymes which contain the SH group in their active sites classified the pure compounds according to their antifungal activity towards seven fungi, this activity decreases according to the type of chemical functions of compound: phenols>alcohols>aldehydes>acetones>ethers> eydrocarbures (Bouchra et al. 2003, 167).

The antifungal activity of oregano essential oil was tested against *Botrytis cinere*, and the inhibition was IC50=35.1ppm). While the antifungical effect of carvacrol and thymol, the main compound of oregano essential oil, was IC_{50}=18.6ppm and IC_{50}=18.9ppm against the same species respectively (Bouchra et al. 2003, 168). The oregano antifungal effect may also be attributed to essential oil and phenolic compounds that are known to cause cell membranes damage, causing leakage of cellular materials and ultimately the microorganism death (Cox et al., 2000). The antimicrobial, e.g., antifungal property of myrtle is suspected to be associated with their high contents of polyphenols and oxygenated monoterpenes.

ANTIMICROBIAL ACTIVITY OF *ORIGANUM MINUTIFLORUM*

The composition of *O. minutiflorum* extracts is known to include thymol, carvacrol, pinene, terpinene, and cymene which are known to have antimicrobial, antifungal, and antioxidant properties (Oke and Aslim 2010, 1728; Dadalioglu and Evrendilek 2004, 5256; Askun et al. 2008, 688).

Several researchers have generally reported that the aqueous extracts of plants do not have much antibacterial activity (Paz et al. 1995, 67; Vlietinck et al. 1995, 31). The antibacterial activity of the *O. minutiflorum* extracts was in the range of 5.0±0.1-20.2±0.2 (mm, inhibition zone diameter). The n-hexane extract had a broad spectrum of activity against both the gram-positive and gram negative bacteria. In general, *L. monocytogenes* ATCC 7644 was the most resistant bacterium, while *S. sonnei* RSKK 878 was the most sensitive. Among all extracts, the n-hexane extract was the most active against *S. sonnei* (20.2±0.2mm). The ethanol and the methanol extracts exhibited the least antimicrobial activity as compared to the other three *O. minutiflorum* extract. As expected, the control treatment (solvents) had no inhibitory effect on any of the test bacteria. MIC values were determined for n-hexane and acetone extracts of *O. minutiflorum* which showed highest inhibition zones in the agar diffusion method. MIC values for bacterial strains which were sensitive to the n-hexane and the acetone extracts of *O. minutiflorum* were in the range of 125-2000μg/ml. The highest inhibitory activity for the n-hexane extract was against *S. sonnei* RSKK 878 which showed the lowest MIC (125μg/ml) and largest growth inhibition halos for agar well diffusion assay (20.2±0.2mm). On the other hand, the acetone extract exhibited the highest inhibitory activity against *S. aureus* ATCC 25923 which showed the lowest MIC (250μg/ml) and largest growth inhibition halos (14.8±0.2mm). *L.*

monocytogenes ATCC 7644 was the most resistant bacterium and exhibited highest MIC (2000μg/ml) for both of the extracts. The inhibition zones of the extracts on test bacteria showed a significant correlation with MIC values ($p<0.05$). Control treatment (DMSO) did not show an inhibitor effect on any of the bacteria (Oke and Aslim 2010, 1730).

Shigella dysenteriae and *S. sonnei* are the predominant species in the tropics, while *S. sonnei* is the predominant species in industrialized countries (Preston and Borczyk, 1994). Controlling the numbers and growth of *S. sonnei* therefore remains an important objective for sectors of the food production industry. *O. minutiflorum* is a well-known aromatic plant which is frequently used as a spice and as a traditional medicinal herb in Anatolia and may be used as a natural preservative against *S. sonnei* for the food production industry (Oke and Aslim 2010, 1728-1731).

Twenty-one *Campylobacter* spp. (12 *C. jejuni*, 5 *C. lari* and 4 *C. coli*) strains using in this study were selected among 300 isolates according to their resistance to ciprofloxacin. The minimum inhibitory concentration (MIC) values for bacterial strains, which were sensitive to the essential oil of *O. minutiflorum*, were in the range of 7.8–800μg/ml. The essential oil obtained showed strong antimicrobial activity against all of the tested ciprofloxacin-resistance *Campylobacter* spp. These results suggest that the essential of *O. minutiflorum* may be used as a natural preservative in food against food-born disease, such as campylobacteriosis (Aslim and Yucel 2008, 602).

Aqueous extracts of *O. minutiflorum* did not show any antimicrobial activity against *H. pylori* J99 at a concentration of 2 mg/ml. While, both methanol and ethanol extracts at the same concentration showed weak inhibitory effects, no significant difference was observed with regards to their antimicrobial activities (Ozen et al. 2014, 329). Recently, plant extracts have been used as an alternative treatment, encouraging the development of novel phytotherapeutic treatments against many microbial infections, including *H. pylori.* Such therapies may aid in overcoming the problems of antibiotic resistance and the non-availability of some of the drugs in rural areas (Geethangili et al. 2010, 150; Rao et al. 2012, 782). Extracts of *O. minutiflorum* have previously been tested for their antioxidant activity and antimicrobial effect on food pathogens. These include; *Escherichia coli* O157:H7, *Listeria monocytogenes*, *Salmonella typhimurium*, *Staphylococcus aureus*, *Campylobacter* spp., *Shigella sonnei*, *Pseudomonas aeruginosa*, *Staphylococcus epidermidis*, *Enterococcus faecalis*, *Bacillus cereus*, *Enterobacter aerogenes*, and *Klebsiella pneumoniae* (Askun et al. 2009, 688; Oke and Aslim 2010, 1728; Aslim and Yucel 2008, 602; Dadalioglu and Evrendilek 2004, 5256).

Application of Oregano Essential Oil in Food Science

The oxidation process is one of the major causes of food spoilage, which results in rancidity and deterioration of the nutritional quality, colour, flavour, texture, and safety of food. A significant number of herbs is used as natural preservatives in food industry. Besides being used to achieve the proper flavour and to intensify the flavorus some spices and herbs exhibit antioxidant effects which is of great importance for food industry (Stanković and Stanojević 2014, 113; Tongnuanchan et al. 2014, 1235).

Origanum vulgare L. is one of the most widely species among all the species within the genus which is distributed all over the Europe, also from the western to central Asia. It is one of the most important culinary herbs in the world. Leaves and flowers of oregano are traditionally used for illnesses such as cough and sore throat and for the relieve of gastrointestinal disorders (Stanojevič et al. 2016, 131).

The results of Stanojevič et al. (2016, 135) indicate that the oregano essential oil could be used as a potential source of natural antioxidants for the food, pharmaceutical and chemical industry. Therefore, oregano essential oil represents the alternative to synthetic additives that exhibit toxic and carcinogenic effects. So, it is interesting to investigate its application as a natural antioxidant additive in some final food and pharmaceutical products, for preservation and/or extension the shelf-life of raw and processed foods as well as pharmaceuticals. In addition, the results of antioxidant activity in the present study suggested that use of oregano is not just reasonable but it should be even favored in the traditional Serbian cuisine.

Several techniques are explored to facilitate the addition of OEO as antimicrobial food additive has been explored. The use of antimicrobial edible film could be a tool for improving food safety and extending the shelf-life of food systems by controlling the release of antimicrobials on food surfaces. Antimicrobial properties of whey protein isolate based or cellulose-based filter paper films containing oregano EOs (5, 10, 20, 40, and 80g/kg) were tested against *Listeria innocua, Staphylococcus aureus,* and *Salmonella enteritidis*, and the highest inhibition zones (aproximately 3750 mm^2) were found against *L. innocua* (Royo et al., 2010, 1513-1519). The addition of essential oil of oregano in tomato-based edible film was effective to inhibit the bacterial growth of *S. enterica* and *Listeria monocytogenes.* Moreover, this edible film showed good physical properties for food applications (Du et al. 2009, 390). The application of oregano films on meat surfaces containing 10^3CFU/cm^2 of *Eschericia coli* O157:H7 or *Pseudomonas* spp. showed that oregano film was effective against both bacteria, showing a 0.95 log reduction of *Pseudomonas* spp. levels and 1.12 log reduction of *E. coli* O157:H7 (Oussalah et al. 2004, 5600).

Incorporation of oregano oil (1%) to a whey protein-edible film was effective at inhibiting the bacterial growth of *L. innocua*, *S. aureus*, *S. enteritidis*, and *Pseudomonas fragi.* Low concentrations of OEO have shown a wide spectrum of action against both pathogen and spoilage bacteria (Fernández-Pan et al. 2012, 383). Promising opportunities are presented by these films with direct application on food systems. In another study, the use of oregano essential oil (500ppm) was effective to effectively reduce populations of *Salmonella* spp. inoculated on iceberg lettuce until 2.28CFU/g, but showed browning and softening of the lettuce leaf surface after 10 min of treatment with oregano oil (Gündüz et al. 2012, 414).

OEO and its principal compounds have been applied also as antimicrobials in fruit and vegetable production. OEO and carvacrol (0.67 and 0.067%) were used to treat apple, mango, orange, and tomato juices inhibiting the growth of *E. coli* O157:H7 (Friedman et al. 2007, 207). Treatments of apples with EOs from oregano (1 and 10%) showed significant efficacy at reducing *Botrytis cinerea* and *Penicillium expansum* growth (Lopez-Reyes et al. 2010, 171). EOs from *O. vulgare* L. (80-0.003μl/ml) inhibited bacterial microflora associated with minimally processed vegetables (De Azeredo et al. 2011, 1543). Carvacrol and thymol (10, 25, 50, 100, 250, and 500μl/l of carvacrol, thymol or the mix (1:1) of carvacrol + thymol) applied into lemon, resulted in low fungal decay induced by *Penicillium digitatum* and *Penicillium italicum* (Pérez-Alfonso et al. 2012, 101). OEO (400ppm) combined with thyme (6000ppm) was evaluated for control of *Enterobacter cloacae* on lettuce (Gutierrez et al. 2009, 142). *Listeria* strains were more sensitive than spoilage bacteria, and oregano and thyme were the most active EOs. The average efficacy of EOs against *Listeria* spp. was in the following order: oregano ≥ thyme > lemon balm, while the efficacy order of EOs against the spoilage bacteria was: oregano ≥ thyme > marjoram.

OEO (0.2% v/w) or its principal components have also been used in conjunction with other technologies, such as vacuum-packaging with ethylenediaminetetraacetic acid (1.5% w/w) and lysozyme solution (1.5% w/w) on semicooked coated chicken meat, extending shelf-lives by 7-8 days compared with controls (Ntzimani et al. 2010, 190). In another investigation carvacrol (0.3-0.5%), caprylic acid (0.25-1.0%), and ε-polylysine (0.125-1.0%) were applied on breaded chicken products and showed a reduction in *Salmonella* populations (Moschonas et al. 2012, 405). Pectin edible films that contained carvacrol (0.5, 1.5, and 3%) and cinnamaldehyde (0.5, 1.5, and 3%) caused the inactivation of *L. monocytogenes* on ham and bologna (Ravishankar et al. 2012, 377). Dipped carp fillets with carvacrol (0.5%) and thymol (0.5%) delayed bacterial growth and extended the shelf-life of the fillets (Mahmoud et al. 2004, 657). The studies of the antimicrobial activity of *Origanum majorana* (1.15, 2.3, 5.75mg/g) in fresh sausage showed that its addition to fresh sausage exerted a bacteriostatic effect at concentrations lower (1.15mg/g) than the minimum inhibitory concentration (2.3mg/g) (Busatta et al. 2008, 209). EO of *Origanum syriacum* var. *bevanii* (0.4, 0.8 1.6, 2.4, and 3.2μg/ml) had a marked antifungal effect against soil contamination with *Sclerotinia sclerotiorum*, both oils reduced sclerotial viability, increasing the number of surviving tomato seedling by 69.8 and 53.3%, respectively (Soylu et al. 2007, 1021). In other study, four pathogenic bacteria (*E. coli* O157:H7, *S. enterica*, *B. cereus*, and *S. aureus*) were inoculated in a dough made from corn flour with carvacrol (0.5, 2, and 5%) and all the strains were completely inactivated within 24 h (Ortega Morente et al. 2010, 274). This information reveals the antimicrobial potential of OEO to be used as a food additive.

Table 6. Antimicrobial, Antioxidant, and Sensorial Effects of Origanum spp. Essential Oils Added to Food products (Ortega-Ramirez et al., 2016)

		Effects			
Oregano Species	**Food Treated**	**Antimicrobial**	**Antioxidant**	**Flavor**	**References**
Origanum vulgare	Cotton seed/ potatoes	ND	Protection against oxidation	Enhancing stability	Houhoula et al. (2003, 1499-1503)
Origanum vulgare ssp. *hirtum*	Extra virgin olive oil	ND	Reduce oxidative rancidity	Preserved sensory quality	Asensio et al. (2012, 294–301)
Origanum syriacum var. *bevanii*	Tomato seedling	Antifungal	ND	ND	Soylu et al. (2007, 1021-1030)
Origanum vulgare	Peanuts	ND	Higher oxidative stability	Oxidized and cardboard flavor intensities increased	Olmedo et al. (2009, 2128-2136)
Origanum marjorana	Sausage	Bacteriostatic	ND	ND	Busatta et al. (2008, 209-211)
Origanum vulgare	Vegetables Salad	Antimicrobial	ND	ND	De Azeredo et al. (2011, 1541-1548)
Origanum onites	Lettuce	Antibacterial	ND	ND	Gündüz et al. (2012, 412-415)
Origanum vulgare	Tuna salad	ND	Increased the oxidative stability	ND	Sørensen et al. (2010, 476-487)
Coridothymus capitatus	Protein edible film	Antibacterial	ND	ND	Fernández-Pan et al. (2012, 383-390)
Origanum vulgare	Sea bream	ND	Strong antioxidant activity	Acceptable sensory scores	Goulas and Kontominas (2007, 287-296)
Origanum onites L.	Chicken	ND	ND	Desirable and compatible	Oral et al. (2009, 1459-1465)
Origanum vulgare	Sausages	Bacteriostatic	ND	Increase sensorial appeal	Busatta et al. (2007, 610-616)
Origanum onites L.	Fresh cut tomatoes and cucumbers	Sanitizers	ND	Without sensorial defect	Sagdic et al. (2012, 7-14)
Origanum vulgare subsp *hirtum*	Sheep meat	ND	ND	Acceptable	Govaris et al. (2010, 175-180)
Oregano sp.	Bolognese sausages	ND	ND	Increased the shelf-life and not found unpleasant by the panellists	Viuda-Martos et al. (2010, 9063-9070)
Origanum vulgare	Rainbow trout	ND	ND	Pleasant	Pyrgotou et al. (2010, 406-411)
Origanum vulgare	Tomato	Antibacterial	ND	ND	Du et al. (2009, 390-397)
Oregano Species	Food Treated	Antimicrobial	Antioxidant	Flavor	References
Origanum vulgare	Apple	ND	ND	ND	Lopez-Reyes et al. (2010, 171-177)
Origanum vulgare	Lettuce	Antibacterial	ND	ND	Gutierrez et al. (2008, 91-97)
Oregano sp.	Chicken	ND	ND	Shelf-life extension	Ntzimani et al. (2010, 187-196)
Origanum vulgare	Beef	Antibacterial	Stabilized lipid oxidation		Oussalah et al. (2004, 5598-5605)

Origanum vulgare EO possesses natural antimicrobial properties; its use to control *L. monocytogenes* in meat has been reported (Fasseas et al. 2008, 1188; Mazzarrino et al. 2015, 794; Petrou et al. 2012, 264). A multiple-hurdle strategy would be useful to reduce the effective EOs concentrations and also to decrease the occurrence of resistant strains (Camo et al. 2011, 174). In this respect, chitosan could be considered a good candidate, as it is regarded a safe food additive at a daily dose up to 3g (Commission Regulation EU 432/2012). Chitosan is the derivative form of chitin, water insoluble, non toxic, biodegradable and biocompatible, showing antioxidant and antimicrobial activity (Rhoades and Roller 2000, 80; Roller et al. 2002, 165).

The effect of chitosan in combination with essential oils has been investigated on chicken fillets (Khanjari et al. 2013, 94; Petrou et al. 2012, 264), cured chicken meat (Shekarforoush et al. 2015, 303), minced pork meat (Bonilla et al. 2014, 2443), bologna (Zivanovic et al. 2005, 45) and other pork cured meats (Ouattara et al. 2000, 139) while, to the best of our knowledge, the combined effect of chitosan and essential oils on pork meat under modified atmosphere, that is the most applied packaging condition for this product in the industry, has not been documented in literature.

The effect of oregano essential oil on the growth of *L. monocytogenes* was evaluated in pork meat in modified atmosphere at refrigeration temperature. The used gas mixture was 70% O_2, 20% CO_2 and 10% N_2, commonly used to preserve the colour of red meat during storage. In untreated control samples, starting from a load of 4.6log CFU/g, the counts of *L. monocytogenes* were almost stable during the first 10 days of storage, afterwards a growth up to 5.3log CFU/g was observed until day 15. Literature data on the development of *L. monocytogenes* in meat under refrigerated storage conditions (4-6°C) are contrasting, as some authors reported that this species was not able to grow in roast beef during 16 days of refrigerated storage (Broady et al. 2014, 482), while others reported its growth at 4°C in aerobic conditions, respectively until 28 days in cubed roast beef (Beverlya et al. 2008, 534) or until 10 days in raw chicken fillets (Khanjari et al. 2013, 94). Coma (2008, 90) described that *L. monocytogenes* was minimally affected by CO_2 level lower than 50%. The growth of *L. monocytogenes* in meats is influenced by different factors, and namely the physiological state of the cells, the strains, atmospheric conditions and competition with other microorganisms (Chen and Shelef 1992, 574; Paparella et al. 2013, 1230). In particular, while the presence of autochtonous microbiota did not affect the survival and growth of *L. monocytogenes* in beef meat (de Aguiar Ferreira Barros et al. 2007, 603), the competition with specific microorganisms such as *Pseudomonas fluorescens* seemed to have distinct and sometimes contrasting behaviors (Buchanan and Bagi 1999, 523). In a previous *in vitro* study (Mazzarrino et al. 2015, 794), 0.06% of the same commercial oregano essential oil (OEO) was able to decrease the load of *L. monocytogenes*. OEO concentrations of 2.0 and 4% OEO were applied in this work just for this reason, considering the well known need to increase the quantities in real systems to achieve in situ the same effect observed *in vitro*. Pork meat samples treated with OEO concentration of 0.5 and 1.0% previously showed the same values of controls, both at T0 and during storage at 4 °C). The application of OEO 2% determined a *L. monocytogenes* reduction of about 0.62 Log after 3 h from the treatment. However, this reduction was lost starting from day 2, with counts comparable to those of the control. A more stable reduction of about 0.50 Log was instead observed in samples treated with OEO 4%, with counts from 4.04 to 4.38 until day 15, suggesting a bacteriostatic effect of the essential oil. These results are in accordance with other authors (Dussault et al. 2014, 514) who evaluated the effect of different essential oils on ham inoculated with *L. monocytogenes*, proving the efficacy of oregano EO in extending the Lag phase and reducing the maximum growth rate of the pathogen. It is important to underline that food structure and nutrients may reduce the effectiveness of EOs (Campos et al. 2011, 1112) since most of the published studies on the antilisterial activity of *Origanum vulgare* essential oil were performed *in vitro*. In this respect, Shekarforoush et al. (2015, 303-309) reported that the inhibitory effect of OEO against *L. monocytogenes* in chicken meat was observed for only 24 h of storage at 8 °C, in spite of the strong activity observed *in vitro*. In this work, we observed that OEO, used alone in a real meat system, was not effective in decreasing the load of the inoculum of *L. monocytogenes*, but it was able to contain the pathogen growth only when used in concentration of 4%. In contrast, a strong reduction of *L. monocytogenes* counts was observed in samples treated with chitosan both alone and in combination with OEO 2 and 4%, although with different effectiveness.

Considering the technological use of oregano essential oil, a wider range of food matrices could be treated to take advantage of its antimicrobial efficacy, like fresh meat, seafood, and several types of whole and fresh-cut fruits and vegetables. Several technologies must be contemplated: nanoemulsions, nanocapsules, vapors, edible films based in different polymers; in conjunction with other preserving technologies like low temperatures, modified atmosphere packaging, and irradiation to achieve a more effective treatment of food products using OEO. The generation of this information will profound on the antimicrobial knowledge and effective uses of the OEO.

CONCLUSION

In conclusion, several industries are now looking for sources of new, natural and safe agents. Essential oil from *Origanum* spp. has shown efficacy retarding lipid oxidation in food matrices. Oregano essential oil possesses strong antimicrobial activity against food pathogen bacteria highlighting its potential as a tool to achieve food safety. Oregano essential oil has shown efficacy in reducing microbial growth of deteriorative microorganisms (bacteria, yeast, molds), representing the potential to increase shelf-life of food. Oregano essential oil can be considered as a rich source of bioactive compounds and its addition to food matrices transmit these benefits; this approach can be use as a tool to generate functional foods. Results obtained from lots of study can help to exploit the use of the *Origanum* EOs studied as the functional food and pharmacological ingredients for promoting health.

REFERENCES

Abdelouaheb, Djilani. Amadou, Dicko. 2012. *The therapeutic benefits of essential oils*. USA: Nutrition Well Being Health.

Abdullah, I. Anwar, H. Rasheed, S. Nigam, P. S. Janneh, O. Sarker, S. D. 2011. Composition, antioxidant and chemotherapeutic properties of the essential oils from two *Origanum* species growing in Pakistan. *Revista Brasileira de Farmacognosia* 21: 943-952.

Adigüzel, A. Medine, G. Meryem, B. Hatice, U. Fikrettin, A. Usa, K. 2005. Antimicrobial effects of *Ocimum basilicum* (*Labiatae*) extract. *Turkish Journal of Biology* 29: 155-160.

Akrayi, Héro F. S. Salih, Rebwar M. H. Hamad, Pishtiwan A. 2015. *In vitro* screening of antibacterial properties of *Rhus coriaria* and *Origanum vulgare* against some pathogenic bacteria. *Science Journal of Koya University* 3: 35-41.

Alagawany, M. El-Hack, Abd M. E. Farag, M. R. Shaheen, H. M. 2018. The usefulness of oregano and its derivates in poultry nutrition. *World's Poultry Science Journal* 74: 463-474.

Al-Howiriny, T. Alsheik, A. Alqasoumi, S. Al-Yahya, M. El-Tahir, K. Rafatullah, S. 2009. Protective effect of *Origanum majorana* L. "Marjoram" on various models of gastric mucosal injury in rats. *American Journal of Chinese Medicine* 37: 531-545.

Al-Mariri, A. Safi, M. 2013. The Antibacterial Activity of Selected Labiatae (Lamiaceae) Essential Oils against *Brucella melitensis*. *Iran Journal of Medical Sciences* 38: 44-50.

Al-Mariri, A. Safi, M. 2014. *In Vitro* Antibacterial Activity of Several Plant Extracts and Oils against Some Gram-Negative Bacteria. *Iran Journal of Medical Sciences* 39: 36-43.

Altundag, S. Aslin, B. 2011. Effect of the endemic plants essential oils on bacterial spot of tomato. *Journal of Plant Pathology* 93: 37-41.

Alzoreky, S. Nakahara, K. 2003. Antimicrobial activity of extracts from some edible plants commonly consumed in Asia. *International Journal of Food Microbiology* 80: 223-230.

Amakran, A. Hamoudane, M. Ramdan, B. Ben Mehdi, N. Ben, R. 2014. Etude des propriétés antioxydants, antiglyquantes et photochimiques de l'huileessentielle *d'Origanum. compactum* de Tétouan/Study of the antioxidant, antiglycemic and photochemical properties of the Origanum compactum essential oil of Tétouan. *Science Library Editions Mersenne* 6: 2111-4706.

Amar, E. C. Faisan Jr. J. P. Apines-Amar, M. J. S. Pakingking Jr. R. V. 2017. Temporal changes in innate immunity parameters, epinecidin gene expression, and mortality in orange-spotted grouper, *Epinephelus coioides* experimentally infected with a fish pathogen, *Vibrio harveyi* JML1. *Fish Shellfish Immunology* 69: 153-163.

Amarowicz, A. Zegarska, Z. Rafałowski, R. Pegg, R. B. Karamac, M. Kosinska, A. 2009. Antioxidant activity and free radical scavenging capacity ofethanolic extracts of thyme, oregano, and marjoram. *European Journal of Lipid Science and Technology* 111: 1111-1117.

Andrews, R. E. Parks, L. W. Spence, K. D. 1980. Some effects of Douglas fir terpenes on certain microorganisms. *Applied Environmental Microbiology* 40: 301-304.

Aristatile, B. Al-Numair, K. S. Veeramani, C. Pugalendi, K. V. 2009. Antihyperlipidemic effect of carvacrol on D-galactosamine-induced hepatoxic rats. *Journal of Basic Clinical Physiology and Pharmacology* 20: 15-27.

Asensio, C. M. Nepote, V. Grosso, N. R. 2012. Sensory attribute preservation in extra virgin olive oil with addition of oregano essential oil as natural antioxidant. *Journal of Food Science* 77: 294-301.

Ashraf, Z. Muhammad, A. Imran, M. Tareq, A. H. 2011. *In vitro* antibacterial and antifungal activity of methanolic, chloroform and aqueous extracts of *Origanum vulgare* and their comparative analysis. *International Journal of Organic Chemistry* 1: 257-261.

Askun, T. Tumen, G. Satil, F. A. Ates, M. 2008. Characterization of the phenolic composition of five plant methanol extracts and their antimicrobial activities. *Pharmacological Biology* 46: 688-694.

Aslim, B. Yucel, N. 2008. *In vitro* antimicrobial activity of essential oil from endemic Origanum minutiflorum on ciprofloxacin-resistant *Campylobacter* spp. *Food Chemistry* 107: 602–606.

Baser, K. H. C. Tümen, G. Selik, E. 1991. The essential oil of *Origanum minutiflorum* O. Schwarz and P.H. Davis. *Journal of Essential Oil Research* 3: 445-446.

Baricevic, D. and Bartol, T. 2002. The biological/pharmacological activity of the oregano genus. In *Oregano: the genera Origanum and Lippia, medicinal and aromatic plants – industrial profiles* edited by Kintzios, S. 177-214. London: Taylor &Francis.

Bellakhdar, J. Passannanti, S. Paternostro, M. P. Piozzi, F. 1988. Constituents of *Origanum compactum*. *Planta Medica* 54: 94.

Betts, G. D. Linton, P. Betteridge, R. J. 1999. Food spoilage yeasts: Effects of pH, NaCl and temperature on growth. *Food Control* 10: 27-33.

Beverlya, R. L. Janes, M. E. Prinyawiwatkul, W. No, H. K. 2008. Edible chitosan films on ready-to-eat roast beef for the control of *Listeria monocyotgenes*. *Food Microbiology* 25: 534-537.

Bezić, N. Skočibušić, M. Dunkić, V. 2005. Phytochemical composition and antimicrobial activity of *Satureja montana* L. and *Satureja cuneifolia* ten essential oils. *Acta Botanica Croatica* 64: 313-322.

Bonilla, J. Vargas, M. Atarés, L. Chiralt, A. 2014. Effect of chitosan essential oil films on the storage-keeping quality of pork meat products. *Food Bioprocessing and Technology* 7: 2443-2450.

Borisutpeth, M. P. Kanbutra, P. Weerakhun, S. Sarachoo, K. Porntrakulpipat, S. 2005. Antibacterial activity of Thai medicinal plant extracts on *Aeromonas hydrophila* and *Streptococcus Agalactiae* isolated from diseased tilapia (*Oreochromis niloticus*) 31st Congress on Science and Technology of Thailand, 2005.

Botanická Fotogalérie cz [*Botanical Gallery cz*] [online, 2018 11 28]. Available from: URL: http:// www.botanickafotogalerie.cz/ fotogalerie.php? lng=en& latName= Origanum%20vulgare&czName=dobromysl%20obecn%C3%A1&title=Origanum%20vulgare%20|%20dobromysl%20obecn%C3%A1&showPhoto_variant=photo_description&show_sp_descr=true&spec_syntax=species&sortby=lat.

Botany Online [online, 2018 12 05]. Available from: http://irapl.altervista.org/botany/main.php?taxon=Origanum+vulgare.

Botsoglou, E. Taitzoglou, I. A. Botsoglou, E. Lavrentiadou, S. N. Kokoli, A. N. Roubies, N. 2008. Effect of long-term dietary administration of oregano on the alleviation of carbon tetrachloride-induced oxidative stress in rats. *Journal of Agricultural and Food Chemistry* 56: 6287-6293.

Botsoglou, N. A. Florou-Paneri, P. Christaki, E. Giannenas, I. Spais, A. B. 2004. Performance of rabbits and oxidative stability of muscle tissues as affected by dietary supplementation with oregano essential oil. *Archives of Animal Nutrition* 58: 209-218.

Bouchra, C. Achouri, M. Idrissi Hassani, L. M. Hmamouchi, M. 2003. Chemical composition and antifungal activity of essential oils of seven Moroccan Labiatae against *Botrytis cinerea* Pers: Fr. *Journal of Ethnopharmacology* 89: 165-169.

Bouhdid, S. Abrini, J. Zhiri, A. Espunsy, M. J. 2009. Manresa, A. Investigation of functional and morphological changes in *Pseudomonas aeruginosa* and *Staphylococcus aureus* cells induced by *O. compactum* essential oil. *Journal of Applied Microbiology* 106: 1558-1568.

Bouhdid, S. Skali, S. N. Idaomar, M. Zhiri, A. Baudoux, D. Amensour, M. Abrini, J. 2008. Antibacterial and antioxidant activities of *Origanum compactum* essential oil. *African Journal of Biotechnology* 7: 1563-1570.

Bouyahya, A. Edoaudi, F. Dakka, N. 2016. *Origanum compactum* Benth.: A review on phytochemistry and pharmacological properties. *Medicinal and Aromatic Plants* 5: 2-3.

Broady, J. Liles, M. Bratcher, C. Schwartz, E. Wang, L. 2014. Survival and growth of *Listeria monocytogenes* on deli roast beef during refrigeration storage. Meat Science 96: 482-483.

Bubueanu, C. Nicu, I. Pirvu, L. 2015. Cromatographic fingerprint analysis and biactivity of *Origanum vulgare* exracts. *Malaysian Journal of Medicinal Biology Research* 2: 157-160.

Buchanan, R.L. Bagi, L.K.1999. Microbial competition: effect of *Pseudomonas fluorescens* on the growth of *Listeria monocytogenes. Food Microbiology* 16: 523-529.

Burt, S. 2004. Essential oils: their antibacterial properties and potential applications in foods-A review. *International Journal of Food Microbiology* 94: 223-253.

Busatta, C. Mossi, A. J. Rodrigues, M. R. A. Cansian, R. L. Oliveira, J. V. D. 2007. Evaluation of *Origanum vulgare* essential oil as antimicrobial agent in sausage. *Brazilian Journal of Microbiology* 8: 610-616.

Busatta, C. Vidal, R. Popiolski, A. Mossi, A. Dariva, C. Rodrigues, M. Corazza, F. Corazza, M. Vladimir Oliveira, J. Cansian, R. 2008. Application of *Origanum majorana* L. essential oil as an antimicrobial agent in sausage. *Food Microbiology* 25: 207-211.

Camo, J. Lorés, A. Djenane, D. Beltrán, J. A. Roncàles, P. 2011. Display life of beef packaged with an antioxidant active film as a function of the concentration of oregano extract. *Meat Science* 88: 174-178.

Campos, C. A. Castro, M. P. Gliemmo, M. F. Schelegueda, L. I. 2011. Use of natural antimicrobials for the control of *Listeria monocytogenes* in foods. *Communicating Current Research and Technological Advances* 2: 1112-1123.

Canbeck, M. Uyanoglu, M. Bayramoglu, G. Senturk, H. Erkasap, N. Koken, T. Uslu, S. Demirustu, C. Aral, E. Husnu Can Baser, K. 2008. Effects of carvacrol on defects of ischemia-reperfusion in the rat liver. *Phytomedicine* 15: 447-452.

Carocho, M. Ferreira, I. C. F. R. 2013. A review on antioxidants, prooxidants and related controversy: Natural and synthetic compounds, screening and analysis methodologies and future perspectives. *Food and Chemical Toxicology* 51: 15-25.

Carson, F. C. Mee, B. J. Rylei, T. V. 2002. Mechanism of action of *Melaleuca alternifolia* (Tea tree) oil on *Staphylococcus aureus* determined by Time-Kill, lysis, leakage, and salt tolerance assays and electron microscopy. *Antimicrobial Agent Chemotherapy* 46: 1914-1920.

Castillo-Juárez, I. González, V. Jaime-Aguilar, H. Martínez, G. Linares, E. Bye, R. Romero, I. 2009. Anti-Helicobacter pylori activity of plants used in Mexican traditional medicine for gastrointestinal disorders. *Journal of Ethnopharmacology* 122: 402-405.

Charles, D. J. 2013. *Antioxidant properties of spices, herbs and other sources*. USA: Springer.

Chaudry, N. M. A. Saeed, S. Tariq, P. 2007. Antibacterial effects of oregano (*Origanum vulgare*) against gram negative bacilli. *Pakistan Journal of Botany* 39: 609-613.

Chen, N. Shelef, L. A. 1992. Relationship between water activity, salts of lactic acid, and growth of *Listeria monocytogenes* in a meat model system. *Journal of Food Protection* 55: 574-578.

Chou, T. H. Ding, H. Y. Hung, W. J. Liang, Ch. 2010. Antioxidative characteristics and inhibition of alpha-melanocyte-stimulating hormone-stimulated melanogenesis of vanillin and vanilic acid from *Origanum vulgare*. *Experimental Dermatology* 19: 742-750.

Cimanga, K. Kambu, K. Tona, L. Apers, S. De Bruyne, T. Hermans, N. Totte, J. Pieters, L. Vlietinck, A. J. 2002. Correlation between chemical composition and antibacterial activity of essential oils of some aromatic medicinal plants growing in the Democratic Republic of Congo. *Journal of Ethnopharmacology* 79: 213-220.

Citarasu, T. 2010. Herbal biomedicines: a new opportunity for aquaculture industry. *Aquaculture International* 18: 403-414.

Cleff, M. B. Meinerz, A. R. Xavier, M. Schuch, L. F. Meireles, M. C. A. Rodrigues, M. R. A. de Mello, J. R. B. 2010. *In vitro* activity of *Origanum vulgare* essential Oil against *Candida* species. *Brazilian Journal of Microbiology* 41: 116-123.

Coccimiglio, J. Alipour, M. Jiang, Z. H. Gottardo, C. Suntres, Z. 2016. Antioxidant, antibacterial, and cytotoxic activities of the ethanolic *Origanum vulgare* extract and its major constituents. *Oxidative Medicine and Cellular Longevity* 2: 1-8.

Coma, V. 2008. Bioactive packaging technologies for extended shelf life of meat-based products. *Meat Science*m 78: 90-103.

Commission Regulation (EU) No 432/2012. *Official Journal of the European Union* L136/1-L136/40.

Cosentino, S. Tuberoso, C.I. Pisano, B. Satta, M. Mascia, V. Arzedi, E. Palmas, F. 1999. *In vitro* antimicrobial activity and chemical composition of Sardinian *Thymus* essential oils. *Letters of Applied Microbiology* 29: 130-135.

Cox, S. D. Mann, C. M. Markham, J. L. Bell, H. C. Gustafson, J. E. Warmington, J. R. Wyllie, S. G. 2000. The Mode of Antimicrobial Action of the Essential Oil of *Melaleuca Alternifolia* (Tea Tree Oil). *Journal of Applied Microbiology* 88 : 170-175.

Dadalioglu, I. Evrendilek, G.A. 2004. Chemical compositions and antibacterial effects of essential oils of Turkish oregano (*Origanum minutiflorum*), bay laurel (*Laurus nobilis*), Spanish lavender (*Lavandula stoechas* L.), and fennel (*Foeniculum vulgare*) on common foodborne pathogens. *Journal of Agriculture and Food Chemistry* 52: 8255-8260.

Daferera, D. J. Ziogas, B. N. Polissiou, M. G. 2000. GC-MS analysis of essential oils from some Greek aromatic plants and their fungitoxicity on *Penicillium digitatum*. *Journal of Agriculture and Food Chemistry* 48: 2576-2581.

Davidson, P. M. 1997. Chemical preservatives and natural antimicrobial compounds. In *Food Microbiology: Fundamentals and Frontiers* edited by Doyle M. P. and Beuchat L. R, Montville, 520-556. Washington: ASM.

Davis, J. 1994. Inactivation of antibiotics and the dissemination of resistance genes. *Science* 264: 375-382.

De Aguiar Ferreira Barros, M. Nero, L .A. Villas-Bôas Manoel, A. d'Ovídio, L. Cavalletti da Silvia, L. Gombossy de Melo Franco, B. D. Beloti, V. 2007. *Listeria* spp. associated to different levels of autochtonous microbiota in meat, meat products and processing plants. *Brazilian Journal of Microbiology* 38: 603-609.

De Azeredo, G. A. Stamford, T. L. M. Nunes, P. C. Neto, G. De Oliveira, M. E. G. De Souza, E. L. 2011. Combined application of essential oils from *Origanum vulgare* L. and *Rosmarinus officinalis* L. to inhibit bacteria and autochthonous microflora associated with minimally processed vegetables. *Food Research International* 44: 1541-1548.

De Falco, E. Mancini, E. Roscigno, G. Mignola, E. Taglialatela-Scafati, O. Senatore, F. 2013. Chemical composition and biological activity of essential oils of *Origanum vulgare* L. subsp *vulgare* L. under different growth conditions. *Molecules* 18: 14948-14960.

De Falco, E. Roscigno, G. Landolfi, S. Scandolera, E. Senatore, F. 2014. Growth, essential oil characterization, and antimicrobial activity of three wild biotypes of oregano under cultivation condition in Southern Italy. *Industrial Crops and Production* 62: 242-249.

De Martino, L. De Feo, V. Formisano, C. Mignola, E. Senatore, F. 2009. Chemical composition and antimicrobial activity of the essential oils fromt chemotypes of *Origanum vulgare* L. ssp *hirtum* (Link) Ietswaart growing wild in Campania (Southern Italy). *Molecules* 14: 2735-2746.

Deak, T.; Beuchat, L. R. 1996. *Handbook of food spoilage*. New York, USA: CRC Press, 1996.

Deans, S. G. Svoboda, K. P. Gundidza, M. Brechany, E. Y. 1992. Essential oil profiles of severe temperate and tropical aromatic plants: their antimicrobial and antioxidant activities. *Acta Horticulture* 306: 229-232.

Dearlove, R. P. Greenspan, P. Hartle, D. K. Swanson, R. B. Hargrove, J. L. 2008. Inhibition of protein glycation by extracts of culinary herbs and spices. *Journal of Medicinal Foods* 11: 275-281.

Dimitrijevic, S.I. Mihajlovski, K. R. Antonovic, D. G. Milanovic-Stevanovic, M. R. Mijina, D. Z. 2007. A study of the synergistic antilisterial effects of a sublethal dose of lactic acid and essential oils from *Thymus vulgaris* L., *Rosmarinus officinalis* L. and *Origanum vulgare* L. *Food Chemistry* 104: 774-782.

Direkbusarakom S. 2014. Application of medicinal herbs to aquaculture in Asia. *Walailak Journal of Science and Technology* 1: 7-14.

Discover Life Online [online, 2018 12 05]. Available from: https://www.google.sk/search?biw=1440&bih=764&tbm=isch&sa=1&ei=nMIHXMxt76uuBMi7mpAP&q=origanum+majorana+distribution+on+worls&oq=origanum+majorana+distribution+on+worl

s&gs_ l= img. 3... 3719. 8246.. 8421... 0. 0.. 0. 97. 1798. 21...... 0.... 1.. gws- wiz-img. CJoe38sIy7A#imgrc=GnT6AIlgIqJKtM.

Djenane, D. Yanguela, J. Montanes, L. Djerbal, M. Roncales, P. 2011. Antimicrobial activity of *Pistacia lentiscus* and *Satureja montana* essential oils against *Listeria monocytogenes* CECT 935 using laboratory media: efficacy and synergistic potential in minced beef. *Food Control* 22: 1046-1053.

Dorman, H. J. Deans, S. G. 2000. Antimicrobial agents from plants: antibacterial activity of plant volatile oils. *Journal of Applied Microbiology* 88: 308-316.

Du, W. X. Olsen, C. W. Avena-Bustillos, R. J. McHugh, T. H. Levin, C. E. Mandrell, R. Friedman, M. 2009. Antibacterial effects of allspice, garlic, and oregano essential oils in tomato films determined by overlay and vapor-phase methods. *Journal of Food Science* 74: 390-397.

Dubber, D. Harder, T. 2008. Extracts of *Ceramium rubrum, Mastocarpus stellatus* and *Laminaria digitata* inhibit growth of marine fish pathogenic bacteria at ecologically realistic concentrations. *Aquaculture* 274: 196-200.

Dussault, D. Dang Vu, K. Lacroix, M. 2014. *In vitro* evaluation of antimicrobial activities of various commercial essential oils, oleoresin and pure compounds against food pathogens and application in ham. *Meat Science* 96: 514-520.

Economakis, C. Demetzos, C. Anastassaki, T. Papazoglou, V. Gazouli, M. Loukis, A. Thanos C. A. Harvala, C. 1999. Volatile constituents of bracts and leaves of wild and cultivated Origanum dictamnus. *Planta Medica* 65: 189-191.

Economakis, C. D. Skaltsa, H. Demetzos, C. Sokovic, M. Thanos, C. A. 2002. Effect of phosphorus concentration of the nutrient solution on the volatile constituents of leaves and bracts of Origanum dictamnus. *Journal of Agricultural and Food Chemistry* 50: 6276-6280.

El-Ashmawy, I. M. El-Nahas, A. I. Salama, O. M. 2005. Protective effect of volatile oil, alcoholic and aqueous extracts of *Origanum majorana* on lead acetate toxicity in mice. *Basic&Clinical Pharmacology and Toxicology* 97: 238-243.

El Babili, F. Bouajila, J. Souchard, J. P. Bertrand, C. Bellvert, F. 2011. Oregano: chemical analysis and evaluation of its antimalarial, antioxidant, and cytotoxic activities. *Journal of Food Science* 76: 512-518.

El Gendy, A. N. Leonardi, M. Mugnaini, L. Bertelloni, F. Valentina V. Ebani, V. V. Nardoni, S. Mancianti, F. Hendawy, S. Omer, E. Pistelli, L. 2015. Chemical composition and antimicrobial activity of essential oil of wild and cultivated *Origanum syriacum* plants grown in Sinai, Egypt. *Industrial Crops and Products* 67: 201-207.

Elmastas, M. Celik, S. M. Genc, N. Aksit, H. Erenler, R. Gulcin, I. 2018. Antioxidant activity of an Anatolian herbal tea *Origanum minutiflorum*: isolation and characterisation of its secondary metabolite. *International Journal of Food Properties* 21: 374-384.

Ennajar, M. Bouajila, J. Lebrihi, A. Mathieu, F. Abderraba, M. Raies, A. Romdhane, M. 2009. Chemical composition, antimicrobial and antioxidant activities of essential oils and various extracts of *Juniperus phoenicea* L. (cupressacees). *Journal of Food Science* 74: 364-371.

Esen, G. Azaz, A. D. Kurkcuoglu, M. Baser, K. H. C. Tinmaz, A. 2007. Essential oil and antimicrobial activity of wild and cultivated *Origanum vulgare* L. subsp. *hirtum* (Link) letswaart from the Marmara region. *Flavour and Fragrance Journal* 22: 371-376.

Fadel, F. Ben Hmamou, D. Salghi, R. Chebli, B. Benali, O. Zarrouk, A. Ebenso, E. E. Chakir, A. Hammouti, B. 2013. Antifungal Activity and Anti-Corrosion Inhibition of OriganumCompactum Extracts. *International Journal of Electrochemical Science* 8: 11019-11032.

Faleiro, L. Miguel, G. Gomes, S. Costa, L. Venâncio, F. Teixeira, A. Figueiredo, A. C. Barroso, J. G. Pedro, L. G. 2005. Antibacterial and antioxidant activities of essential oils isolated from *Thymbra capitata* L. (Cav.) and *Origanum vulgare* L. *Journal of Agricultural and Food Chemistry* 53: 8162-8168.

Fasseas, M. K. Mountzouris, K. C. Tarantilis, P. A. Polissiou, M. Zervas, G. 2008. Antioxidant activity in meat treated with oregano and sage essential oils. *Food Chemistry* 106: 1188-1194.

Fernández-Pan, I. Royo, M. Ignacio Maté, J. 2012. Antimicrobial activity of whey protein isolate edible films with essential oils against food spoilers and foodborne pathogens. *Journal of Food Science* 77, 383-390.

Frans, I. Michiels, C. W. Bossier, P. Willems, K. A. Lievens, B. Rediers, H. 2011. *Vibrio anguillarum* as a fish pathogen: virulence factors, diagnosis and prevention. *Journal of Fish Disease* 34: 643-661.

Friedman, M. Henika, P. R. Levin, C. E. Mandrell, R. E. 2007. Recipes for antimicrobial wine marinades against *Bacillus cereus*, *Escherichia coli* O157:H7, *Listeria monocytogenes*, and *Salmonella enterica*. *Journal of Food Science* 72: 207-213.

García-Beltrán, J. M. Esteban, M. A. 2016. Properties and applications of plants of *Origanum* sp. Genus. *SM Journal of Biology* 2, 1006. https://www.researchgate.net/publication/316740994_Properties_and_Applications_of_Plants_of_Origanum_SpGenus

Geethangili, M. Fang, S. H. Lai, C. H. Rao, Y. K. Lien, H. M. Tzeng, Y. M. 2010. Inhibitory effect of *Antrodia camphorata* constituents on the *Helicobacter pylori*-associated gastric inflammation. Food Chemistry 119: 149-153.

Goel, P. Vasudeva, N. 2015. *Origanum majorana* L. – Phytochemical review. *Indian Journal of Nature Products and Resources* 64: 261-267.

Gortzi, O. Lala, S. Chinou, I. Tsaknis, J. 2007. Evaluation of the antimicrobial and antioxidant activities of *Origanum dictamnus* extracts before and after encapsulation in liposomes. *Molecules* 12: 932-945.

Goulas, A. E. Kontominas, M. G. 2007. Combined effect of light salting, modified atmosphere packaging and oregano essential oil on the shelf-life of sea bream (*Sparus aurata*): biochemical and sensory attributes. *Food Chemistry* 100: 287-296.

Govaris, A. Botsoglou, N. Papageorgiou, G. Botsoglou, E. Ambrosiadis, I. 2004. Dietary versus post mortem use of oregano oil and/or alpha-tocopherol in turkeys to inhibit development of lipid oxidation in meat during refrigerated storage. *International Journal of Food Science and Nutrition* 55: 115-123.

Govaris, A. Solomakos, N. Pexara, A. Chatzopoulou, P. 2010. The antimicrobial effect of oregano essential oil, nisin and their combination against *Salmonella Enteritidis* in minced sheep meat during refrigerated storage. *International Journal of Food Microbiology* 137: 175-180.

Goze, I. Cetin, A. Goze, A.2010. Investigation of effects of essential oils of *Origanum minutiflorum* O. Schwarz and P. H. Davis and *Cyclotrichium niveum* (*Labiateae*) plants an angiogenesis in schell-less chick embryo culture. *African Journal of Biotechnology* 9: 2156-5160.

Gündüz, G. T. Niemira, B. A. Gönül, Ş.A. Karapinar, M. 2012. Antimicrobial activity of oregano oil on iceberg lettuce with different attachment conditions. *Journal of Food Science* 77: 412-415.

Gupta, S. M. Arif, M. Ahmed, Z. 2011. Antimicrobial activity in leaf, seed extract and seed oil of *Jatropha curcas* L. plant. *Journal of Applied and Natural Science* 3: 102-105.

Gutierrez, J. Barry-Ryan, C. Bourke, P. 2009. Antimicrobial activity of plant essential oils using food model media: efficacy, synergistic potential and interactions with food components. *Food Microbiology* 26: 142-150.

Gutierrez, J. Barry-Ryan, C. Bourke, P. 2008. The antimicrobial efficacy of plant essential oil combinations and interactions with food ingredients. *International Journal of Food Microbiology* 124: 91-97.

Hajlaoui, H. Mighri, H. Aouni, M. Gharsallah, N. Kadri, A. 2016. Chemical composition and *in vitro* evaluation of antioxidant, antimicrobial, cytotoxicity and anti-acetylcholinesterase properties of Tunisian *Origanum majorana* L. essential oil. *Microbial Pathogenesis* 95: 86-94.

Hajlaoui, H. Trabelsi, N. Noumi, E. Snoussi, M. Fellah, H. Ksouri, R. Bakhrouf, A. 2009. Biological activities of the essential oils and methanol extract of two cultivated mint species (*Mentha longifolia* and *Mentha pulegium*) used in the Tunisian folkloric medicine. *World Journal of Microbiology and Biotechnology* 25: 2227-2238.

Hakki, H. Mavi, A. A. Yildrim, A. Digrak, M. Hirata, T. 2003. Screening Chemical Composition and *in Vitro* Antioxidant and Antimicrobial Activities of the Essential Oils from *Origanum syriacum* L. Growing in Turkey. *Biological and Pharmaceutical Bulletin* 26: 1725- 1729.

Harpaz, S. Glatman, L. Drabkin, V. Gelman, A. 2003. Effects of herbal essential oils used to extend the shelf life of freshwater reared Asian sea bass fish (Latescalcarifer). *Journal of Food Protection* 66: 410-417.

Haworth, J. E. 2003. Nature antioxidants review. In *Proceeding of the 56th American meat science association reciprotal meat conference.* Colombia: Missouri.

Hazzit, M. Baaliouamer, A. Leonor-Faleiro, M. Graca, M. M. 2006. Composition of the essential oils of Thymus and Origanum species from Algeria and their antioxidant and antimicrobial activities. *Journal of Agriculture and Food Chemistry* 54: 6314-21.

Heo, H. J. Cho, H. Y. Hong, B. Kim, H. K. Kim, S. K. Kim, C. J. Shin, D. H. 2002. Ursolic acid of *Origanum majorana* L. Reduces Abeta-induced oxidative injury. *Molecular Cells* 13: 5-11.

Hernández-Hernández, E. Regalado-González, C. Vázquez-Landaverde, P. Guerrero-Legarreta, I. García-Almendárez, B. E. 2014. Microencapsulation, Chemical Characterization, and Antimicrobial Activity of Mexican (*Lippia graveolens* H.B.K.) and European (*Origanum vulgare* L.) Oregano Essential Oils. *Scientific World Journal*, ID 641814. doi: 10.1155/2014/641814.

Hili, P. Evans, C. S. Veness, R. G. 1997. Antimicrobial action of essential oils: the effect of dimethylsulphoxide on the activity of cinnamon oil. *Letters of Applied Microbiology* 24: 269-275.

Houhoula, D. P. Oreopoulou, V. Tzia, C. 2003. Antioxidant efficiency of oregano during frying and storage of potato chips. *Journal of Science and Food Agriculture* 83: 1499-1503.

Hristova, Y. Gochev, V. Wanner, Z. Jirovetz, L. Schmidt, E. Girova, T. Kuzmanov, A. 2013. Chemical composition and antifungal activity of essential oil of *Salvia sclarea* L. from Bulgaria against clinical isolates of *Candida* species. *Journal of Bioscience and Biotechnology* 2: 39-44.

Hsieh, P. C. Mau, J. L. Huang, S. H. 2001. Antimicrobial effect of various combinations of plant extracts. *Food Microbiology* 18: 35-43.

Imai, H. Osawa, K. Yasuda, H. Hamashima, H. Arai, T. Sasatsu, M. 2001. Inhibition by the essential oils of peppermint and spearmint of the growth of pathogenic bacteria. *Microbios* 106: 31-39.

Juliano, C. Mattana, A. Usai, M. 2000. Composition and *in vitro* antimicrobial activity of the essential oil of Thymus herba-barona Loisel growing wild in Sardinia. *Journal of Essential Oil Research* 12: 516-22.

Kalpoutzakis, E. Aligiannis, N. Mentis, A. Mitaku, S. Charvala, C. 2001. Composition of the essential oil of two *Nepeta* species and in vitro evaluation of their activity against *Helicobacter pylori*. *Planta Medica* 67: 880-883.

Karaboduk, K. Karabacak, O. Karaboduk, H. Tekinay, T. 2014. Chemical analysis and antimicrobial activities of the *Origanum vulgare* subsp. *Hirtum. Journal of Environmental Protection and Ecology* 15: 1283-1292.

Karakaya, S. El, S. N. Karagözlü, N. Şahin, S. 2011. Antioxidant and antimicrobial activities of essential oils obtained from Oregano (*Origanum vulgare* ssp. *hirtum*) by using different extraction methods. *Journal of Medicinal Food* 14: 645-652.

Karaman, I. Sahin, F. Gulluce, M. Ogutcu, H. Sengul, M. Adoguzel, A. 2003. Antimicrobial activity of aqueous and methanol extracts of *Juniperus oxycedrus* L. *Journal of Ethnopharmacology* 85: 231-235.

Karanika, M.S. Komaitis, M. Aggelis, G. 2001. Effect of aqueous extracts of some plants of Lamiaceae family on the growth of *Yarrowia lipolytica*. *International Journal of Food Microbiology* 64: 175-181.

Khanjari, A. Karabagias, I. K. Kontominas, M. G. 2013. Combined effect of N, O-carboxymethyl chitosan and oregano essential oil to extend shelf life and control *Listeria monocytogenes* in raw chicken meat fillets. *LWT Food Science and Technology* 53: 94-99.

Khosravi, A. R. Shokri, H. Kermani, S. Dakhili, M. Madani, M. Parsa, S. 2011. Antifungal properties of *Artemisia sieberi* and *Origanum vulgare* essential oils against *Candida glabrata* isolates obtained from patients with vulvovaginal candidiasis. *Journal de Mycologie Medicale* 21: 93-99.

Kiferle, C. Lucchesini, M. Mensuali-Sodi, A. Maggini, R. Raffaelli, A. Pardossi, A. 2011. Rosmarinic acid content in basil plants grown in vitro and in hydroponics. *Central European Journal of Biology* 6: 946-957.

Kikuzaki, H. Nakatani, N. 1989. Structure of a new antioxidative phenolic acid from oregano (*Origanum vulgare* L.). *Agricultural and Biological Chemistry* 53: 519-524.

Kilicgün, H. Korkmaz, M. 2014. Hepatoprotective and antidiabetic activity of *Origanum minutiflorum* O. Schwarz and P.H. Davis grown wild Turkey. *Bothalia Journal* 44: 260-267.

Klūga, A. Terentjeva, M. Kántor, A. Kluz, M. Puchalski, C. Kačániová, M. 2017. Antibacterial activity of *Melissa officinalis* L., *Mentha piperita* L., *Origanum vulgare* L. and *Malva mauritiana* against bacterial microflora isolated from fish. *Advances Research of Life Sciences* 1: 75-80.

Koukoulitsa, C. Zija, C. Geromichalos, G. D. Demopoulus, V. J. Skaltsa, H. 2006. Evaluation of aldose reductase inhibition and docking studies of some secondary metabolites, isolated from *Origanum vulgare* L. spp. *hirtum*. *Bioorganic and Medicinal Chemistry* 14: 1653-1659.

Kulisić, T. Krisko, A. Dragović-Uzelac, V. Milos, M. Pifat, G. 2007. The effects of essential oils and aqueous tea infusions of oregano (*Origanum vulgare* L. *spp. hirtum*), thyme (*Thymus vulgaris* L.) and wild thyme (*Thymus serpyllum* L.) on the copper-induced oxidation of human low-density lipoproteins. *International Journal of Food Science and Nutrition* 58: 87-93.

Kumar, S. 2011. Free radicals and antioxidants: human and food system. *Advances in Applied Science Research* 2: 129-135.

Kunicka-Styczyńska, A. 2011. Activity of essential oils against food-spoiling yeast. A review. *Flavour and Fragrance Journal* 26: 326-328.

Kurşat, M. Emre, I. Yilmaz, Ö. Erecevit, P. 2011. Antioxidant and antimicrobial activity in the seeds of *Origanum vulgare* L. subsp. *gracile* (C. Koch) letswaart and *Origanum acutidens* (Hand. - Mazz.) letswaart from Turkey. *Grasas y Aceites* 62: 410-417.

Kustrak, D. Kuftinec, J. Blazevic, N. Maffei, M. 1996. Composition of the essential oil composition of two subspecies of *Satureja montana*. *Journal of Essential Oil Research* 8: 7-13.

Kuttappagari, K. K. Teja, C. S. R. Rommalapati, R. K. Poosarla, C. H. Gonzu, S. R. Reddy, B. V. R. 2015. Role of antioxidant un facilitating the body function: A review. *Journal of Orofacial Sciences* 157: 71-75.

Lambert, R. J. Skandamis, P. N. Coote, P. J. Nychas, G. J. 2001. A study of the minimum inhibitory concentration and mode of action of oregano essential oil, thymol and carvacrol. *Journal of Applied Microbiology* 91: 453-462.

Leung, A. Y. and Foster, S. 1996. *Encyclopaedia of common natural ingredients used in foods, drugs, and cosmetics* (2nd ed.). New York: Wiley.

Leyva-López, N. Gutiérrez-Grijawa, E. P. Vasquez, G. Heredia, J. B. 2017. Essential oils of oregano: Biological activity beyond their antimicrobial properties. *Molecules* 22: 1-24.

Li, Z. Henning, S. M. Zhang, Y. Zerlin, A. Li, L. Gao, K. Lee, R. P. Karp, H. Thames, G. Bowerman, S. Heber, D. 2010. Antioxidant-rich spice added to hamburger meat during cooking results in reduced meat, plasma, and urine malondialdehyde concentrations. *The American Journal of Clinical Nutrition* 91: 1180-1184.

Ličina, B. Z. Stefanović, O. D. Vasić, S. M. Radojević, I. D. Dekić, M. S. Čomić, L. R. 2013. Biological activities of the extracts from wild growing Origanum vulgare L. *Food Control* 33: 498-504.

Lin, Y. T. Kwon, Y. I. Labbe, R. G. Shetty, K. 2005. Inhibition of *Helicobacter pylori* and associated urease by oregano and cranberry phytochemical synergies. *Applied and Environmental Microbiology* 71: 8558-8564.

Liolios, C. C. Gortzi, O. Lalas, S. Tsaknis, J. Chinou, I. 2009. Liposomal incorporation of carvacrol and thymol isolated from the essential oil of *Origanum dictamnus* L. and *in vitro* antimicrobial activity. *Food Chemistry* 112: 77-83.

Liolios, C. C. Graikou, K. Skaltsa, E. Chinou, I. 2010. Dittany of Crete: A botanical and ethnopharmacological review. *Journal of Ethnopharmacology* 131: 229-241.

Lis-Balchin, M. Deans, S. G. 1997. Bioactivity of selected plant essential oils against *Listeria monocytogenes*. *Journal of Applied Microbiology* 82: 759-762.

Lolos, M. Oreopoulou, V. Tzia, C. 1999. Oxidative stability of potato chips: effect of frying oil type, temperature and antioxidants. *Journal of Food and Agriculture* 79: 1524-1528.

Loper, J. E. Henkels, M. D. Roberts, R. G. Grove, G. G. Willett, M. J. Smith, T. J. 1991. Evaluation of streptomycin, oxytetracycline, and copper resistance of *Erwinia amylovora* isolated from pear orchards in Washington State. *Plant Disease* 75: 287-290.

Lopez-Reyes, J. G. Spadaro, D. Gullino, M. L. Garibaldi, A. 2010. Efficacy of plant essential oils on postharvest control of rot caused by fungi on four cultivars of apples *in vivo*. *Flavour and Fragrance Journal* 25: 171-177.

Lu, Y. Gao, B. Chen, P. Charles, D. Yu, L. 2014. Characterisation of organic and conventional sweet basil leaves using chromatographic and flow-injection mass spectrometric (FIMS) fingerprints combined with principal component analysis. *Food Chemistry* 154: 262-268.

Mahmoud, B. S. Yamazaki, K. Miyashita, K. Il-Shik, S. Dong-Suk, C. Suzuki, T. 2004. Bacterial microflora of carp (*Cyprinus carpio*) and its shelf-life extension by essential oil compounds. *Food Microbiology* 21: 657-666.

Mancini, E. Camele, I. Elshafie, H. S. De Martino, L. Pellegrino, C. Grulova, D. De Feo, V. 2014. Chemical composition and biological activity of the essential oil of *Origanum vulgare* ssp. *hirtum* from different areas in the southern Apennines (Italy). *Chemical Biodiversity* 11: 639-651.

Manohar, V. Ingram, C. Gray, J. Talpur, N. A. Echard, B. W. Bagchi, D. 2001. Antifungal activities of origanum oil against *Candida albicans*. *Molecular and Cellular Biochemistry* 228: 111-117.

Marrelli, M. Confortia, F. Formisano, C. Rigano, D. Arnold, N. A. Menichini, F. Senatore, F. 2016. Composition, antibacterial, antioxidant and antiproliferative activities of essential oils from three *Origanum* species growing wild in Lebanon and Greece. *Natural Product Research* 30: 735-739.

Martins, N. Barros, L. Santos-Buelga, C. Henriques, M. Silva, S. Isabel Ferreira, C. F. R. 2014. Decoction, infusion and hydroalcoholic extract of *Origanum vulgare* L.: different performances regarding bioactivity and phenolic compounds. *Food Chemistry* 158: 73-80.

Masood, N. Chaudhry, A. Saeed, S. Tariq, P. 2007. Antibacterial effects of oregano (*Origanum vulgare*) against gram negative bacilli. *Pakistan Journal of Botany* 39: 609-613.

Mazzarrino, G. Paparella, A. Chaves-López, C. Faberi, A. Sergi, M. Sigismondi, C. Compagnone, D. Serio, A. 2015. *Salmonella enterica* and *Listeria monocytogenes* inactivation dynamics after treatment with selected essential oils. *Food Control* 50: 794-803.

McCue, P. P. Shetty, K. 2004. Inhibitory effects of rosmarinic acid extracts on porcine pancreatic amylase *in vitro*. *Asia Pacific Journal of Clinical Nutrition* 13: 101-106.

Mead, P. S. Slutsker, L. Dietz, V. McCaig, L. F. Breese, J. S. Shapiro, C. Griffin, P. M. Tauxe, R. V. 1995. Food related illness and dead in the United States. *Emerging Infectious Diseases* 5: 607-625.

Mechergui, K. Jaouadi, W. Coelho, J. A. Serra, M. C. Khouja, M. L. 2015. Biological activities and oil properties of *Origanum glandulosum* Desf: A Review. *Phytothérapie* 14: 102-108.

Melo, A. D. Amaral, A. F. Schaefer, G. Luciano, F. B. de Andrade, C. Costa, L. B. Rostagno, M. H. 2015. Antimicrobial effect against different bacterial strains and bacterial adaptation to essential oils used as feed additives. *Canadian Journal Veterinary Research* 79: 285-289.

Milos, M. Mastelic, J. Jerkovic, I. 2000. Chemical composition and antioxidant effect of glycosidically bound volatile compounds from oregano (*Origanum vulgare* L. ssp. *hirtum*. *Food Chemistry* 71: 79-83.

Mitropoulou, G. Fitsiou, E. Stavropoulou, E. Papavassilopoulou, E. Vamvakias, M. Pappa, A. Oreopoulou, A. Kourkoutas, Y. 2015. Composition, antimicrobial, antioxidant, and antiproliferative activity of *Origanum dictamnus* (dittany) essential oil. *Microbial Ecology in Health Disease* 6, 26543. doi: 10.3402/mehd.v26.26543

Morshedloo, M. R. Mumivand, H. Crailer, L. E. Maggi, F. 2017. Chemical composition and antioxidant activity of essential oils in *Origanum vulgare* subs. *gracil*e at different phenological stages and plant parts. *Journal of Food Processing and Preservation* 42: doi: 10.1111/jfpp.13516.

Moschonas, G. Geornaras, I. Stopforth, J. D. Wach, D. Woerner, D. R. Belk, K. E. Smith, G. C. Sofos, J. N. 2012. Activity of caprylic acid, carvacrol, ε-polylysine and their combinations against salmonella in not-ready-to-eat surface-browned, frozen, breaded chicken products. *Journal of Food Science* 77: 405-411.

Muller-Riebau, F. Berger, B. Yegen, O. 1995. Chemical composition and fungitoxic properties to phytopathogenic fungi of essential oils of selected aromatic plants growing wild in Turkey. *Journal of Agriculture Food Chemistry* 43: 2262-2266.

Muniruzzaman, M. Chowdhury, M. B. R. 2009. Sensitivity of fish pathogenic bacteria to various medicinal herbs. *Bangladesh Journal of Veterinary Medicine* 2: 75-82.

Nakhaei, M. M., Malekzadeh, F. Khaje-Karamoddin, M. Ramezani, M. 2006. *In vitro* anti-*Helicobacter pylori* effects of sweet basil (*Ocimum basilicum* L.) and purple basil (*Ocimum basilicum* var. *purpurascens*). *Pakistan Journal of Biological Sciences* 9: 2887-2891.

Nardoni, S. Giovanelli, S. Pistelli, L. Mugnaini, L. Profili, G. Pisseri, F. 2005. *In Vitro* Activity of Twenty Commercially Available, Plant-Derived Essential Oils against Selected Dermatophyte Species. *Nature Product Communication* 10: 1473-1478.

Nazzaro, F. Fratianni, F. De Martino, L. Coppola, R. De Feo, V. 2013. Effect of Essential oils on Pathogenic Bacteria. *Pharmaceuticals (Basel)* 12: 1451-1474.

Nguyen, A. N. Jacq, A. 2014. Small RNAs in the *Vibrionaceae*: an ocean still to be explored. *Wiley Interdisciplinary Review* 5: 381-392.

Ntzimani, A. G. Giatrakou, V. I. Savvaidis, I. N. 2010. Combined natural antimicrobial treatments (EDTA, lysozyme, rosemary and oregano oil) on semi cooked coated chicken meat stored in vacuum packages at 4°C: microbiological and sensory evaluation. *Innovative Food Science and Emerging Technologies* 11: 187-196.

Ohno, T. Kita, M. Yamaoka, Y. Imamura, S. Yamamoto, T. Mitsufuji, S. Kodama, T. Kashima, K. Imanishi, J. 2003. Antimicrobial activity of essential oils against *Helicobacter pylori*. *Helicobacter* 83: 207-215.

Oke, F. Aslim, B. 2010. Biological potentials and cytotoxicity of various extracts from endemic *Origanum minutiflorum* O. Schwarz & P.H. *Food and Chemical Toxicology* 48: 1728-1733.

Olmedo, R. H. Asensio, C. Nepote, V. Mestrallet, M. G. Grosso, N. R. 2009. Chemical and sensory stability of fried-salted peanuts flavored with oregano essential oil and olive oil. *Journal of Science and Food Agriculture* 89: 2128-2136.

Oral, N. Vatansever, L. Sezer, Ç. Aydın, B. Güven, A. Gülmez, M. Başer, K. Kürkçüoğlu, M. 2009. Effect of absorbent pads containing oregano essential oil on the shelf life extension of overwrap packed chicken drumsticks stored at four degrees Celsius. *Poultry Science* 88: 1459-1465.

Ortega Morente, E. Abriouel, H. López, R. L. Ben Omar, N. Gálvez, A. 2010. Antibacterial activity of carvacrol and 2-nitro-1-propanol against single and mixed populations of foodborne pathogenic bacteria in corn flour dough. *Food Microbiology* 27: 274-279.

Ortega-Ramirez, L. A. Rodriguez-Garcia, I. Silva-Espinoza, B. A. Ayala-Zavala, J. F. 2016. Chapter 71 Oregano (*Origanum* spp.) *Oils. Essential Oils in Food Preservation, Flavor and Safety*. USA: Elsevier 625-631.

Ouattara, B. Simarad, R. E. Piette, G. Bégin, A. Holley, R. A. 2000. Inhibition of surface spoilage bacteria in processed meats by application of antimicrobial films prepared with chitosan. *International Journal of Food Microbiology* 62: 139-148.

Oussalah, M. Caillet, S. Salmiéri, S. Saucier, L. Lacroix, M. 2004. Antimicrobial and antioxidant effects of milk protein-based film containing essential oils for the preservation of whole beef muscle. *Journal of Agriculture and Food Chemistry* 52: 5598-5605.

Ozen, F. Ekinci, F. Y. Korachi, M. 2014. The inhibition of *Helicobacter pylori* infected cells by *Origanum minutiflorum*. *Industrial Crops and Products* 58: 329-334.

Ozkalp, B. Sevgi, F. Ozcan, M. Ozcan, M. M. 2010. The antibacterial activity of essential oil of oregano (*Origanum vulgare* L.). *Journal of Food and Agriculture Environment* 8: 272-274.

Paparella, A. Serio, A. Chaves-López, C. Mazzarrino, G. 2013. *Plant-based intervention strategies for Listeria monocytogenes control in foods* Science, Technology and Education, Formatex Research Center 1230-1246.

Paz, E. A. Cerdeiras, M. P. Fernandez, J. Ferreira, F. Moyna, P. Soubes, M. Vázque, A. Vero, S. Zunino, L. 1995. Screening of Uruguayan medicinal plants for antimicrobial activity. *Journal of Ethnopharmacology* 45: 67-70.

Pelczar, M. J. Chan, E. C. S. Krieg, N. R. 1988. *Microbiology*. New York: McGraw- Hill International.

Pérez-Alfonso, C. Martínez-Romero, D. Zapata, P. Serrano, M.; Valero, D. Castillo, S. 2012. The effects of essential oils carvacrol and thymol on growth of *Penicillium digitatum* and *P. italicum* involved in lemon decay. *Internatinal Journal of Food Microbiology* 58: 101-106.

Periago, P. M. Conesa, R. Delgado, B. Fernández, P. S. Palop, A. 2006. *Bacillus megaterium* spore germination and growth inhibition by a treatment combining heat with natural antimicrobials. *Food Technology and Biotechnology* 44: 17-23.

Petr, J. Vítková, K. Ranc, V. Znaleziona, J. Maier, V. Knob, R. Sevcík, J. 2008. Determination of some phenolic acids in *Majorana hortensis* by capillary electrophoresis with online electrokinetic preconcentration. *Journal of Agricultural and Food Chemistry* 56: 3940-3944.

Petrou, S. Tsiraki, M. Giatrakou, V. Savvaidis, I. N. 2012. Chitosan dipping or oregano oil treatments, singly or combined on modified atmosphere packaged chicken breast meat. *International Journal of Food Microbiology* 156: 264-271.

Pinterest [online, 2018 12 05]. Available from: https://sk.pinterest.com/pin/317574211199128515/.

Pinterest [online, 2018 12 05]. Available from: https://www.google.sk/search?q=origanum+majorana+botanical+picture&source=lnms&tbm=isch&sa=X&ved=0ahUKEwiAqpGA94jfAhWNZ1AKHcp8ADYQ_AUIDigB&biw=1440&bih=764#imgrc=wBOvIbluB5rQxM.

Pitt, J. I. Hocking, A. D. 1997. *Fungi and food spoilage* (2nd ed.). London, UK: Blackie Academic and Professional.

Preston, M. A. Borczyk, A. A. 1994. Genetic variability and molecular typing of *Shigella sonnei* strains isolated in Canada. *Journal of Clinical Microbiology* 32: 1427-1430.

Pyrgotou, N. Giatrakou, V. Ntzimani, A. Savvaidis, I. N. 2010. Quality assessment of salted, modified atmosphere packaged rainbow trout under treatment with oregano essential oil. *Journal of Food Science* 75: 406-411.

Rahbar, N. Shafaghat, A. Salimi, F. 2012. Antimicrobial activity and constituents of the hexane extracts from leaf and stem of *Origanum vulgare* L. ssp. *viride* (Boiss.) Hayek. growing wild in Northwest Iran. *Journal of Medicinal Plants Research* 6: 2681-2685.

Rao, Y. K. Lien, H. M. Lin, Y. H. Hsu, Y. M. Yeh, C. T. Chen, C. C. Lai, C. H. Tzeng, Y. M. 2012. Antibacterial activities of *Anisomeles indica* constituents and their inhibition effect on *Helicobacter pylori*-induced inflammation in human gastric epithelial cells. *Food Chemistry* 132: 780-787.

Ravishankar, S. Jaroni, D. Zhu, L. Olsen, C. McHugh, T. Friedman, M. 2012. Inactivation of *Listeria monocytogenes* on ham and bologna using pectin-based apple, carrot, and hibiscus edible films containing carvacrol and cinnamaldehyde. *Journal of Food Science* 77: 377-382.

Rhoades, J. Roller, S. 2000. Antimicrobial actions of degraded and native chitosan against spoilage organisms in laboratory media and foods. *Applied Environmental Microbiology* 66: 80-86.

Rivas, A. J. Lemos, M. L. Osorio, C. R. 2013. *Photobacterium damselae* subsp. *damselae*, a bacterium pathogenic for marine animals and humans. *Frontiers in Microbiology* 25: 283.

Roller, S. Sagoo, S. Board, R. O' Mahony, T. Caplice, E. Fitzgerald, G. Fogden, M. Owen, M. Fletcher, H. 2002. Novel combinations of chitosan, carnocin and sulphite for the preservation of chilled pork sausages. *Meat Science* 62: 165-177.

Rosato, A. Vitali, C. Piaruli, M. Mazzotta, M. Maria, P. A. Rosanna, M. 2009. *In vitro* synergic efficacy of the combination of nystatin with the essential oils of *Origanum vulgare* and *Pelargonium graveolens* against some *Candida species. Phytomedicine* 16: 972-975.

Royo, M. Fernández-Pan, I. Maté, J. I. 2010. Antimicrobial effectiveness of oregano and sage essential oils incorporated into whey protein films or cellulose-based filter paper. *Journal of Science and Food Agriculture* 90: 1513-1519.

Sadikoglu, N. Ozhatay, N. 2015. Morphological characteristics of exported taxa as oregano from Turkey I: *Origanum. Journal of Pharmacy of Istanbul University* 45: 87-126.

Saeed, S. Tariq, P. 2009. Antibacterial activity of oregano (*Origanum vulgare* Linn.) against gram positive bacteria. *Pakistan Journal of Pharmaceutical Science* 22: 421-424.

Sagdıc, O. Ozcan, M. 2003. Antibacterial activity of Turkish spice hydrosols. *Food Control* 14: 141-143.

Sagdic, O. Ozturk, I. Tornuk, F. 2012. Inactivation of non-toxigenic and toxigenic *Escherichia coli* O157: H7 inoculated on minimally processed tomatoes and cucumbers: utilization of hydrosols of *Lamiaceae* spices as natural food sanitizers. *Food Control* 30: 7-14.

Şahin, F. Güllüce, M. Daferera, D. Sökmen, A. Sökmen, M. Polissiou, M. Agar, G. Ozer, H. 2004. Biological activities of the essential oils and methanol extract of *Origanum vulgare* ssp. *vulgare* in Eastern Anatolia region of Turkey. *Food Control* 15: 549-557.

Saito, Y. Kimura, Y. Sakamoto, T. 1976. Studies on the antioxidant properties of spices III. The antioxidant effects of petroleum ether soluble and insoluble fractions from spices. *Journal of Japanese Society of Food and Nutrition* 29: 505-510.

Sari, A. B. Ustuner, O. 2018. Antioxidant and immunostimulant effects of *Origanum minutiflorum* O. Schwarz and P.H. Davis in rainbow trout. *Fresenius Environmental Bulletin* 27: 1013-1021.

Sarikurkcu, C. Zengin, G. Oskay, M. Uysal, S. Ceylan, R. Aktumsek, A. 2015. Composition, antioxidant, antimicrobial and enzyme inhibition activities of two *Origanum vulgare* subspecies (subsp. *vulgare* and subsp. *hirtum*) essential oils. *Industrial Crops and Products* 70: 178-184.

Saxena, D. Jayant, S. K. Soni, K. Neekhra, K. 2016. *Origanum majorana*: A potential herb for functional food. *European Journal of Pharmaceutical and Medical Research* 3: 321-325.

Sbayou, H. Oubrim, N. Bouchr, F. B. Ababou, B. Boukachabine, K. Amghar, S. 2014. Chemical composition and antioxidant activity of essential oil of *Origanum compactum* against foodborne bacteria. *International Journal of Engineering Research* 3: 3562-3567.

Shati, A. A. 2011. Effects of *Origanum majorana* L. on cadmium induced hepatoxicity and nephrotoxicity in albino rats. *Saudi Medical Journal* 32: 797-805.

Shekarforoush, S. S. Basiri, S. Ebrahimnejad, H. Hosseinzadeh, S. 2015. Effect of chitosan on spoilage bacteria, *Escherichia coli* and *Listeria monocytogenes* in cured chicken meat. *International Journal of Biological Macromolecules* 76: 303-309.

Sikkema, J. de Bont, J. A. Poolman, B. 1995. Mechanisms of membrane toxicity of hydrocarbons. *Microbiol Review* 59: 201-222.

Sivropoulou, A. Papanikolaou, E. Nikolaou, C. Kokkini, S. Lanars, T. Arsenakis, M. 1996. Antimicrobial and cytotoxic activities of *Origanum*essential oils. *Journal of Agriculture and Food Chemistry* 4: 1202-1205.

Soares, I. H. Loreto, É. S. Rossato, L. Mario, D. N. Venturini, T. P. 2015. *In vitro* activity of essential oils extracted from condiments against fluconazole-resistant and -sensitive *Candida glabrata*. *Journal de Mycologie Medicale* 25: 213-217.

Sökmen, M. Serkedjieva, J. Daferera, D. Gulluce, M. Polissiou, M. Tepe, B. Akpulat, H. A. Sahin, F. Sokmen, A. 2004. *In vitro* antioxidant, antimicrobial, and antiviral activities of the essential oil and various extracts from herbal parts and callus cultures of Origanum acutidens. *Journal of Agricultural and Food Chemistry* 52: 3309-3312.

Soliman, K. M. Badeaa, R. I. 2002. Effect of oil extracted from some medicinal plants on different mycotoxigenic fungi. *Food and Chemical Toxicology* 40: 1669-1675.

Sørensen, A. D. M. Nielsen, N. S. Jacobsen, C. 2010. Oxidative stability of fish oil-enriched mayonnaise-based salads. *European Journal of Lipid Science and Technology* 112: 476-487.

Soro, D. Kone, M. W. Kamanzi, K. 2010. Evaluation des activités antimicrobiennes et anti-radicaux libres de quelques taxons bioactifs de Côte d'Ivoire [Evaluation of the antimicrobial and free radical-free activities of some bioactive taxa of Côte d'Ivoire]. *European Journal of Scientific Research* 40: 307-317.

Soylu, S. Yigitbas, H. Soylu, E. Kurt, Ş. 2007. Antifungal effects of essential oils from oregano and fennel on *Sclerotinia sclerotiorum*. *Journal of Applied Microbiology* 103: 1021-1030.

Srihari, T. Sengottuvelan, M. Nalini, N. 2008. Dose-dependent effect of oregano (*Origanum vulgare* L.) on lipid perocidation and antioxidant status in 1,2-dimethylhydrazibe-induced rat colon carcinogenesis. *Journal of Pharmacy and Pharmacology* 60: 787-794.

Stamatis, G. Kyriazopoulos, P. Golegou, S. Basayiannis, A. Skaltsas, S. Skaltsa, H. 2003. *In vitro* anti-Helicobacter pylori activity of Greek herbal medicines. *Journal of Ethnopharmacology* 88: 175-179.

Stanković, M. Z. Stanojević, L.P. 2014. *Tehnologija lekovitog i začinskog bilja* [*Medicinal and spice technology*] Tehnološki fakultet, Leskovac 113.

Stanojević, L. P. Stanojević, J.S. Cvetković, D.J. Ilić, D.P. 2016. Antioxidant activity of oregano essential oil (*Origanum vulgare* L.). *Biologica Nyssana* 7: 131-139.

Stefanakis, M. K. Touloupakis, E. Anastasopoulos, E. Ghanotakis, D. Katerinopoulos, H. E. Makridis, P. 2013. Antibacterial activity of essential oils from plants of the genus *Origanum. Food Control* 34: 539-546.

Suresh, P. Ingle, V. K. Vijayalakshima, V. 1992. Antibacterial activity of eugenol in comparison with other antibiotics. *Journal of Food Science and Technology* 29: 254-6.

Tabanca, N. Kirimer, N. Demirci, B. Demirci, F. Baser, K. H. C. 2001. Composition and antimicrobial activity of the essential oils of *Micromeria cristata* subsp. *Phyrgia* and the enantiomeric distribution of borneol. *Journal of Agriculture and Food Chemistry* 49: 4300-4303.

Teixeira, B. Marques, A. Ramos, C. Serrano, C. Matos, O. Neng, N. R. Nogueira, J. M. Saraiva, J. A. Nunes, M. L. 2013. Chemical composition and bioactivity of different oregano (*Origanum vulgare*) extracts and essential oil. *Journal of Science and Food Agriculture*, 93: 2707-2714.

Tongnuanchan, P. Benjakul, S. 2014. Essential oils: extraction, bioactivities, and their uses for food preservation. *Journal of Food Science* 79: 1231–1249.

Topdag, S. Aslaner, A. Tataroglu, C. Ilce, Z. 2005. Evaluation of antioxidant capacity in lung carcinoma. *Indian Journal of Thoracic and Cardiovascular Surgery* 21: 269-71.

Triantaphyllou, K. Blekas, G. Boskou, D. 2001. Antioxidative propertoes of water extracts obtained from herbs of the species *Lamiaceae. International Journal of Food Science and Nutrition* 52: 313-317.

Tsai, P. J. Tsai, T. H. Yu, C. H. Ho, S. C. 2007. Evaluation of NO-supressing activity of several Mediterranean culinary spices. *Food Chemistry and Toxicology* 45: 440-447.

Ultee, A. Bennik, M. H. Moezelaar, R. 2002. The phenolic hydroxyl group of carvacrol is essential for action against the food-borne pathogen *Bacillus cereus. Applied Environmental Microbiology* 68: 1561-1568.

Ultee, A. Kets, E. P. Smid, E. J. 1999. Mechanisms of action of carvacrol on the food-borne pathogen *Bacillus cereus. Applied Environmental Microbiology* 65: 4606-4610.

Vagi, E. Rapvi, E. Hadolin, M. Vasarhelyine Perdei, K. Balazs, A. Blazovics, A. Simandi, B. 2005. Phenolic and triterpenoid antioxidants from *Origanum majorana* L., herb and extracts obtained with different solvents. *Journal of Agricultural and Food Chemistry* 53: 17-21.

Valero, M. Salmeron, M. C. 2003. Antibacterial activity of 11 essential oils against *Bacillus cereus* in tyndallized carrot broth. *International Journal of Food Microbiology* 85: 73-81.

Vazirian, M. Mohammadi, M. Farzaei, M. H. Amin, G. Amanzadeh, Y. 2015. Chemical composition and antioxidant activity of *Origanum vulgare* subsp. *vulgare* essential oil from Iran. *Research Journal of Pharmacognosy* 2: 41-46.

Veres, K. Varga, E. Schelz, Z. Molnar, J. Bernáth, J. Máthé, I. 2007. Chemical composition and antimicrobial activities of essential oils of four lines of *Origanum vulgare* subsp. *hirtum* (link) Ietswaart grown in Hungary. *Natural Product Communication* 2: 1155-1189.

Viuda-Martos, M. Ruiz-Navajas, Y. Fernández-López, J. Pérez-Álvarez, J. 2010. Effect of orange dietary fibre, oregano essential oil and packaging conditions on shelf-life of bologna sausages. *Food Control* 2: 436-443.

Viuda-Martos, M. El Gendy, Ael-N. Sendra, E. Fernández-López, J. Abd El Razik, K. A. Omer, E. A. Pérez-Alvarez, J. A. 2010. Chemical Composition and Antioxidant and Anti-Listeria Activities of Essential Oils Obtained from Some Egyptian Plants. *Journal of Agricultural and Food Chemistry* 58: 9063-9070.

Vlietinck, A. J. van Hoof, L. Totté, J. Lasure, A. Vanden Berghe, D. Rwangabo, P. C. 1995. Mvukiyumwami, J. Screening of hundred Rwandese medicinal plants for antimicrobial and antiviral properties. *Journal of Ethnopharmacology* 46: 31-47.

Walker, S. J. 1988. Major spoilage micro-organisms in milk and dairy products. *Journal of the Society of Dairy Technology* 41: 91-92.

Weerakkody, S. N. Caffin, N. Turner, S. M. Dukes, A. G. 2010. *In vitro* antimicrobial activity of less-utilized spice and herb extracts against selected food-borne bacteria. *Food Control* 21: 1408-1414.

Williams, P. Cifuentes, X. Velasrov, V. Campos, J. Bórquez, F. Allende, R. 2018. Can dietary dried oregano improve the digestible nutrient intake of growing goats? *Chilean Journal of Agricultural Research* 34: 19-25.

Young, J. F. Stagsted, J. Jensen, S. K. Karlsson, A. H. Henckel, P. 2003. Ascorbic acid, alpha tocopherol, and oregano supplements reduce stress-induced deterioration of chicken meat quality. *Poultry Science* 82: 1343-1351.

Zaidi, S. F. H. Yamada, K. Kadowaki, M. Usmanghani, K; Sugiyama, T. 2009. Bactericidal activity of medicinal plants, employed for the treatment of gastrointestinal ailments, against Helicobacter pylori. *Journal of Ethnopharmacology* 121: 286-291.

Zhang, X. L. Guo, Y. S. Wang, C. H. Li, G. Q. Xu, J. J. Chung, H. Y.; Ye, W. C. Li, Y. L. Wang, G. C. 2014. Phenolic compounds from *Origanum vulgare* and their antioxidant and antiviral activities. *Food Chemistry* 152: 300-306.

Zilberg, D. Tal, A. Froyman, N. Abutbul, S. Dudai, N. Golan-Goldhirsh, A. 2010. Dried leaves of *Rosmarinus officinalis* as a treatment for streptococcosis in tilapia. *Journal of Fish Disease* 33: 361-369.

Zivanovic, S. Chi, S. Draughon, A. F. 2005. Antimicrobial activity of chitosan films enriched with essential oils. *Journal of Food Sciences* 70: 45-51.

In: Oregano: Properties, Uses and Health Benefits
Editor: Gema Nieto Martínez
ISBN: 978-1-53616-284-4

Chapter 2

IMPROVEMENT OF OREGANO USE THROUGH THE BIOREFINERY CONCEPT

Paula Andrea Marín Valencia, José Andrés González Aguirre and Carlos Ariel Cardona Alzate*
Departamento de Ingeniería Química, Universidad Nacional de Colombia, Manizales, Colombia

ABSTRACT

Along the years, cosmetics, fragrances and health care industry have been the basis for developing huge research on aromatic plants as a fundamental raw material for natural products. The demand for these products as well as the possibility to enhance the growing of strategic crops in isolated rural areas is very well connected with the idea of exploiting industrially all valuable compounds in the aromatic plants resulting in new profitable feedstocks. Colombia has been characterized as a potential natural products producer due to its large biodiversity. So many aromatic plants are cultivated in this country (e.g., basil, cilantro, laurel, oregano, rosemary, sage, calendula, etc.) being European oregano (Origanum vulgare) and American oregano (Lippia graveolens) two of the most commercialized oregano types. However, the bioactive compounds (carvacrol and thymol in case of oregano) are not totally used despite their renowned application in natural care and health industry as antioxidants, fungicidal and bactericidal compounds. The main industrial use of oregano is for culinary purposes, but technological extraction of polyphenols and antioxidants from leaves and flowers represent a great opportunity. Besides, the stem of the plant is obtained as a residue and it can be used as lignocellulosic substrate for anaerobic digestion in order to produce biogas, electricity and steam as integral products. This chapter states an opportunity of using Origanum vulgare as potential platform for producing polyphenols, biogas and energy under biorefinery approach. A techno-economic assessment will be carried out in order to compare the feasibility of stand-

* Corresponding Author's E-mail: ccardonaal@unal.edu.co.

alone and biorefinery processes. Biorefinery approach enhances the economic performance at high scales and the stand-alone process is profitable at low scales, the environmental impact using all residues generated by the oregano processing is comparable with other biorefineries.

Keywords: oregano, biorefineries, technoeconomic analysis, environmental analysis

1. Introduction

As a biomass source, herbs and spices have great potential for producing chemical platforms and added value compounds for food, cosmetic and pharmaceutical industries. The current global trade in spices is US$ 38 billion, where India, China and Vietnam are the major producers (Jambor, Toth, and Koroshegyi 2015). Since 1991 this market has grown US$ 30 billion. This growth goes in line with the agricultural products growth, showing a significant increasing trend led by biotechnological and renewable sectors. About 85% of traded spices are in whole form, with processing and packaging in the final destination for the retail market or food industry (Shylaja 2004). The market for added-value compounds from herbs grows equally as the whole plant market given the requirements from big companies to replace synthetic compounds in cosmetics, food and health. However, the competition against petro-based market becomes tougher due to the lack of consolidated extraction processes and the low yields usually reached. Regarding this, it is opened the door of researching about techno-economic analysis of herbs-based bio-compounds, with added value properties. This chapter considers the current situation of one of the most popular aromatic herbs used as food additive: Oregano. It will be described in this introduction the main aspects related to real cultivation, chemical composition and extraction, biorefinery possibilities and a case of study showing the technical, economic and environmental assessment of an oregano-based biorefinery in the Colombian context.

1.1. Aromatic Herbs and Spices

The role of aromatic plants and herbs in human history have been significant for the development of the civilization and culture (Shylaja 2004). The knowledge of aromatic plants has been handed down from generation to generation for thousands of years (Bown 1996). Nowadays, many newest medicines, chemicals and flavors depend on herbs and spices for flavoring, smelling and functional properties given by inner chemical compounds inside the matrix of the herb. In many parts of the world, herbs are being grown as field crop due to their great demand. However, small-scale production as catch-crop among other vegetables and ornamentals, still remains as they were for thousands of years ago.

Table 1. Conventional classification of spices based on (Shylaja 2004)

Classes	Spices
Hot spices	Capsicum (chilies), Cayenne pepper, black and white peppers, ginger, mustard
Mild spices	Paprika, coriander
Aromatic spices	Allspice (pimento), cardamom, cassia, cinnamon, clove, cumin, dill, fennel, fenugreek, mace and nutmeg
Herbs	Basil, bay, dill leaves, oregano, tarragon, thyme, marigold
Aromatic vegetables	Onion, garlic, shallot, celery

The term 'herb' has more than one meaning. The Geneva-based International Standards Organization (ISO) defines spices and condiments as: "Vegetable products or mixtures thereof, free from external matter, used for flavoring, seasoning, and imparting aroma in foods.

The term 'spice' is thus used to cover the use of spices, herbs and certain aromatic vegetables to add flavor and odor to foods. Even the term 'spice' incorporate herbs, the distinction of herbs and spices can be described as follows: "Herbs may be defined as the dried leaves of aromatic plants used to impart flavor and odor to foods with, sometimes, the addition of color. The leaves are commonly traded separately from the plant stems and leaf stalks" (Shylaja 2004). "Spices may be defined as the dried parts of aromatic plants with the exception of the leaves. This definition is wide-ranging and covers virtually all parts of the plant" (Shylaja 2004) The commonly classification of spices is based on degree of taste as is shown in Table 1.

Herbs and spices have strong importance in daily life, as ingredients in food, alcoholic beverages, medicine, perfumery, cosmetics, dye and also as garden plants. They are used in foods for flavoring (parsley, cinnamon, oregano, vanilla, mint, etc.), deodorizing (garlic, rosemary, sage, onion, etc.), pungency (garlic, savory, bay, leek, etc.), dye (paprika, turmeric, saffron) purposes (Shylaja 2004)(Shylaja 2004). Taking into account the antioxidant and antimicrobial activity of herbs and spices, they have a dual function: adding flavor and taste and delaying the spoilage of food. Besides all of this, many herbs and spices have been used in cosmetics, perfumery and beauty since ancient times. Their essential compounds are important for manufacturing soaps, toothpastes and lotions, as well as cleansing agents, infusions, skin toners, eye lotions, shampoos and antiseptic and antitanning lotions (Westland 1987). In health care, herbs and spices have played an important role through ages. China and India have their own herbal systems of medicine (Ayurvedic). All herbs and spices have medical properties such as anti-inflammatory, diuretic, antiseptic, anticoagulant, laxative, fungicidal, among many others (Shylaja 2004). One of the most recognized herbs around the world is oregano (Origanum vulgare) due to its leaves are a favorite seasoning for pizza and other Italian dishes. Besides that, oregano contains phenolic compounds such as flavonoids that may help to protect humans from health diseases like cardiovascular and intestinal cancer. Based on the matter of this book, it will be introduced some general aspects about oregano, cultivation and potential uses as biorefinery feedstock.

1.2. Oregano

Oregano is the name for a culinary and medicinal herb derived from Lamiaceae family. It has been used for years in cooking and medicine for its flavoring and medicinal benefits. It is considered as a perennial herb, with creeping roots, branched woody stems and petiolate and hairy leaves (Grieve and Leyel 1992). The overall market of oregano is increasing and undoubtedly it is the biggest-selling herb today. Latest estimates put worldwide production at about 12000 metric tones (Trumpy and James 2012). Turkey commands the world production and trade (over two-thirds of the total production), followed by Mexico and Greece. Though Italy cultivates large amounts of oregano, they consume it internally. USA is the principal importer of oregano with 40% of the total production. In the regular Turkish market, pure oregano price is about 2575 US$ per metric ton. In other markets, the price goes from 3200 to 5510 US$/mt (Peru and Mexico respectively) (Trumpy and James 2012).

The herb is often sold by mesh size, depending on the customer requirements, indicating the particle size. After cleansing, Mediterranean oregano is milled and grinded into a size of 30 or 60 mesh (Shylaja 2004). The original fresh material is a fundamental fact that determines the quality of the dried herb. Nonetheless, the milling and drying method, the type of packaging and storage conditions also have certain effects on the shelf life and microbial quality of the herbs. Blending of oregano with another spices is very common, in particular for increasing the essential oil concentration (> 3%). Quality evaluation consists usually in a test of color of the traded spice, but it could also include the number of glandular hairs. Leaves should be uniform and have less than 15% of moisture. The essential oil concentration should not be lower than 0,5% (w/w). Final product should be free of impurities such as insects, animal hair or excretions (Shylaja 2004).

2. Oregano Cultivation

Oregano is a perennial plant that grows spontaneously in areas across the Mediterranean region, preferably in high lands with cool summer (Kintzios 2002). The reported optimal condition crop of oregano is 6 - 28°C with annual precipitation of 0.5 - 2.7 m and a soil pH of 4.9 – 8.7 (Shylaja 2004). When oregano is cultivated in cold climates it can be treated as an annual crop. When it is grown as perennial, roots should be divided every three years for enhancing the flavor. In order to avoid the exploitation of oregano from the wild forest, domestication and cultivation practices are being carried out.

For cultivation, oregano is seeded and transplanted into fields. It has a spreading root system that can be expanded by seed or cuttings, the latter are placed 30 cm separated one each other. If seeds are used, they have to be sown in a seedbox in spring and planted outside when seedling are 7.5 cm high. Every four years plants should be replaced to prevent legginess (Shylaja 2004). Ploughing and fertilization of the soil with ammonium phosphate, during the last two-month period of the year is sufficient for oregano cultivation under normal conditions, pest control is done at least four times in the year (manually or using pesticides) (Kintzios 2002) and mechanical weed control (Padulosi 1996). The lifespan of oregano is about five or six years and most times, one harvest is done in the first year and two in the following years (Shylaja 2004) (Shylaja 2004). The yield ranges from 2.5 to 3.5 T/ha and the essential oil yield ranges from 0.5 to 1.5% of dry weight (Kitiki 1996).

Two or three harvests of the crop are allowed annually depending on the irrigation frequency and yield. The leaves and stem should be harvested when the plant is at full bloom, beginning 10 cm from the ground. In small plantations, harvesting is done manually, mechanical harvesting is only able for large field (Shylaja 2004). After harvesting, plant material is dried in drying sheets to avoid the direct sunlight in order to preserve the color and aroma (Kintzios 2002). Although natural drying is often recommended, for industrial purposes drying ovens operating at 30 - 35°C are most used. According to quality standards, moisture content of 7% (minimum) and 12% (maximum) is required (Kitiki 1996). Leaves should be dried in warm, shaded place, at moderate temperatures (> 37°C); preferably using freeze-drying processes in order to conserve volatile compounds and aroma.

Nowadays, crop improvements are highly looked for producers in order to overcome difficulties related with yield parameters, e.g., growth habit, leaf/steam ratio, stress (salt, cold) tolerance and resistance to diseases and quality parameters, e.g., better aromatic characteristics, color (green is preferred to grey), essential oil content (usually more than 2%) and composition providing the antioxidant and antimicrobial properties (Shylaja 2004). To complete these objectives, short time of breeding, selection and hybridization methods, combined with analytical controls on the variability of the material, are some proper techniques for enhancing the crop issue.

3. Chemical Composition and Extraction Methods

Concerning to the structural composition of leaves and stem, the chemical profile is based on a lignocellulosic matrix, which enhance the structural properties of the plant. The typical composition of this type of biomass is 40 - 50% cellulose, 25 - 30% hemicellulose and 15 - 20% lignin and extractable components (Knauf and Moniruzzaman 2004). Cellulose is a linear syndiotactic (alternating spatial arrangement of the side chains) biopolymer of glucose linked together by β-(1→4)-glycosidic bonds, whereas hemicellulose is a branched heteropolymer of D-xylose, L-arabinose, D-mannose, D-glucose, D-galactose and D-glucuronic acid. Lignin is a complex hydrophobic, cross-linked aromatic biopolymer composed of three major phenolic components, namely p-coumaryl alcohol, coniferyl alcohol and sinapyl alcohol (Menon and Rao 2012). Table 2 shows a general composition of oregano essential oil.

The extractives are a group of volatile compounds that confer aroma and color to biomass. They can be extracted via water solubilization that may include inorganic material, non-structural sugars and nitrogenous material, among others. Inorganic material in the water may come from both the biomass and any soluble compound associated with biomass such as soil or fertilizers. Ethanol soluble material includes chlorophyll, waxes or other minor components (Sluiter et al. 2008). Essential oil extraction is basically performed through steam distillation in order to obtain a terpenoids matrix (Table 2 for oregano), but it may vary significantly depending on the type of biomass. Some other polyphenolic compounds, which have added-value in industry due to their antioxidant properties, can be extracted through other techniques such as solvent extraction (sometimes non-polar solvents), microwaves, ultrasound and supercritical fluids extraction.

The most important group of compounds from a commercial and application point of view in oregano, refers to its volatile matrix, basically composed of terpenoids. However, composition can vary significantly among species and regions. Oregano species can be rich in phenolic monoterpenoids such as carvacrol, thymol, while species rich in bicyclic monoterpenoids cis- and trans-sabinene hydrate are commercially designated as marjoram (Shylaja 2004) (Shylaja 2004). As an example, the chemical profile of oregano essential oil from Colombia for four different species evaluated previously are: O. vulgare L. ssp. hirtum showed the highest value of carvacrol (90,3%), while thymol (78%) was the highest in L. origanoides, which is an endemic specie in south of Colombia (Patia region). O. majorana was principally represented by bicyclic monoterpenoids sabinene (4,3%) and cis- and trans- sabinene hydrates (17.1%). In contrast, the major volatile compounds found in O. vulgare was thymol (21,5%) and carvacrol showed the lowest value (4,3%) (Betancourt et al. 2014). All of those compounds can be found in the 'standard' review of the composition of the oregano essential oil (Table 2) (Shylaja 2004), the difference lies in the amount of each component according with the specie.

Table 2. Comprehensive composition of oregano essential oil based on (Shylaja 2004)

Cymyl- compounds	Sabinyl-compounds	Acyclic compounds	Bornyl- compounds	Sesqui-terpenoids	Di-terpenoids	Tri-terpenoids
p-cymene	Sabinene	Geraniol	Borneol	allo-aromadendrene	Akhdarenol	β-amyrin
p-cymenene	Sabinene hydrate	Geranyl acetate	Bornylacetate	β-bisabolene	Akhdardiol	Betulic acid
p-cymen-8-ol	cis-sabinene hydrate	Linalool	Camphene	β-bourbonene	Akhdartriol	Betulin
Carvacrol	trans-sabinene hydrate	Linalyl acetate	Camphor	γ-cadinene	Iso-akhdartriol	Uvaol
Carvacrol acetate	cis-sabinene hydrate acetate	β-myrcene	Isoborneol	α-cadinol		Ursolic acid
Carvacrol methylether	trans-sabinene hydrate acetate		Isobornyl aceate	β-caryophyllene		Oleanolic acid
γ-terpinene	cis-sabinol			Caryophyllene oxide		
Thymol	trans-sabinol			α-copaene		
Thymol acetate	Sabina ketone			β-cubonene		
Thymohydro-quinone	Sabinyl acetate			Germacrene-D		
Thymoquinone	Thujene			Germacrene-D-ol Bicyclogermacrene α-humulene α-muurolene γ-muurolene		

Several extraction techniques for obtaining essential oil and added-value polyphenolic compounds from oregano have been developed through years. The classical and conventional methods for extracting essential oil from oregano are: Hydrodistillation (HD), Steam distillation (SD), Solvent extraction, and Enfleurage. HD consists in evaporating essential oil by heating a mixture of water and other solvent (normally ethanol) and plant materials, followed by the liquefaction of vapor in a condenser (Rassem, Nour, and Yunus 2016). SD is one of the ancient and official approved methods for obtaining essential oils from herbaceous materials. The plant materials charged in a container are subjected to the steam without maceration or contact to liquid water. The injected steam passes through the plant and breaks up the pores of the raw material releasing the essential oil. Solvent extraction consists in an extracting unit loaded with perforated trays of essential oil plant material and repeatedly washed with the solvent (Rassem, Nour, and Yunus 2016). The choice of the solvent is based on the chemical characteristics of the essential oil components. Enfleurage consists in a large frame plate glass smeared with a layer of animal fat, usually lard or tallow. Plant material is placed on the fat and its scent is allowed to diffuse in to the fat over course of 1-3 days.

All of these techniques are not so friendly with environment and their yields are not so high. New types of extraction methods have been developed with the aim of improve the environmental performance and reach higher yields. Supercritical fluid extraction (SFE), Microwave assisted hydrodistillation (MAHD), ultrasound-assisted extraction (UAE), solvent-free microwave extraction (SFME), microwave hydro-diffusion and gravity (MHG). From above mentioned methods, SFE is the most researched because of its high yield production, wide range of applications and easy and low cost technology implementation. In practice, more than 90% of all analytical SFE extractions are performed with carbon dioxide due to its relatively low critical pressure (74 bars) and temperature (32°C), CO_2 is non-toxic, nonflammable, noncorrosive, safe, available in high purity at relatively low cost and is easy removed from the extract (Rozzi et al. 2002). Sometimes, CO_2 may be modified by co-solvents such as ethanol and methanol. This method is normally used at laboratory scale to extract certain compounds with high antioxidant activity. Nevertheless, SFE becomes very expensive in industrial scale due to the high capital investment for the equipment. The modus operandi of SFE consists in cooling the carbon dioxide under - 30°C in order to increase the pressure to the desired one (>100 bar) without a huge temperature increasing. After this, the plant material is placed in a chamber at moderate temperatures (< 40°C) with the co-solvent if it is required (depends on the solubility of the analyte in carbon dioxide), with the aim of being permeated by CO_2 performing the extraction by releasing the essential oils or polyphenolic components. Finally a depressurization tank is required to evaporate all the carbon dioxide and purifying the analyte.

4. Use of Wastes for Anaerobic Digestion

The growth of horticulture industries worldwide has generated huge quantities of wastes. In the fruit and vegetable industry, the preparation and processing procedures could lead to one third of the product being discarded (Ece and Utku 2014). There is need to consider wastes as potential resources rather than undesirable and unwanted materials, to avoid contamination of air, water, and land resources, and to avoid transmission of hazardous materials (Obi, Ugwuishiwu, and Nwakaire 2016). Nevertheless, transformation of waste products with high value-added allows companies to reduce the global treatment costs, sometimes even to take some profits and thus improve their competitiveness. Moreover, the recovery process of byproducts is part of the current existing sustainable development and environmental protection (Sahraoui et al. 2011).

The "unavoidable food waste" is animal or vegetal waste that origins from food but it is not likely that humans will eat it (Stenmarck et al. 2011), food wastes are residues of high organic load and result in liquid or solid form. There are several biological and chemical processes applied for food waste treatment such as composting, aerobic and anaerobic digestion, thermophilic anaerobic digestion, sequencing batch reactor, electrodialysis, wet oxidation, pyrolysis, incineration, solid state fermentation, and ozonation (Deepanraj, Vijayalakshmi, and Ranjitha 2015). Some characteristics of food wastes that have been reported in the literature indicating moisture content of 74 – 90%, volatile solids to total solids ratio of 80 – 97%, and carbon to nitrogen ratio of 14.7 – 36.4. Due to relatively high moisture content of food waste, bioconversion technologies, such as anaerobic digestion, are more suitable compared to thermochemical conversion technologies, such as combustion and gasification (Zhang et al. 2007).

In some studies, the use of food and agriculture wastes for biogas production through anaerobic digestion has been studied, includes animal wastes, industrial wastes, food processing wastes, plant residues, etc. Recently, scientists have proposed withered flowers and vegetable wastes as a potential feedstock for the biogas production (Deepanraj, Vijayalakshmi, and Ranjitha 2015). A study revealed that, flower waste had shown a faster rate of biogas production and then, higher biogas production per unit weight of the substrate than vegetable waste. These vegetable and flower wastes are feasible to be used as feedstocks to take advantage for energy generation and to be used as a gas for domestic purpose (Deepanraj, Vijayalakshmi, and Ranjitha 2015). Rolando et al. studied the biogas production from wastes generated in the extraction of coriander essential oil, which are wet and must be treated to avoid contamination (Rolando, Díaz, and Puerta 2007). The results exposed a reduction of volatile solids between 45 - 50%.

5. Oregano as Biorefinery Platform

Nowadays, the biorefinery concept has gained a lot of importance for biotechnological industry around the world. The need for replacing fossil fuels and chemicals and reducing the environmental impacts, it has led the researchers and manufacturers since 2000's to make several efforts in developing sustainable processes from biomass. The biorefinery concept is referred as: "Biorefining is the sustainable processing of biomass into a spectrum of marketable products and energy" (Cherubini 2010). The biorefinery concept includes a wide range of technologies able to separate biomass resources (wood, grasses, corn, etc.) into their building blocks (carbohydrates, proteins, triglycerides, etc.), which can be converted to value added products, biofuels and chemicals. A biorefinery is a facility (or network of facilities) that integrates biomass conversion processes and equipment to produce transportation biofuels, power and chemicals from biomass (Cherubini 2010). All the sub-streams and by-products in a biorefinery are used to generate added value outputs.

Aromatic plants do not escape from the concept mentioned above, indeed they have great potential as biorefinery raw material due to its wide range of valuable products for pharmaceutic, cosmetic and food industries. As one of the most valuable products that can be obtained from biomass, essential oils are bio-based clusters of compounds that are useful in so many industries such as food, pharmaceutics and cosmetics (Burt 2004). Certain herbs may have great potential in polyphenolic extraction too, generating at least essential oils and one or two added value compound with antioxidant properties. Meanwhile, the byproducts generated by cultivation, pretreatment and extraction may be used as substrate for anaerobic digestion in order to produce biogas. Figure 1 shows a schematic representation of this process. The biogas generated may be used in a combined heat and power cycle (CHP) for supplying the energy requirements of the process. Based on the descriptions presented previously, and taking into account that this technology model has not been implemented in industry so far, a technical, economic and environmental assessment of an aromatic plant-based biorefinery becomes crucial in order to determine the feasibility of the process in the current market conditions.

In this sense, Oregano as one of the most recognized herbs, has been cultivated in tropical regions over thousands of years and has influenced the culture and the food practices. Colombia, located in the center of the America's tropical region, surrounded by Atlantic and Pacific oceans, represents perfectly the tropical region, having high levels of biomass production. On this country, there is a great interest on the development of the agricultural sector to increase its productivity and adopt emerging approaches such as biorefining (J. Moncada, Cardona, and Pisarenko 2013).

Colombia is a net importer for essential oils with 6.95 USD millions in 2017 principally from Brazil. Nevertheless, is a net exporter of spices and herbs with 2.6 USD million (Intracen 2013). This means that improvements have to be done in order to leverage the aromatic compounds from herbs production. As one of the most popular herbs in Colombia, oregano share 10% of the total aromatic plants market. The following study case is based on the needing of Colombia for improving the polyphenols and essential oil production from aromatics herbs, performing a techno-economic and environmental assessment of this biorefinery approach.

6. Case Study

6.1. Simulation Procedure

The process to obtain phenolic compounds from oregano leaves, and their subsequent use for biogas production was performed in the software aspen plus (ASPEN TECHNOLOGY INC.). This software allowed the mass and energy balance calculations, which were needed to estimate the technical, economic and environmental feasibility of the process.

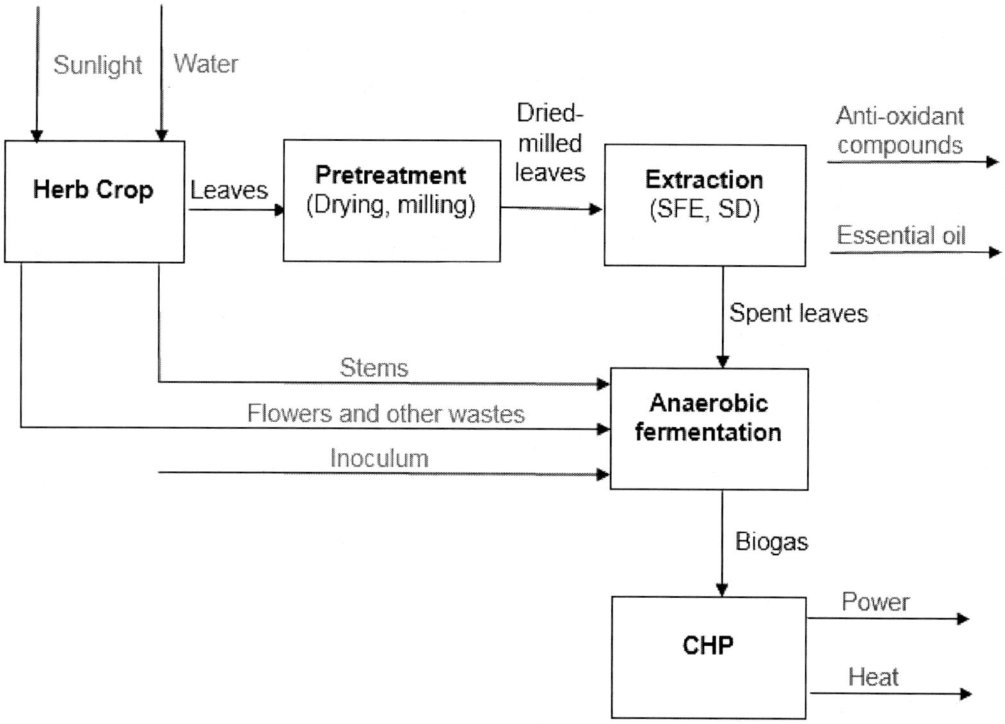

Figure 1. Basic block diagram of a biorefinery from aromatic herbs.

6.1.1. Supercritical Fluid Extraction

For the extraction of phenolic compounds with supercritical fluid technology, the Redlich-Kwong-Aspen thermodynamic model (RKA) was used, based on previous work in which this model was used and good results were obtained (Manan, Siang, and Mustapa 2009) (Zamudio, Schwarz, and Knoetze 2013). Furthermore, as it is mentioned in the Aspen models manual "the RK-ASPEN property method can be used for hydrocarbon processing applications. It is also used for more polar components and mixtures of hydrocarbons, and for light gases at medium to high pressures" (Aspen Technology Inc 2010).

To carry out the simulation, it is necessary the chemical characterization of the oregano leaves. The cellulose, hemicellulose and lignin reported by Martinez (Martinez 2006), the essential oil yield reported by Busatta et al. (Busatta et al. 2017), and the moisture and ash reported by Tévez (Tevez 2017) was taking into account. To define the essential oil composition, the two major phenolic components of the oil were taken into account in equal fractions, which are reported and correspond to thymol and carvacrol (Busatta et al. 2017). The characterization of the oregano leaves is shown in Table 3.

Due to both the stems and leaves of oregano were used, initially an amount of 10 T/h of oregano leaves was taking into account and the whole amount of plant used was calculated regarding the proportion of leaves, stems and inflorescences reported for the plant (Sotiropoulou and Karamanos 2010)(Gerami et al. 2016). The oregano leaves inlet in an oven to be dried until reach a moisture of 10% this process was carried out at 40°C, since in other studies have been reported that at this temperature the best extraction yields are obtained (Sarmiento Pérez 2016). Then, the solid is grinded to particle size below 500 μm in order to expose the oily fraction and to allow a proper extraction condition.

Subsequently, the reduced size and dried solid entry in the extraction vessel. The conditions of carbon dioxide input were considered as the normally pipe conditions, which are close to 57 bar and 20°C (The Linde Group 2018). To reach supercritical conditions, the carbon dioxide initially is cooling to approximately − 30°C, ensuring liquid phase. The cooling fluid used for this stage is ethylene glycol-water coolant (70:30) mixture (Jonathan Moncada, Tamayo, and Cardona 2015). After, the CO_2 pressure is increased until 200 atm in a pump and it is heating at 40°C (extraction conditions), the CO_2 flow was calculated according to the ratio raw material:CO_2 reported previously (Busatta et al. 2017). Then, the supercritical fluid passes through the extraction vessel previously filled with the solid material. After the extraction process, two streams are obtained: one including the exhausted solid and a second one, including the essential oil diluted in supercritical CO_2. The extract was depressurized in a valve and in a flash separator two streams were obtained, the CO_2 and essential oil. The amount of CO_2 recycled to the process was 97%. In Figure 2, the supercritical fluid extraction process is shown.

Table 3. Chemical composition of Oregano leaves

Component	Value (%)
Moisture	67.45
Cellulose	9.44
Hemicellulose	15.16
Lignin	4.30
Ash	0.87
Thymol	1.39
Carvacrol	1.39

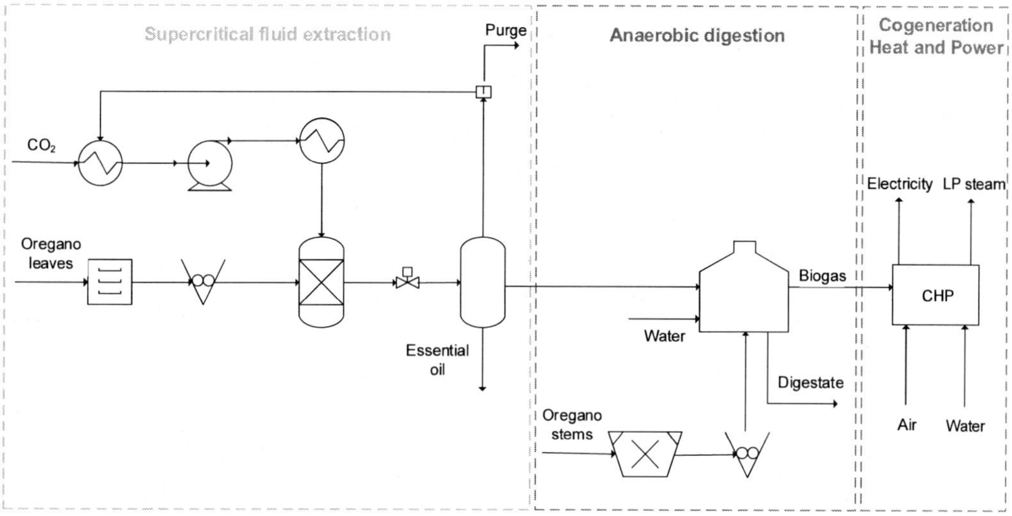

Figure 2. Process flow diagram.

6.1.2. Anaerobic Digestion

The anaerobic digestion process for the production of biogas was carried out with the exhausted oregano leaves and the stems separated previously from the raw material. The characterization of the oregano stems was taken from the work reported by Yanik et al. (Yanik et al. 2007). Due to the oregano plant have a height of approximately 70 cm, two mills were considered for stems pretreatment, one to obtain a particle size of around 1.5 cm and the other to reach 500 μm.

The whole raw material for digestion was charged in the reactor, the amount of water required was calculated taken into account a percentage of 15% (w/v) over the raw material, based on wet continuous system for which less than 20% of dry matter is needed (International Renewable Energy Agency IRENA 2018). The inoculum inlet was not regarding, assuming that the reactor start time has already passed, which can be 6 months later (Manrique-Losada, Vera-Barragán, and Peláez 2012), to do a self-sustainable process. The temperature for the anaerobic reactor was 37°C for anaerobic digestion in mesophilic conditions.

The mathematical model of Buswell was used to determine the yield of biogas production in anaerobic digestion. The Buswell equation starts from the chemical or elemental composition of a generic organic compound and calculates stoichiometrically the main products of an anaerobic digestion by means of the oxidation-reduction reaction in which water intervenes (Buswell and Mueller 1952; Reyes and Echeverr 2017). Within these formed compounds described by the Buswell equation are methane, carbon dioxide, ammonia and hydrogen sulfide. In this case study, both ammonia as hydrogen sulfide was not considered. The Buswell equation estimates the theoretical maximum methane production, assuming the complete decomposition of the biomass implemented. For this case study, only the fraction of volatile solids reported by Rolando et al. (Rolando, Díaz, and Puerta 2007) was used for the calculation in order to obtain more real and approximate experimental results.

These results offer a theoretical yield of biogas, which only consider methane and CO_2 as digestion products. From these results, the 80% of yield was regarding to use a more realistic value. Finally, one stream containing feedstock exhausted, named digestate was obtained and a second one corresponding to biogas. The biogas purification was not considered because the amount of sulphur reported (Yanik et al. 2007) is low and the sulphur compounds production was assumed to be negligible. In Figure 2, the anaerobic digestion process is shown.

6.1.3. Cogeneration

To simulate the cogeneration system, the Peng Robinson thermodynamic package was used according to previously reported paper (Ekwonu, Perry, and Oyedoh 2013), for this process the amount of stoichiometric oxygen necessary for the combustion of biogas was calculated according to the equation:

$$CH_4 + 2O_2 \rightarrow CO_2 + 2H_2O \qquad (6.1)$$

The above considers that only methane will offer the calorific power resulting from combustion, it was considered 1% of oxygen excess to ensure complete combustion and the amount of air that must enter to the combustion reactor was calculated. The air was compressed to reach 10 bar as reported by Solarte-Toro et al. (Solarte-Toro, Chacón-Pérez, and Cardona-Alzate 2018) and the combustion temperature was 1000°C (an average of the combustion temperature) (Basu 2013). The combustion gases passess through a turbine where the pressure was decreased until 1 bar and generates work as product, then the hot gases passess through a simultaneous heat exchanger to heat up the pressurized water and to produce low pressure steam with 10% temperature excess to avoid condensation.

6.2. Economic Assessment

The economic analysis was performed using the Aspen Process Economic Analyzer software (ASPEN TECHNOLOGY INC). This software allows to calculate the equipment cost and the energy requirements. The capital depreciations, maintenance costs, labor costs, fixed charges, general and administrative costs and the plant overhead were calculated based on the percentages described for the economic assessment of chemical processes of Peters and Timmerhaus (Peters and Timmerhaus 1991). To evaluate the economic viability, Colombia's data were used, a tax rate and interest rate values taken were 25 and 17%, respectively. Additionally, the straight-line method was selected for depreciation and a period of 10 years was choosen. The process was evaluated considering 330 days and 24 h/day of operation, this means 7920 h/year (Pereira and Meireles 2007).

Due to both stems and oregano leaves were used in the process, the cost of oregano as a total raw material was considered as the production cost of the oregano crop in the first year (Pezotti 2014). To define the sale price of oregano oil, some articles were taken into account, in which supercritical fluids extractions were made to obtain oils from herbs as Rosemary and Cupuassu (Shariaty-Niassar et al. 2009)(Cavalcanti, Albuquerque, and Meireles 2016). In other report, the change in the selling price is demonstrated for the raw material and extraction method (Range products 2018). Finally, the selling price reported by ultra international B.V. (B.V. 2018) was considered but only a percentage, regarding that the oregano oil of this report is unrefined. Respect to equipment cost estimation, two extractor vessels was considered to simulate a continuous process, sbince for the extraction yield used was necessary an extraction time close to 80 minutes. In Table 4, the costs of raw materials, products, utilities and the operation data used for the economic assessment are shown.

Table 4. Data used for the economic assessment

Feature	Value	Unit	Reference
Raw materials			
Oregano	0.42	USD/kg	(Pezotti 2014)
Water	2*10-3	USD/kg	(Ministerio de Tecnologías de la Información y las Comunicaciones 2018)
CO_2	1.55	USD/kg	(Jonathan Moncada, Tamayo, and Cardona 2015)
Product			
Essential oil of oregano leaves	38	USD/kg	-
Operation			
Low pressure steam	1.57	USD/T	(Cardona Alzate, Solarte Toro, and Gómez 2018)
Electricity	0.14	USD/kWh	(Cardona Alzate, Solarte Toro, and Gómez 2018)
Fuel	24.58	USD/MW	(Cardona Alzate, Solarte Toro, and Gómez 2018)
Operator labor cost	2.14	USD/h	(Cardona Alzate, Solarte Toro, and Gómez 2018)
Supervisor labor cost	4.29	USD/h	(Cardona Alzate, Solarte Toro, and Gómez 2018)

6.3. Environmental Analysis

The potential environmental impact (PEI) is a quantitative indicator of the environmental friendliness or unfriendliness of a process. The PEI is defined as the effect that a chemical would have if it were simple emitted into the environment. This indicator provides an insight of the negative or positive effect of the overall material and energy balance in the environment. For this purpose, the simulation tool Waste Reduction Algorithm (WAR) developed by Environmental Protection Agency EPA, USA, was used in order to evaluate the mass and energy balance of the process and to determine whether or not the process is environmentally friendly. WAR algorithm evaluates the PEI in terms of eight categories: Human Toxicity Potential by Ingestion (HTPI), Human Toxicity Potential by Exposure (HTPE) dermal or inhalation, Terrestrial Toxicity Potential (TTP) Aquatic Toxicity Potential (ATP), Global Warming Potential (GWP), Ozone Depletion Potential (ODP), Photo-Chemical Oxidation Potential (PCOP) and Acidification Potential (AP) (García-Velásquez and Cardona Alzate 2018).

7. Results

7.1. Economic Analysis of the Stand-Alone and Bio-Refinery Process

In Table 5, the comparison between the stand alone and the biorefinery processes using oregano as a raw material is shown. These results correspond to a base case of 10 T/h of oregano leaves, which corresponds to 24 T/h of the whole plant. First, the results of the utilities requirements needed for the plant operation are observed, in which the biorefinery approach can be self-sustainable in terms of the cooling water and energy requirements, since the use of biogas in the cogeneration allows to supply the energetic requirement and the cooling water can be used coming from the wastewater treatment. For the steam requirement, cogeneration in the biorefinery approach supplies 94% of the requirement, so it is possible to affirm that the process with a biorefinery approach can to be self-sustainable.

The results of the Table 5 show that the biorefinery approach requires a value close to twice with respect to the stand-alone process, both in Capital expenditures (Capex) and Operation expenses (Opex). This is because for the biorefinery it is necessary to take into account the expense of the equipment for anaerobic digestion and cogeneration, and therefore in operating costs. However, it is necessary to remember that the same process can cover the entire operation expense. For the stand-alone process, the base case is profitable in the first year with a present value (VPN) in the project lifetime of 29.94 mUSD/year. The minimum raw material flow in which the stand alone process can operate, this means, the flow in which neither losses nor profits are generated, is 17 T/day. Figure 3 shows the VPN for different raw material flows evaluated in the stand alone process over the project lifetime.

For the biorefinery process, the base case is profitable in the second year with a present value (VPN) in the project lifetime of 21.43 mUSD/year. The minimum raw material flow in which the biorefinery process can operate is 40 T/day. Figure 4 shows the VPN for different raw material flows evaluated in the biorefinery process over the project lifetime. The payback periods for both exposed processes are in agreement to those reported by other authors, whose values are around two years and re-affirm the viability of the process (Prado, Veggi, and Meireles 2014)(Development Studies Associates (DSA) 2008).

The results shown allow affirming that both the stand alone and in biorefinery process are profitable. This is due to although the extraction yields of the interest compounds are low, because this substances are present in small proportions in the plants, its sale price is high due to the beneficial effects of the compounds. As the feasibility of both processes has already been demonstrated, the selection of the type of process to be implemented must be based on different perspectives. As it was initially considered, the flow of raw material takes into account the whole plant, including the leaves, stem and flowers, for the stand alone process only the leaves were used, considering the stem and the flowers as a waste to which treatment should be given. Since, the direct disposition of wastes remaining are watered continuously and allows as it is for several months, which may sometimes cause not controlled anaerobic condition and leads to bad smell, attracts flies and spread epidemic diseases. In some cases, the wastes are used for livestock feeding or dried and burned in the field. Therefore, proper management of solid waste in the agricultural field is necessary (Lokeshwari and Swamy 2010).

Table 5. Economic assessment results

	Stand alone	Biorefinery		
		Requirements	Generated	Net
Requirements				
Energy (kW)	268.54	348.96	354.19	0
LP steam (kg/h)	2285.24	2366.84	2230	136.84
Cooling water (kg/h)	-	55848.56	59643.44 (reused water)	0
Economic				
Opex (mUSD)	0.53	0.98		
Capex (mUSD)	2.46	5.57		

For the biorefinery approach both the leaves and stems are taken into account as raw material, so the flowers remain. However, the disposition of the stems is avoided (in comparison with the stand alone process), which represent a large percentage of the whole plant. The oregano flowers can be taken into account in future studies, evaluating the value added compounds that can be extracted or considering it as feedstock for anaerobic digestion and thus be able to supply the remaining 6% requirement of low pressure steam, which was not able to supply with the exposed biorefinery process. In addition, since the biorefinery process is prone to be completely self-sustaining, this process can be proposed for use in non-interconnected areas, since unlike the stand-alone process, this process would not need the provision of public utilities.

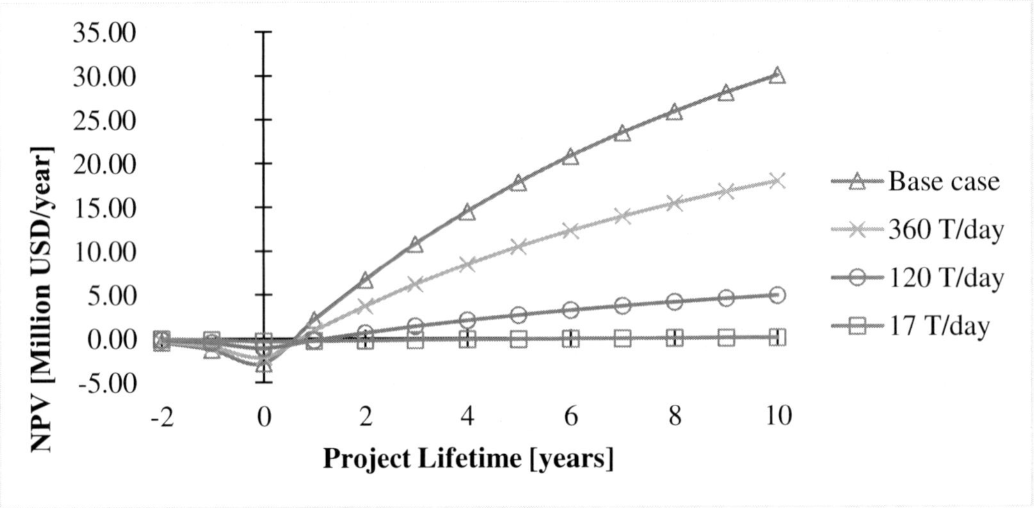

Figure 3. VPN over project lifetime for stand alone process.

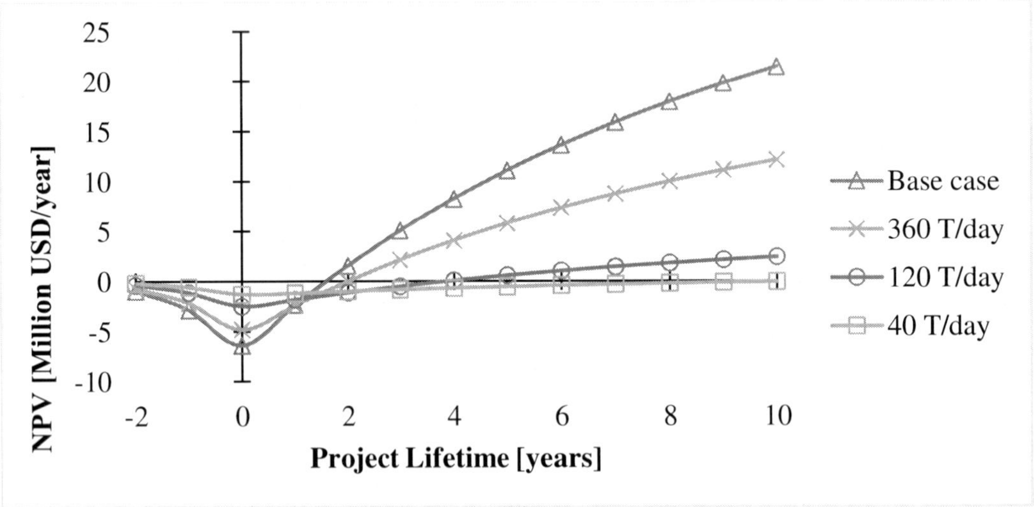

Figure 4. VPN over project lifetime for biorefinery process.

In order to make even more profitable the two processes shown, and due that to supply the carbon dioxide represents the highest raw materials cost. It is possible to consider the implementation of the process in the proximity of fermentation plants, since in these processes the release of carbon dioxide takes place as by-product of the transformation. Thus, only the conditioning cost of this raw material would be taken into account as have been reported previously (Albarelli et al. 2018). Furthermore, the biorefinery process can evaluated the use of the digestate generated in the anaerobic digestion for composting or burning as have been reported in other studies (Moller and Muller 2012) to increase the profitability. Another key point to increase the profitability of the process could be to reduce the costs associated with the drying of the raw material. In this way, it can propose the sunlight drying, which may be feasible depending on the thermal floor where the process will be installed.

7.2. Environmental Analysis of the Oregano Biorefinery

Figure 5 shows a comparison between the stand-alone and the biorefinery approaches. For the biorefinery approach, HTPI and TTP are the major contributors to the environmental impact and a lesser degree HTPE with values of 0.19, 0.18 and 0.04 PEI/kg of product, respectively. This is due the releasing of "digestate", which is a sludge that has high bacterial and organic charge, besides it contains damaging compounds for life such as heavy metals and sulphur. As it is dangerous for humans (HTPI and HTPE categories), is dangerous for terrestrial beings too, such as fauna and flora (TTP). The other outlet streams do not contribute significantly to the environmental impact of the process. The global warming potential (GWP) and acidification potential (AP) do not have a relevant impact because they are often related with energy consumption, which in this case is totally provided by the cogeneration system through power and heat generation.

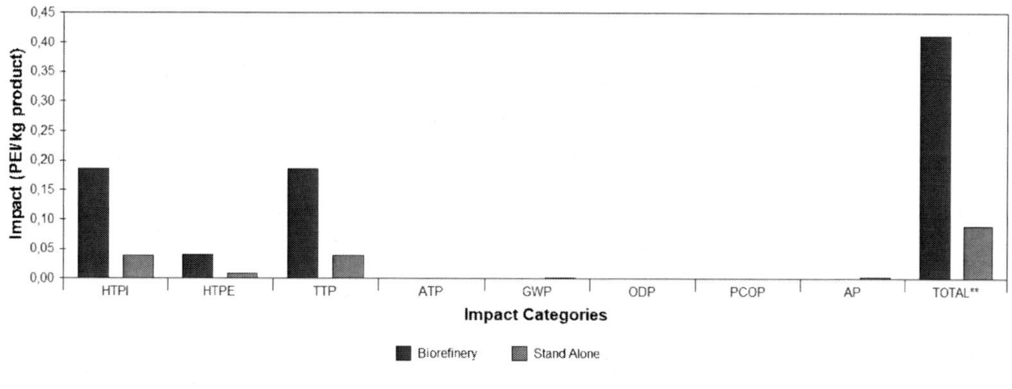

Figure 5. Potential environment impacts of the biorefinery and stand-alone process based on oregano.

For the stand-alone approach, HTPI, TTP and HTPE categories are mostly affected as the biorefinery approach, but the PEI of each one is four times lower (0.04, 0.04, 8*10-3 PEI per kg of product respectively). The PEI of stand-alone is lower than biorefinery due to the impact generated by anaerobic digestion wastes. An alternative for adding value to this stream is producing solid manure after for oregano crop from digestate through stabilization processes. In this case, exists a trade-off between the benefits achieved by cogeneration in terms of energy and cost savings and the environmental impact involved.

The total PEI of the stand-alone scenario is 0.09 PEI/kg. Moncada et al. (Jonathan Moncada, Tamayo, and Cardona 2014; Jonathan Moncada, Tamayo, and Cardona 2015) report an overall environmental impact of 0.03 PEI/kg and 0.02 PEI/kg for essential oil SFE from oregano and citronella respectively. These values are not too far each other and represent a good approach of the transformation process environmental impact. The total PEI of the biorefinery scenario is 0.40 PEI/kg of product that means 1700 PEI/h. Martinez-Ruano et al. (Martínez-Ruano et al. 2018) report 95.000 PEI/h for a biorefinery from banana peel that produces biogas, ethanol and xylitol. In this sense, the biorefinery scenario presents higher environmental impact than stand-alone scenario for oregano, it represents lower PEI per hour than other biorefineries using anaerobic digestion technology. It is important to note that this environmental assessment was made only for the transformation step, meaning gate to gate approach, without the crop or the distribution steps.

Conclusion and Recommendations

The results showed that it is possible to extract polyphenols from Oregano as raw material by SFE through biorefinery approach. Oregano, as the most traded aromatic herb in the world due to its importance on food, is a promising platform for producing antioxidant chemicals such as thymol and carvacrol. The technological development of new extraction technologies has allowed obtaining high yield and better selectivity for polyphenolic compounds from aromatic herbs, in this oregano case.

From the economic point of view, the stand alone and biorefinery processes are viable for the raw material costs and sale prices proposed. However, there are different ways of making the processes more economically viable. In addition, the total use of raw materials is essential to avoid generating contamination and more profitability process.

The effect of energy integration drives to a decrease in the production cost of the technology. Other important aspect assessed in this study case, is the potential environment impact (PEI) as environmental indicator. It was achieved less PEI in the stand-alone scenario than biorefinery scenario. It is important to note that efforts have to be made for valorizing the waste generated in the anaerobic digestion which is the core of cogeneration system in the biorefinery scenario. Manure for oregano crop is an alternative, but future studies have to be made in order to validate this possibility. On the other hand, further researches have to head up the LCA (Life Cycle Assessment) of the whole chain (cradle to grave approach) of biorefinery based on aromatic herbs.

REFERENCES

Albarelli, Juliana., Diego, Santos., María, Cocero. & Maria, Meireles. (2018). "Perspectives on the Integration of a Supercritical Fluid Extraction Plant to a Sugarcane Biorefinery: Thermo-Economical Evaluation of CO2 Recycle Systems." *Food Science and Technology*, *38* (1), 13–18. doi:10.1590/1678-457x.33516.

Aspen Technology Inc. (2010). "Thermodynamic Property Models." In *Aspen Physical Property System - Physical Property Models*, 12–184. doi:10.1063/1.464553.

B. V., Ultra International. (2018). "Essential Oils Market Report." http://ultranl.com/ultracms/wp-content/uploads/MR-SPRING-2018-DIGITALVERSION_new.pdf.

Basu, Prabir. (2013). *Biomass Gasification, Pyrolysis and Torrefaction: Practical Design and Theory. Biomass Gasification, Pyrolysis and Torrefaction: Practical Design and Theory*. 2nded. doi:10.1016/C2011-0-07564-6.

Betancourt, Liliana., Fernando, Rodriguez., Vienvilay, Phandanouvong., Claudia, Ariza-Nieto., Michael, Hume., David, Nisbet., German, Afanador-Téllez., et al. (2014). "Composition and Bactericidal Activity against Beneficial and Pathogenic Bacteria of Oregano Essential Oils from Four Chemotypes of Origanum and Lippia Genus." *Journal of Analytical Methods in Chemistry*, 2015, (1–2 SPEC. ISS.), 831238. doi:10.1155/2015/831238.

Bown, Deni. (1996). *Encyclopedia of Herbs and Their Uses*. Dorling Kindersley.

Burt, Sara. (2004). "Essential Oils: Their Antibacterial Properties and Potential Applications in Foods—a Review." *International Journal of Food Microbiology*, *94* (3). Elsevier: 223–53. doi:10.1016/J.IJFOODMICRO.2004.03.022.

Busatta, Cassiano., Juliana, Barbosa., Rafael, Imlau Cardoso., Natalia, Paroul., Maria, Rodrigues., Débora, De Oliveira., José, Vladimir De Oliveira. & Rogério, Luis Cansian. (2017). "Chemical Profiles of Essential Oils of Marjoram (Origanum Majorana) and Oregano (Origanum Vulgare) Obtained by Hydrodistillation and Supercritical CO2." *Journal of Essential Oil Research*, *29* (5), 367–74. doi:10.1080/10412905.2017.1340197.

Buswell, A. M. & Mueller, H. F. (1952). "Mechanism of Methane Fermentation." *Industrial & Engineering Chemistry*, *44* (3), 550–52. doi:10.1021/ie50507a033.

Cardona, Alzate., Carlos, Ariel., Juan, Camilo Solarte Toro. & Álvaro, Gómez. (2018). "Fermentation, Thermochemical and Catalytic Processes in the Transformation of Biomass through Efficient Biorefineries." *Catalysis Today*, *302*, 61–72. doi:10.1016/j.cattod.2017.09.034.

Cavalcanti, Rodrigo N., Carolina, L. C. Albuquerque. & Angela, A. Meireles M. (2016). "Supercritical CO2 Extraction of Cupuassu Butter from Defatted Seed Residue: Experimental Data, Mathematical Modeling and Cost of Manufacturing." *Food and Bioproducts Processing*, 48–62. doi:10.1016/j.fbp.2015.10.004.

Cherubini, Francesco. (2010). "The Biorefinery Concept: Using Biomass instead of Oil for Producing Energy and Chemicals." *Energy Conversion and Management*, *51* (7). Elsevier Ltd: 1412–21. doi:10.1016/j.enconman.2010.01.015.

Deepanraj, A., Vijayalakshmi, S. & Ranjitha, J. (2015). "Production of Bio Gas from Vegetable and Flowers Wastes Using Anaerobic Digestion." *Applied Mechanics and Materials*, *787*, 803–8. doi:10.4028/www.scientific.net/AMM.787.803.

Development Studies Associates (DSA). (2008). "Project Profile on the Establishment of Essential Oils Producing Plant." Adis abeba. http://www.ethiopianembassy.org/AboutEthiopia/InvestmentProjectProfiles/Manufacturing/Agro-processing/ Essential_Oils.pdf.

Ece, Canan. & Omer, Utku. (2014). "Development of Value-Added Products from Food Wastes." *Food Processing: Strategies for Quality Assessment*, 453–75. doi:10.1007/978-1-4939-1378-7_18.

Ekwonu, M. C., Perry, S. & Oyedoh, E. A. (2013). "Modelling and Simulation of Gas Engines Using Aspen HYSYS." *Journal of Engineering Science and Technology Review*, *6* (3), 1–4. www.jestr.org.

García-Velásquez, Carlos Andrés. & Carlos, Ariel Cardona Alzate. (2018). "Biochemical Pathway for Hydrogen Production Using Coffee Cut-Stems as Raw Material." *European Journal of Sustainable Development Research*, no. November. doi:10.20897/ejosdr/3949.

Gerami, Farzad., Parviz, R Moghaddam., Reza, Ghorbani. & Abbas, Hassani. (2016). "Effects of Irrigation Intervals and Organic Manure on Morphological Traits, Essential Oil Content and Yield of Oregano (Origanum Vulgare L.)." *Annals of the Brazilian Academy of Sciences*, *88* (4), 2375–85. doi:10.1590/0001-3765201620160208.

Grieve, M. (Maud). & Leyel, C. F. (1992). *A Modern Herbal: The Medicinal, Culinary, Cosmetic and Economic Properties, Cultivation and Folklore of Herbs, Grasses, Fungi, Shrubs and Trees with All Their Modern Scientific Uses*. Tiger Books International.

International Renewable Energy Agency IRENA. (2018). *Biogas for Road Vehicles: Tehnology Brief*. Abu Dhabi.

Intracen. (2013). "*Spices Market*." http://www.intracen.org/uploadedFiles/intracenorg/Content/Exporters/Market_Data_and_Information/Market_information/Market_Insider/Spices/ITC Market Insider Spices report September 2016 .pdf.

Jambor, A., Toth, A. T. & Koroshegyi, D. (2015). *Competitiveness in the Trade of Spices : A Global Evidence*, no. 119669.

Kintzios, Spiridon. (2002). *Oregano: The Genera Origanum and Lippia*. Greece: Taylor & Francis. doi:http://dx.doi.org/10.1016/j.seizure.2008.05.010.

Kitiki, A. (1996). "Status of Cultivation and Use of Oregano in Turkey." *Oregano Proceedings of the IPGRI International Workshop on Oregano, 8-12 May 1996, CIHEAM, Valenzano, Bari, Italy*, October, 76–93.

Knauf, M. & Moniruzzaman, M. (2004). *International Sugar Journal. International Sugar Journal*. Vol. *106*. International Sugar Journal.

Lokeshwari, M. & Nanjunda Swamy, C. (2010). "Waste to Wealth - Agriculture Solid Waste Management Study Copyright." *Pollution Research*, *29* (3), 129–33. https:// www. researchgate. net/ publication/ 289615034_ Waste_ to_ wealth_-_ Agriculture_solid_waste_management_study.

Manan, Zainuddin A., Lim, C. Siang. & Ana, N. Mustapa. (2009). "Development of a New Process for Palm Oil Refining Based on Supercritical Fluid Extraction Technology." *Industrial & Engineering Chemistry Research*, *48*, 5420–26. doi:10.1021/ie801735y.

Manrique-Losada, Lis., Marcela, Vera-Barragán. & Marlon, Peláez. (2012). "Inoculum Evaluation for Anaerobic Digestion of Domestic Wastewater in Conditions of the Amazonian Piedmont." *Momentos de Ciencia*, *9* (2). Urban and Fischer.

Martínez-Ruano, Jimmy Anderson., Ashley, Sthefanía Caballero-Galván., Daissy, Lorena Restrepo-Serna. & Carlos, Ariel Cardona. (2018). "Techno-Economic and Environmental Assessment of Biogas Production from Banana Peel (Musa Paradisiaca) in a Biorefinery Concept." *Environmental Science and Pollution Research*, no. Weiland 2010: 1–10. doi:10.1007/s11356-018-1848-y.

Martinez, Ricardo. (2006). "Evaluation of Shrub Leaves and Pods Consumed by the Goats by *In Vitro* Technique of Gas Production." *Estado de México*. doi:10.7868/ S002636561705010X.

Menon, Vishnu. & Mala, Rao. (2012). "Trends in Bioconversion of Lignocellulose: Biofuels, Platform Chemicals and Biorefinery Concept." *Progress in Energy and Combustion Science*, *38* (4). Pergamon: 522–50. doi:10.1016/J.PECS.2012.02.002.

Ministerio de Tecnologías de la Información y las Comunicaciones. (2018). "Tarifa Servicio De Acueducto Y Alcantarillado | Datos Abiertos Colombia." ["Aqueduct and Sewer Service Rate | Open Data Colombia"]. https:// www.datos.gov.co/Ambiente-y-Desarrollo- Sostenible/ Tarifa- Servicio-De-Acueducto-Y-Alcantarillado/ 75he-jkve/ data.

Moller, Kurt. & Torsten, Muller. (2012). "Effects of Anaerobic Digestion on Digestate Nutrient Availability and Crop Growth: A Review." *Engineering in Life Sciences*, *12* (3), 242–57. doi:10.1002/elsc.201100085.

Moncada, J., Cardona, C. A. & Pisarenko, Yu. A. (2013). "Solubility of Some Phenolic Acids Contained in Citrus Seeds in Supercritical Carbon Dioxide: Comparison of Mixing Rules, Influence of Multicomponent Mixture and Model Validation." *Theoretical Foundations of Chemical Engineering*, *47* (4), 381–87. doi:10.1134/ S0040579513040234.

Moncada, Jonathan., Jhonny, A. Tamayo. & Carlos, A. Cardona. (2015). "Techno-Economic and Environmental Assessment of Essential Oil Extraction from Oregano (Origanum Vulgare) and Rosemary (Rosmarinus Officinalis) in Colombia." *Journal of Cleaner Production*. Elsevier Ltd. doi:10.1016/j.jclepro.2015.09.067.

Moncada, Jonathan., Jhonny, Tamayo. & Carlos, Cardona. (2014). "Techno-Economic and Environmental Assessment of Essential Oil Extraction from Citronella (Cymbopogon Winteriana) and Lemongrass (Cymbopogon Citrus): A Colombian Case to Evaluate Different Extraction Technologies." *Industrial Crops and Products*, *54*. Elsevier B.V.: 175–84. doi:10.1016/j.indcrop.2014.01.035.

Obi, F. O., Ugwuishiwu, B. O. & Nwakaire, J. N. (2016). "Agricultural Waste Concept, Generation, Utilization and Management." *Nigerian Journal of Technology*, *35* (4), 957–64. doi:10.4314/njt.v35i4.34.

Padulosi, S. (1996). *Oregano*. Valenzano, Bari, Italy: International Plant Genetic Resources Institute. https://www.bioversityinternational.org/fileadmin/ _migrated/ uploads/tx_news/Oregano_199.pdf.

Pereira, Camila. & Angela, Meireles. (2007). "Economic Analysis of Rosemary, Fennel and Anise Essential Oils Obtained by Supercritical Fluid Extraction." *Flavour and Fragance Journal*, *22*, 407–13. doi:10.1002/ffj.1813.

Peters, Max S. & Klaus, D. Timmerhaus. (1991). *Plant Design and Economics for Chemical Engineers*. Singapore: McGraw-Hill.

Pezotti, Germán. (2014). *Handbook on the Cultivation of Export Condimentary Plants under Good Agricultural Practices*. Medellín: Gobernación de Antioquia, Secretaría de Agricultura y Desarrollo Rural.

Prado, Juliana., Priscilla, Veggi. & Angela, Meireles. (2014). "Supercritical Fluid Extraction Of Lemon Verbena (*Aloysia Triphylla*): Process Kinetics and Scale-Up, Extract Chemical Composition and Antioxidant Activity, and Economic Evaluation." *Separation Science and Technology*, *49*, 569–79. doi:10.1080/ 01496395. 2013.862278.

Range products. (2018). "*Essential Pure Natural*." Welshpool. Accessed December 10. https://www.rangeproducts.com.au/Price List.pdf.

Rassem, Hesham H. A., Abdurahman, H. Nour. & Rosli, M. Yunus. (2016). "Techniques For Extraction of Essential Oils From Plants: A Review." *Australian Journal of Basic and Applied Sciences*, *10* (16), 117–27.

Reyes, Ileana Pereda. & Antonio, Echeverr. (2017). *El Modelo de Buswell. Aplicación y Comparación* [*The Buswell Model. Application and Comparison*]. no. January 2016.

Rolando, Aída., Roberto, Díaz. & Analía, Puerta. (2007). "Tratamiento Por Digestión Anaeróbica de Los Residuos de La Extracción Del Aceite Esencial Del Coriandro." ["Anaerobic Digestion Treatment of Coriander Essential Oil Extraction Residues"]. *Revista Brasileña de Agroecología*, *2* (1). Buenos Aires: 191–98.

Rozzi, N. L., Phippen, W., Simon, J. E. & Singh, R. K. (2002). "Supercritical Fluid Extraction of Essential Oil Components from Lemon-Scented Botanicals." *LWT - Food Science and Technology*, *35* (4). Academic Press: 319–24. doi:10.1006/ FSTL.2001.0873.

Sahraoui, Naima., Maryline, Abert Vian., Mohamed, El Maataoui., Chahrazed, Boutekedjiret. & Farid, Chemat. (2011). "Valorization of Citrus by-Products Using Microwave Steam Distillation (MSD)." *Innovative Food Science and Emerging Technologies*, *12* (2), 163–70. doi:10.1016/j.ifset.2011.02.002.

Sarmiento, Pérez. & Olga, Isabel. (2016). "Evaluación de La Cinética de Extracción Del Aceite Esencial de Calendula Officinalis L. Mediante Hidrodestilación Y Calentamiento Óhmico Asistido Por Hidrodestilación." [Evaluation of the Kinetics of Essential Oil Extraction from Calendula Officinalis L. Through Hydrodestilation and Ohmic Heating Assisted by Hydrodestilation]. Universidad Nacional Abierta y a Distancia. https://stadium.unad.edu.co/preview/UNAD.php?url=/bitstream/10596/11836/1/1026569480.pdf.

Shariaty-Niassar, Mojtaba., Behdad, Aminzadeh., Pouya, Azadi. & Saeed, Soltanali. (2009). "Economic Evaluation of Herb Extraction Using Supercritical Fluid." *Chemical Industry and Chemical Engineering Quarterly*, *15* (3), 143–48. doi:10.2298/CICEQ0903143S.

Shylaja, M. R. (2004). *Handbook of Herbs and Spices*. Edited by K. V. Peter. *Handbook of Herbs and Spices*. 2nd ed. New York: Woodhead Publishing Limited, Abington Hall, Abington. doi:10.1533/9781855738355.1.11.

Sluiter, A., Ruiz, R., Scarlata, C., Sluiter, J. & Templeton, D. (2008). "*Determination of Extractives in Biomass: Laboratory Analytical Procedure (LAP); Issue Date 7/17/2005*." http://www.nrel.gov/biomass/analytical_procedures.html.

Solarte-Toro, Juan Camilo., Yessica, Chacón-Pérez. & Carlos, Ariel Cardona-Alzate. (2018). "Evaluation of Biogas and Syngas as Energy Vectors for Heat and Power Generation Using Lignocellulosic Biomass as Raw Material." *Electronic Journal of Biotechnology*, *33* (May), 52–62. doi:10.1016/j.ejbt.2018.03.005.

Sotiropoulou, D. E. & Karamanos, A. J. (2010). "Field Studies of Nitrogen Application on Growth and Yield of Greek Oregano (Origanum Vulgare Ssp. Hirtum (Link) Ietswaart)." *Industrial Crops and Products*, *32*, 450–57. doi:10.1016/j.indcrop.2010.06.014.

Stenmarck, Asa., Ole, Jörgen., Kirsi, Silvennoinen., Juha-Matti, Katajajuuri. & Mads, Werge. (2011). "*Initiatives on Prevention of Food Waste in the Retail and Wholesale Trades*." Swedish. http://www.refreshcoe.eu/wp-content/uploads/2017/06/B1988.pdf.

Tevez, Monica. (2017). "Caracterization Oca Snack (Oxalis Tuberosa Mol.) with Cheese and Oreganum Incorporation." *Repositorio Institucional*. http:// repositorio.unap.edu.pe/bitstream/handle/UNAP/6038/Tevez_Huaman_Monica.pdf?sequence=1&isAllowed=y.

The Linde Group. (2018). "*Safety Advice 12-Working with Carbon Dioxide CO2*." Germany. https://www.linde-gas.pt/en/images/Safety_Advice_12_tcm303-25938.pdf.

Trumpy, Stefano. & Webb, James. (2012). “Herbs Market Report.” In *11TH World Spice Congress*, *25*. World spice congress. http://worldspicecongress.com/uploads/files/24/sess01-f.pdf.

Westland, Pamela. (1987). *The Encyclopedia of Herbs and Spices*. Edited by Marshall Cavendish. Omega Books. http://books.google.com.au/books?id=0wzMAAAACAAJ.

Yanik, Jale., Christoph, Kornmayer., Mehmet, Saglam. & Mithat, Yüksel. (2007). “Fast Pyrolysis of Agricultural Wastes: Characterization of Pyrolysis Products.” *Fuel Processing Technology*, *88*, 942–47. doi:10.1016/j.fuproc.2007.05.002.

Zamudio, M., Schwarz, C. E. & Knoetze, J. H. (2013). “Experimental Measurement and Modelling with Aspen Plus® of the Phase Behaviour of Supercritical CO2+(n-dodecane+1-decanol+3,7-Dimethyl-1-Octanol).” *The Journal of Supercritical Fluids*. Vol. *84*. doi:10.1016/j.supflu.2013.09.015.

Zhang, Ruihong., Hamed, M. El-Mashad., Karl, Hartman., Fengyu, Wang., Guangqing, Liu., Chris, Choate. & Paul, Gamble. (2007). “Characterization of Food Waste as Feedstock for Anaerobic Digestion.” *Bioresource Technology*, *98* (4), 929–35. doi:10.1016/j.biortech.2006.02.039.

In: Oregano: Properties, Uses and Health Benefits
Editor: Gema Nieto Martínez
ISBN: 978-1-53616-284-4

Chapter 3

Use of Carvacrol as Antimicrobial in Edible Matrices Based on Starch and HPMC

Lía N. Gerschenson[1,2], PhD, Silvia K. Flores[1,2,*], PhD, Paola C. Alzate[2], PhD and Sofía Miramont[1], MD

[1]Universidad de Buenos Aires, Facultad de Ciencias Exactas y Naturales, Departamento de Industrias, Ciudad Autónoma de Buenos Aires, Argentina
[2]CONICET - Universidad de Buenos Aires, Instituto de Tecnología de Alimentos y Procesos Químicos (ITAPROQ), Ciudad Autónoma de Buenos Aires, Argentina

Abstract

Oregano (*Origanum vulgare L.*) is an herbaceous plant native to the Mediterranean regions that has been used for medicinal purposes, owing to its antimicrobial, antioxidant and antifungal properties. In particular, the essential oil (EO) of this plant is extracted with the aim of being used mainly in pharmaceutical, cosmetic and food industry. Many of these EOs are safe compounds classified as GRAS (generally recognized as safe). The primary components of the oregano EO are:carvacrol and thymol. These main components are phenolic substances, responsible for the antimicrobial properties. The objective of this work was to evaluate the effect of the carvacrol addition (0.10% or 0.5% w/w) on the antimicrobial, mechanical and physical properties of self-supporting edible films based on native cassava starch (2.67% w/w) and hydroxypropyl methylcellulose (HPMC, 0.67% w/w), plasticized with glycerol (1.70% w/w) and additionally added with potassium sorbate (0.30% w/w). Moreover, the effect of different emulsification speeds (6500 rpm or 21500 rpm) on the film properties was analyzed. It was observed that the films were structurally amorphous and prone to yellow color. A high shear rate generated a higher solubility and

* Corresponding Author's E-mail: skflores14@gmail.com.

tensile strength than the film obtained at a lower speed, while the deformation showed no significant differences between studied films. To evaluate the antimicrobial action, films were formulated with 0.50% w/w of carvacrol and the agar diffusion assay was carried out. The spoilage microorganisms of foods such as *Z. bailii, L. plantarum,* and *P. fluorescens* were tested, observing a complete inhibition of the microbial growth in the contact zone of the film with the agar. For this formulation, the physical properties were evaluated and compared with films containing only sorbate. It was evidenced that Elastic Modulus, rupture stress and deformation decreased with respect to those films that did not contain the component of the oregano EO. On the other hand, films did not show differences in color, water solubility and water vapor permeability. The results obtained provide essential information on the carvacrol performance as edible films component to increase the shelf life of food products and improve their quality, helping to optimize their production and behavior and to satisfy consumer demand for more natural and safe products, benign with the environment.

Keywords: edible films, antimicrobials, carvacrol, physical and chemical characterization, antimicrobial performance

Introduction

The development of new food preservation methodologies, in order to obtain food that is safe and has improved its nutritional and organoleptic characteristics, is a research area of constant interest and permanent progress. Among the emerging technologies for the optimization of food preservation, the use of edible films or coatings that can impart specific functional properties to food arises as a novel alternative.

Edible films can be used to support additives such as antimicrobials, thus being used to impart a highly localized functional effect (Flores and Gerschenson, 2007) or to produce a gradual release of the antimicrobial to food (Chang and Seow, 2000). It should be noted that the conditions of formation and the composition of the films, affect the migration of these additives compromising their effectiveness (Flores and Del Nobile, 2007). In general, it is desired that the obtained films are totally neutral with respect to the color and smell of the product. In cases of edible films that are used for antimicrobial support, there is little systematic information concerning the influence on the physicochemical and mechanical properties of films and on the activity and diffusivity of the supported antimicrobial. According to the above, it is highlighted the importance of obtaining information in relation of edible films properties useful to increase the quality of foods, contributing to the optimization of film performance. This information will contribute to deepen the knowledge in the development of these materials. For the formulation of edible films, starches, cellulose derivatives, chitosan, gums, whey proteins, soy protein concentrates as well as fats and oils can be used (Phan and Voilley, 2009; Chillo and Del Nobile, 2008). Furthermore, the use of plasticizers such as glycerol or sorbitol is necessary in order to provide the desired flexibility and extensibility to these films (Fernández Cervera and Yliruusi, 2004).

Edible Films Components

Starch

Starch is a reserve polysaccharide in most vegetables and is widely used in the manufacturing of edible films. It consists of two types of chains: amylose and amylopectin. Amylose is a linear chain polysaccharide of units of α-D-glucopyranose linked by 1- 4 bonds and has a low molecular weight (20 - 800 kg/mol). In contrast, amylopectin is a highly branched polymer with 1- 6 bonds at the branching points and a high molecular weight (5000 - 30000 kg/mol). The amylose content is around 20-25% in most starches (Peressini and Sensidoni, 2003).

The starch granule consists of concentric layers or growth rings. In each layer, the molecules of amylose and amylopectin are intermixed and arranged radially. During heating of the aqueous suspension, the linear amylose molecules and the external side chains of the amylopectin are joined together by hydrogen bridges to form micelles (crystalline areas). These micelles are responsible for holding the granule together, allowing swelling instead of complete granule rupture and solubilization of the molecules. Along a linear chain, or in the external ramifications of amylopectin, there may be several crystalline zones, because of different local intermolecular associations. Between these micellar zones there are amorphous zones. The coupling of the axial-equatorial position of the D-glucopyranosyl units with 1 - 4 bonds in the amylose chains gives the molecules a helix or spiral shape with a right turn. The inside of the helix contains only hydrogen atoms and is therefore lipophilic, while the hydroxyl groups are located on the outside of the helix. Each helix has six units of -D-glucose per turn. When two helixes are associated, they form a double helix structure. Starch granules without heat treatment are birefringent, indicating a high degree of internal order. Birefringence is the ability to refract light in two directions. Under polarized light, the granules present a marked cross of interference. The loss of birefringence indicates the loss of molecular order in the crystalline zones and it is used as a criterion for gelatinization. (Xie and Avérous, 2013).

The formation of edible starch films involves the gelatinization of the starch granules by heating in excess of water. This procedure results in the swelling and disruption of the starch granule, as well as the leaching of soluble compounds (amylose) from the granule. A viscous mass is obtained, consisting of two phases: a continuous phase consisting basically of solubilized amylose and a discontinuous phase of remaining granules, mainly based on amylopectin. The cooling of the hot paste results in the formation of a viscoelastic gel (Flores and Gerschenson, 2007).

During storage of products containing gelatinized starch, amylose tends to crystallize and amylopectin to recrystallize (starch retrogradation) resulting in a partially crystalline product with a much more rigid texture (Wang and Wang, 2015).

Cassava Starch

Cassava is a tuber widely found in Latin America, Asia and South Africa. In Latin America, cassava root is popularly used as food, animal feed or is cooked and ingested as a vegetable. It has been verify that cassava starch is used to a much lesser extent than other starches, such as corn starch, in the food industry. One potential use of cassava starch that has been previously considered is its application as a matrix for the development of edible films (Flores and Gerschenson, 2007).

Coatings based on cassava starch are tasteless, odorless and transparent, they do not change the taste, aroma or appearance of the product. This starch is an abundant and economical material, although it shows a high hydrophilic character, constituting a poor barrier to water vapor. That is why lipids can be added to the formulations of the edible films elaborated with starch, to reduce the permeability to the water vapor (Chiumarelli and Hubinger, 2014). One of the characteristics of the starch films is its swelling capacity, which has a pronounced effect on antimicrobial release kinetics when the films are used to support these additives. In contact with fluids, water diffuses into the film, resulting in a relaxation of the polymer chain with expansion of its volume; consequently, the additive dissolves and diffuses out of the system (Flores and Del Nobile, 2007).

Hydroxypropyl Methylcellulose (HPMC)

Hydroxypropyl methylcellulose (HPMC) is a cellulose derivative that has methyl and hydroxypropyl groups in its chain. They mainly differ from other derivatives in their molecular weight, viscosity, degree of substitution and molar substitution. Along the cellulose chain, methyl groups are hydrophobic zones while hydroxypropyl groups are more hydrophilic. The introduction of these substitutes allows HPMC to behave as a surfactant. The usefulness of non-ionic cellulose ethers is fundamentally based on four attributes: they are efficient thickeners, have surface activity, can form interfacial films and the ability to form thermo-reversible gels. Hydrophobic interactions are responsible for the formation of HPMC gels during heating. As temperature increases, molecules absorb translational energy and gradually lose their hydration, resulting in lower viscosity (Coffey and Henderson 2006, 123-153). Subsequently, polymer-polymer interactions take place, due to interactions between hydrophobic groups, thus causing opacity in the solution and an infinite network that causes an increase in viscosity (gel point) and turbidity if the concentration is relatively high (Sarkar and Walker, 1995).

Mixture of Biopolymers in Film Making

Although edible films based on polysaccharides exhibit good mechanical and oxygen barrier properties, their water vapor barrier and moisture resistance are poor due to their hydrophilic nature. Therefore, advantages are obtained from the combination of polysaccharides and lipids in edible films. Starch-based edible films exhibit physical characteristics like synthetic polymers, such as being transparent, odorless, semi-permeable to carbon dioxide and resistant to the passage of oxygen. On the other hand, they show some disadvantages such as their strong hydrophilic character and poor mechanical properties. This can be overcome with the addition of cellulose to starch, which can help decrease water vapor permeability and increase mechanical strength (Laxmikant and Deka, 2014). It has been reported some studies on the mixing of different polysaccharides in adequate proportions in order to optimize the properties of the resulting biopolymer films or to decrease the costs of producing new materials with innovative properties to be used for specific purposes (Espinel Villacrés and Gerschenson, 2014).

Plasticizers

The most commonly used plasticizers in edible films are polyols such as glycerol, sorbitol, glycerol derivatives and polyethylene glycols or lipids and their derivatives such as phospholipids, fatty acids and surfactants. They are generally required in approximately 10 to 60% in relation to the solids present, depending on the rigidity of the polymer. The main disadvantage of plasticizers is that they decrease the cohesion of the film, causing increased permeability to gases, water vapor and solutes. Plasticizers can be defined as very low molecular weight non-volatile compounds added to different polymers to reduce brittleness, impart flexibility and improve film strength. In the specific case of films, plasticizers reduce cracking and improve flexibility. In general terms, these components reduce intermolecular forces along the polymer chains, which increases free volume and chain movements (Sothornvit and Krochta 2005, 403-428). Glycerol is the most widely used plasticizer to improve the mechanical properties and transparency of edible films. The hydroxyl groups present in glycerol are responsible for inter- and intramolecular interactions (hydrogen bridges) in polymer chains, providing the films with a more flexible structure (Prakash Marana and Thirugnanasambandhamd, 2013).

Edible Films Preparation

In order to obtain edible films, the casting technique has been used in most of the reported works. Generally, in this technique, the materials are adequately dissolved in a solvent such as water, alcohol or solvent mixtures. Additives such as flavorings, antimicrobial agents, colorants and others can also be added to edible films formulation, and these biopolymer structures act as controllers of the location or release speed of these additives in foods.

In detail, the formation of edible films using starch, involves in a first step, the gelatinization of granules by heating in water. As the temperature increases, swelling and disruption of the granule occurs, as well as leaching of the soluble (amylose) components of the granule. As a result, a viscous mass is obtained, which is dispensed in molds, generally plastic or silicone, and dried in an oven with air convection. Subsequently, the already formed films are separated from the mold, stabilized in a controlled humidity atmosphere and finally characterized.

Different authors have reported that the composition, the method of film formation and the conditions in the drying process influence the performance of films based on proteins or starches. Therefore, it is important to study the physical, chemical and mechanical properties of edible films in relation to their formulation and processing. These properties must be adequately controlled in order to obtain films with the desired characteristics and thus be able to evaluate the advantages and disadvantages of their application in food preservation (Flores and Gerschenson, 2007).

Physical Characterization of Edible Films

The physical properties of edible films containing cassava starch and glycerol are affected by gelatinization and drying processes. It has been found that these processes modulate the characteristics of the matrix, determining changes in these properties (Flores and Gerschenson, 2007). On the other hand, the release of potassium sorbate from edible films based on cassava starch with glycerol as plasticizer has been studied and it was concluded that the high drying speed used in the casting technique, determined the obtaining of films with an amorphous structure, which contributed greatly to the relaxation of the matrix for the release of sorbate in a liquid medium (Flores and Del Nobile, 2007).

Crystallinity

The crystalline structure of the starch films can be identified through their X-ray diffraction pattern. Four main types of diffraction patterns of the native starches have been identified: A, B, C and V (Liu 2005, 318-337). The X-ray diffraction pattern reflects the different types of packaging of the double helices of amylopectin. The type A structure has a densely packed arrangement of double helices, while the type B structure consists of a more open packing with a greater amount of inter-helical water. In general, tuber starches have a type B crystal structure. The introduction of other compounds in starch preparations can interrupt the double helix conformations of the starch, forming simple stable strands of the helices type, of conformation V. The conformation V is the resulting, for example, from complexes formed between amylose and substances such as aliphatic fatty acids, surfactants, emulsifiers, n-alcohols, glycerol. When polar lipids and amylose are present, type V structures can result from gelatinization, both during heating and cooling (Flores and Gerschenson, 2007). The crystallinity of the starch films depends on the type of starch and the processing settings, such as the drying conditions (speed and temperature), the moisture content of the films and storage temperature (Mali and Zaritzky, 2002). The effect of different conditions on crystallinity has been studied. The increase in water content increases the degree of crystallinity and the kinetics of crystallization, while a higher content of glycerol slows the kinetics of crystallization (Delville and Bliard, 2003). The crystallinity of the starch films increases with the storage time (Mali and Zaritzky, 2002) due to the retrogradation phenomenon of the starch. The formation of crystals can act as "cross-linking" of the structure, generating internal tensions (Delville and Bliard, 2003). Therefore, while the crystallinity of the matrix increases, its deformability decreases drastically and the tensile strength and modulus of elasticity increase. The crystalline structure of starch films is often analyzed with a diffractometer using X-rays. This diffractometer, called a Powder Diffractometer, has a Bragg-Brentano type geometry in which the electronic counter can form a variable angle ($2\theta = 3°-110°$) with the incident X-ray beam. When the sample rotates an angle θ the counter rotates 2θ.

Color

Color is an important attribute of food quality, since its evaluation strongly condition consumer acceptance. Color is a mental response to the visible spectrum of light reflected or emitted by an object. This radiation interacts with the retina of the eye and then the response signal is transmitted to the brain by the optic nerve, where colors are assigned to that signal. In food, appearance is the primary criterion for making purchasing decisions. Appearance is used throughout the chain of production, storage, marketing and use, as the first judgment of the product's quality. Color is an especially important attribute, since it provides basic appearance information for humans and has a close association with quality factors such as freshness, maturity, variety, attractiveness and food safety (Wu and Sun, 2013).

In the instrumental evaluation of color, a photocolorimeter is commonly used to measure the relationship between the light reflected by the food and a known standard. Measurements are taken through an integrating sphere and a diffraction network, at various points, across the visible range of the electromagnetic spectrum. Different instruments measure at different wavelength intervals, depending on the nature of the spectral analyzer and the control electronics. The reflectance is expressed as a percentage or a fraction. Thus, a perfect reflective diffuser will have a 100% reflectance. A black sample, on the other hand, which absorbs the entire incident light, will have a reflectance of 0%. In the middle of both ends, fall all other visible colors. If the sample absorbs everything but the red light, it will show reflectance values in the red zone of the reflectance spectrum. The photocolorimeter "captures" all the light reflected by the surface across the visible wavelength range and can then graphically analyze and report what the perceived color will be. For color quantification, there are sophisticated systems such as those developed by CIE, the International Commission on Illumination. Among them, is the XYZ system (tristimulus values), whose parameters represent the three theoretical colors red, green and blue that, as experimentally proved, are seen by observers. Another system is the CIELab, in which the value "L*" measures the luminosity of the sample, representing the mathematical approximation of the eye's response to the black-white. A perfect white has a value of one hundred (100) and a perfect black has a value of zero (0) on the L* scale. The value "a*" measures the amount of red/green present and the value "b*" measures the amount of yellow/blue. Thus, positive "a*" values are reddish, negative "a*" values are greenish, positive "b*" values are yellowish and negative "b*" values are bluish. The mixture of all of them, together with the brightness value "L*", makes it possible to identify and define all the shades. The Hunter L, a, b and CIELab systems are similar in organization, but a given product will have different numerical values in these two spaces. The two scales derive mathematically from the values X, Y, Z. Color functions are values that are obtained by mathematical combination of tristimulus values and that represent the color attributes, according to the different chromatic spaces (Wu and Sun, 2013).

Mechanical Properties: Quasi-Static Tests (Tensile)

In accordance with ASTM D 882-10, this test can be used to determine the tensile properties of plastics in the form of thin sheets or films (less than 1.0 mm thick) by means of a Universal Testing Machine. The determined tensile properties are valuable for the identification and characterization of materials regarding control and specification purposes. Tensile properties may vary with specimen thickness, method of preparation, test speed and manner of measuring extension.

Under an applied force, a material may flow or deform. The simplest behavior for fluids is that of ideal or Newtonian liquids. At the opposite end, there are materials that do not flow, but deform elastically, as is the case of ideal or Hookeans solids. Between these two extreme ideal situations, is the viscoelastic behavior corresponding to most foods (Aguilera and Stanley 1999).

To determine the tensile strength of plastic materials, a force is applied to one end of the specimen so it is stretched to rupture and strain and tensile stress is evaluated.

Water Solubility

Solubility is defined as the measure that indicates the amount of solute that can be dissolved in an amount of solvent at a given temperature. This property is of great importance in determining the functionality of edible films. Tongdeesoontorn and Rachtanapun (2011), reported that films made with 5% (w/w) cassava starch and (1.5% w/v) glycerol presented a solubility of 73% which is quite high. Other studies conducted by Chiumarelli and Hubinger (2012) showed that the solubility of films based on cassava starch and added with glycerol varied between 27.50% and 43.14%, concluding that these values are adequate for the application of films on fresh cut fruits. A desirable characteristic in edible films is the water resistance, since it contributes to maintain their integrity, in case they are going to be used for the preservation of high humidity foods. An antimicrobial film with poor water resistance dissolves rapidly in contact with high moisture contents, determining that the film releases the antimicrobial agent. However, these coatings could be used in ready-to-eat food where a high percentage of solubility in the mouth is desirable (Ozdemir et al., 2008).

Water Vapor Permeability (WVP)

According to ASTM E96-00, permeability is defined as the rate at which water vapor is transmitted through an area unit of a flat material with known thickness, induced by a difference in vapor pressure between two compartments separated by the material, under defined atmospheric pressure and temperature. This property can be useful in understanding possible mass transfer mechanisms and the interactions between water vapor and polymer in edible films. The difference in the chemical potential of water is the driving force of water transfer through the film. When the process occurs at constant temperature and pressure, the difference in water's chemical potential is proportional to the difference in water vapor concentration between the two sides. Permeability can be defined as the product of solubility and diffusivity when Fick's and Henry's Laws are fully applied. For most edible films, water vapor interacts strongly with the structure of the biopolymer matrix, resulting in diffusion and solubility coefficients dependent on the driving force (Bertuzzi and Gottifredi, 2007).

Antimicrobial Characterization of Edible Films

Table 1. Bacteria frequently present in food

Foods	Microorganisms
Red meats and poultry	*Enterobacter, Listeria, Campylobacter, Aeromonas*
Processed meats	*Bacillus, Clostridium, Lactobacillus, Pseudomonas, Proteus, Sthapylococcus*
Eggs and by-products	*Aeromonas, Enterobacter, Escherichia, Pseudomonas, Proteus, Salmonella*
Fish and seafood	*Aeromonas, Pseudomonas, Proteus, Vibrio*
Milk	*Bacillus, Clostridium, Lactobacillus, Pseudomonas, Sterptococcus*
Fruits and vegetables	*Bacillus, Clostridium, Pseudomonas*

Food Spoilage Micro-Organisms

Foods are susceptible to alteration by different genera of bacteria and yeasts and, in turn, can serve as vehicles for pathogens or their toxins. Some examples of bacteria usually found in food are shown in Table 1 (USDA, 2012).

Bacteria

Pseudomonas

Some Gram-negative psychotropic bacteria that can multiply in meat, dairy and vegetable products influence the quality and shelf life of these products and can be responsible for considerable economic losses. The main flora responsible for such deterioration during aerobic storage is the genus Pseudomonas (Lebert, et al., 2000). This group of bacteria presents polar flagella and has an important effect on the deterioration of foods preserved at refrigerated temperatures such as fresh eggs, meat, fish and milk (USDA, 2012).

Lactobacillus

They are lactic bacteria, Gram-positive, non-spore forming, facultative anaerobic fermentative and traditionally used for the preservation of a wide variety of fermented products. This genus comprises more than 50 different species. In addition, they are versatile as they are found in a wide range of foods including dairy, meat and fermented vegetables (De Vriesa et al., 2006). The species of the genus Lactobacillus can be anaerobic or microaerophilic. They are divided into homofermentative if they degrade glucose producing only lactic acid and heterofermentative if they form a mixture of lactic acid, CO_2, ethanol and/or acetate. Lactic acid lowers the pH of the medium and inhibits the development of other bacteria, favoring their adaptability to different habitats. Although the genus Lactobacillus does not negatively affect human health, it represents problems and losses for the producer, because of this genus can alter the sensory properties in food products. If the load is very high, they may alter the taste, aroma and consistency and the product may not be edible for the consumer (Fialova and Hrusova, 2008).

Yeast

Being part of the group of fungi, these microorganisms are characterized by being robust and able to grow in all types of foods, including cereals, meats and fruits. They are important altering microorganisms that can cause significant economic losses in the industry (Gerez and Rollán, 2013). The yeasts form pasty colonies on the culture media, which are constituted, mostly, by isolated cells that tend to be spherical, ovoid, ellipsoid or elongated. A few have hyphae. Yeasts are frequently found in leaves and flowers. They are also on the epidermis of fruits and can penetrate the underlying tissues as a result of mechanical damage. Their presence depends on temperature, pH, humidity and the availability of simple sugars. Yeasts are the most common cause of alteration of fruits and juices, as they have fermentable sugars. Among the genera commonly associated with this deterioration are Zygosaccharomyces, Candida, Debaryomyces and Pichia (Snyder and Worobo, 2018). The best-known deteriorative yeasts are facultative anaerobic fermentative organisms that produce ethanol and carbon dioxide from simple sugars. Some fermentative yeasts are osmophilic organisms, which can grow slowly at water activities as low as 0.6. Representative genera include Saccharomyces and Zygosaccharomyces (Ollé and Gerschenson, 2014). The negative effects of yeasts on foods are related to their physiological characteristics, which include their ability to multiply at low temperatures, their metabolic activities and their resistance to various physical-chemical stresses of importance in food preservation (Jakobsen and Narvhus, 1996).

Additives with Antimicrobial Action Used in Edible Films: Active Packaging

Microorganisms, temperature, sunlight, oxygen, humidity, among others, are often the main causes of the loss of quality of packaged food products. These factors could induce microbial growth in foods, degradation of components and alterations in organoleptic properties with consequent consumer rejection. In relation to prevent microbial development, in the last decade research have focused on the formulation and study of antimicrobial packaging (Kurek and Debeaufort, 2013). Edible films that support additives (antioxidants, antimicrobials, etc.), with the objective of reducing their destruction by contact with the medium, ensuring their gradual release and minimizing the amount of the additive to be used, are known as active films (Gerschenson and Flores 2016). The design of an antimicrobial packaging system requires a complete study on how to introduce antimicrobial compounds into films. The application of edible films containing antimicrobials could help to obtain a localized functional effect on the surface of the food product and/or contribute to produce a gradual release of the antimicrobial, controlling its diffusion to the food and/or protecting the additive from interaction with other components or environmental factors, which could promote its destruction or inactivation (Arismendi and Gerschenson, 2013). Different preservatives such as bacteriocins, sorbates, organic acids, salts and essential oils (EO) from various plant extracts have been incorporated into edible films and/or coatings to provide antimicrobial activity (Ollé and Gerschenson, 2014; Flores and Gerschenson, 2007; Choi and Lee, 2016; Alarcón-Moyano and Matiacevich, 2017). Increased bacterial resistance to certain antimicrobials and efforts to use natural preservatives in food production and storage, have increased the interest in possible applications of OEs and their constituents. In addition, these agents have GRAS status defined by the FDA (U.S. Food and Drug Administration).

Carvacrol

Oregano (*Origanum vulgare L.*) is an herbaceous plant native to the Mediterranean regions that has been used as a medicinal plant, owing to its antimicrobial, antioxidant and antifungal properties. In particular, the essential oil of this plant is extracted with the aim of being used mainly in pharmaceutical, cosmetic and food industry. Many of these EOs are safe compounds classified as GRAS (generally recognized as safe). Carvacrol (Figure 1), a phenolic monoterpene, is one of the most important constituents of the oregano essential oil and has been found to be an efficient antimicrobial agent. The antimicrobial and antifungal effects of carvacrol have been proven on many microorganisms including Escherichia coli, Pseudomonas fluorescens, Staphylococcus aureus, Lactobacillus plantarum, Bacillus subtillis, Trichophyton mentagrophytes and Trichophyton rubrum (Homayouni and Nassiri, 2017; Higueras and Hernández-Muñoz, 2015; Tunç and Duman, 2011). The effectiveness of antimicrobial films is determined in part by the rate of release of antimicrobial components. A very slow release would cause microbial growth to be insufficiently inhibited; on the other hand, a very rapid release would prevent inhibition from being sustained over time. The rate of release depends on the type of polymer, the method of film processing, the interactions between antimicrobial and the polymeric material and environmental conditions (Tunç and Duman, 2011). Plant oils and extracts generally have inhibitory activity against certain important microorganisms in food. Considering the large number of chemical compounds present in essential oils, it is important to clarify that their antimicrobial activity is not attributed to a specific mechanism. The components of essential oils: thymol, carvacrol and eugenol, which are phenolic compounds, possess strong antimicrobial properties against various microorganisms of interest in food; their mechanism of action could be compared with that of other phenolic compounds, causing disorder of the cytoplasmic membrane, breaking of the motive force of the proton, flow of electrons and coagulation of the cellular content. Another important characteristic of essential oils is their hydrophobicity, which allows the separation of lipids from the cell membrane and mitochondria, disordering the structure and making it more permeable, which allows the filtration of ions and other cellular contents (García-García and Palou-García 2008, 41-51).

Therefore, the use of carvacrol as an active agent could provide adequate antimicrobial protection. Its inclusion in films is interesting since, as it is not incorporated into the food, interactions with other components of the food and with external factors (oxygen, light, environmental humidity) would be reduced, which would contribute to a greater efficiency of this compound. The use of a smaller quantity would also help to obtain suitable organoleptic properties (Arrieta and Jiménez, 2014).

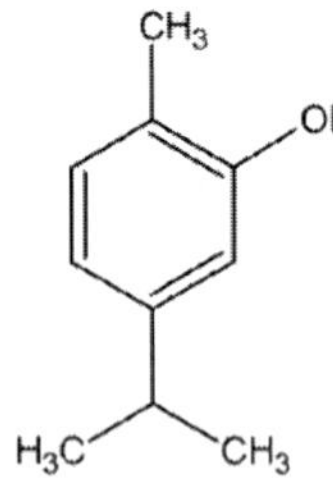

Figure 1. Carvacrol molecule.

Sorbic Acid and Potassium Sorbate

Among the most widely used antifungal additives in foods are sorbic acid (2,4-hexadienoic acid) and its salt (potassium sorbate, Figure 2), collectively referred as sorbates. Sorbates are GRAS compounds with high water solubility. Its inhibitory action is strongly influenced by the type of food, processing and storage conditions and the level of preservative. Sorbates are stable in their dry form, but in aqueous solutions they undergo oxidative degradation depending on pH, water activity, presence of other additives, storage and processing conditions. Sorbate degradation is accompanied by a concomitant increase in carbonyl concentrations, mainly acetaldehydes and β-carboxyacrolein, which influences the development of non-enzymatic browning (Campos and Gerschenson, 2000). Several studies on edible films and coatings containing sorbates were conducted (Vásconez and Gerschenson, 2009; Chillo and Del Nobile, 2008; Flores and Gerschenson, 2007: Flores and Del Nobile, 2007; Famá and Gerschenson, 2005), reporting their physical and antimicrobial properties against yeast.

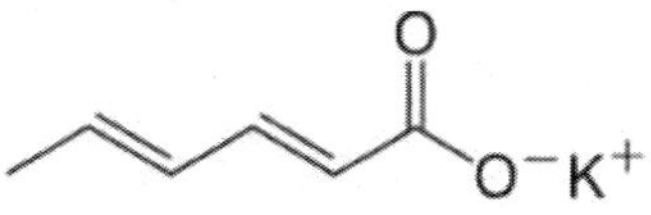

Figure 2. Potassium sorbate molecule.

Flores and Del Nobile (2007) studied the performance of films based on cassava starch carrying sorbate and established that the films were effective in controlling the growth of the *Z. bailii* population, acting as a preservative releasing agent or as a barrier against external yeast contamination. At acid pH, sorbic acid is effective because the undissociated lipophilic molecule is freely permeable through the cell membrane. Subsequently, upon encountering a higher pH inside the cell, the molecule dissociates resulting in the release of anions and protons, which cannot pass through the plasma membrane. It has been proposed that inhibition of microbial growth may be due to different actions such as alteration of the membrane, inhibition of essential metabolic reactions such as glycolysis, induction of a high response to energy stress or accumulation of toxic anions (Kralj and Zupancic-Kralj, 2001).

Characterization of the Antimicrobial Activity of Films

The use of edible films supporting preservatives allows combining the antimicrobial action with the oxygen barrier and, to a lesser extent, with the water vapor barrier exerted by the biopolymer film. The film could also contribute to the cohesiveness of the food (Barzegar and Hamidi-Esfahani, 2014). In the selection of an appropriate antimicrobial, it is important to consider several factors, including its efficacy against the selected microorganism, the amount to be incorporated, the possible interactions between the added antimicrobial and other food components. Interactions of the antimicrobial with the biopolymer constituting the film matrix should also be considered as they could modify the activity of the antimicrobial and the characteristics of the film. Considering that antimicrobial edible packaging is a new technology with the potential to assist in food preservation, its performance is usually studied through the agar diffusion test.

Agar Diffusion Test

Also called the halo test, it consists of placing a film disc containing the antimicrobial to be studied on a plate with inoculated agar and, after incubation under specific conditions, the diameter of the clear inhibition zone is measured where there was no growth. This test is generally applied to check if the preservative can diffuse from the film, thus being available to act as an antimicrobial agent. In this assay, the diffusion of antimicrobials from the film under study to the agar depends on the size, shape and polarity of the antimicrobial molecule, as well as the structural and physicochemical characteristics of the film. This methodology is widely used to determine the susceptibility of different microorganisms to different chemical compounds, including some drugs. This method is simple, economical, requires little preparation and does not need specialized equipment and, a great advantage, is that it uses small quantities of the component to evaluate (Ventura and Coutinho, 2012). In a study carried out by Iturriaga and Martínez de Marañón (2012) the antimicrobial activities of different essential oils were evaluated using the agar diffusion method. The authors demonstrated that the essential oils of oregano and thyme were the most effective in inhibiting *L. innocua*. In the case of the bacteria *P. fluorescens*, the essential oils of thyme, oregano and clove were more active, having the same degree of effectiveness against this strain. In another study carried out by Souza and Trajano (2007), the antimicrobial capacity of the oregano essential oil against different types of yeasts was demonstrated by the diffusion test in inoculated Sabouraud agar. The authors confirmed the observation of important inhibition halos and concluded that the minimum inhibitory concentration (MIC) of this oil was 10μL/mL for most of the strains evaluated.

OBJECTIVE

The objective of the present work was to evaluate the effect of the carvacrol addition on the antimicrobial, mechanical and physical properties of self-supporting edible films based on native cassava starch and HPMC, plasticized with glycerol and added with potassium sorbate. Moreover, the influence of different emulsification speeds (6500 rpm or 21500 rpm) on the film physical properties was analyzed.

METHODS

Materials

Cassava starch (Bernesa S.A., Argentina), hydroxypropyl methylcellulose (HPMC) (Methocel premium® K4M, Dow Chemical, USA) and glycerol (Sintorgan®, Argentina) were used to form the film matrix. The antimicrobials used in the films formulation were carvacrol (Sigma®, USA) and potassium sorbate (Sigma®, USA).

Edible Film Production

A mixture of cassava starch, glycerol, potassium sorbate and distilled water was stirred at 25°C for 15 min in order to humidify the starch granules. Another mixture of distilled water and HPMC was also prepared, and after homogenization, the temperature was increased at a rate of 4.2°C/ min up to 84°C in order to achieve HPMC gelation. Then, the starch suspension was incorporated to HPMC slurry and the global temperature dropped to 75°C. Subsequently, the heating continued at a rate of 4.2°C/min until reaching 93°C in order to achieve the starch gelatinization and the homogenization of the system. Finally, carvacrol was added and proceeded to the emulsification for 2 min using an Ultra Turrax® emulsifier (IKA,Germany) at speeds of 6500 rpm (low speed (LS) films) or 21500 rpm (high speed (HS) films). Bubbles were eliminated by centrifugation (Eppendorf, Germany) for 5 minutes at 500 rpm and 25°C. The final slurry composition was: starch 2.67 g/100g; HPMC 0.67 g/100g; glycerol 1.70 g/100g; potassium sorbate 0.3 g/100g; carvacrol 0.1 g/100g and distilled water 94.56 g/100g. The total amount of prepared slurry was 300 g. Aliquots (20 g) of the film-forming solution were dispensed over 9 cm diameter polystyrene Petri dishes. The drying was carried out at 35ºC during 24 hours in a chamber with forced air convection. Once constituted, the films were separated from the dishes and equilibrated in 57.7% relative humidity (R.H.) atmosphere at 25ºC prior to their characterization.

Physical Characterization of Edible Films

Optical Microscopy

The optical microscopy was performed using a Zeiss Axioskop 2 Plus optical microscope (Zeiss, Germany). The film-forming solution was dispensed on a slide and observed directly. The observations were made with a magnification of 100X.

X-Ray Crystallography

A Philips X-ray diffractometer with vertical goniometer (Cu Kα radiation, λ = 1,542 Å) was used. The determinations were made at 40 kV and 30 mA. The films were mounted on a glass sample holder and placed in the equipment container. The X-ray intensity was recorded with a scintillation counter in a scattering angle range (2θ) of 6-33° using a scanning speed of 1°/min.

Color

A Minolta Colorimeter CM-508d (Tokyo, Japan) with a 1.5 cm opening diameter was used. The colorimeter was calibrated with black and white standard plates. The D-65 illuminant and 2° observer angle were selected for the measurement. The film discs of diameter approximately equal to 8 cm were supported on the white standard plate (Trezza and Krochta, 2000) and any air bubbles were eliminated by lightly pressure on the specimen. The determinations of color were made in three positions on the surface of each films. The measured parameters corresponded to the CIELab system, in which L* indicates brightness (0 corresponds to black and 100 corresponds to white), the positive values of a* indicate red and the negative, green and positive values of b* indicate yellow while the negative one indicates blue. The color difference was also calculated:

$$\Delta E = \sqrt{(L^* - L_0^*)^2 + (a^* - a_0^*)^2 + (b^* - b_0^*)^2} \quad (1)$$

where L*, a*, b* are the values for the films of interest and L_0*, a_0*, b_0*, are the chosen reference values.

The yellow index (YI) was evaluated according to ASTM D1925 (1988) and the color index (CI) was determined using the following equation (Murillo-Martínez and Vernon-Carter, 2011):

$$CI = (a^*1000)/(L^*b^*) \quad (2)$$

IC values between -40 and -20 correspond to the color range from violet to dark green; values between -20 and -2 correspond to samples with colors between dark green and greenish yellow; values between -2 and +2 indicate yellowish green. On the other hand, CI between +2 and +20 correspond to pale yellow to deep orange and between +20 and +40 indicate from deep orange to dark red.

Transparency and Opacity

The light barrier properties of the films were measured at selected wavelengths between 400 and 800 nm, using a UV-160 spectrophotometer (Shimadzu, Japan) according to Fang and Dalgleish (2002). The transparency of the films was obtained from the measured absorbance at 600 nm (Shiku and Tanaka, 2004) and using the following equation:

$$\frac{A_{600}}{x} = \frac{-\log T_{600}}{x} \quad (3)$$

where A_{600} is the absorbance at 600 nm, T_{600} is transmittance at 600 nm, and x is film thickness (mm). A high transmittance value means high transparency; on the contrary, a low value means low transparency.

The opacity was calculated as the area under the curve of the absorbance spectrum of the film between 400 and 800 nm. The opacity is expressed in units of absorbance (UA) per nm (Hewage and Vithanarachchi, 2009).

Water Solubility

The initial percentage of dry matter was determined by drying 2 cm diameter film discs in a vacuum oven at 100°C for 24 hours. At the same time, other discs were cut, weighed and immersed in 50 mL of distilled water for 24 hours at 25°C. The remaining films were recovered by filtration and dried (100°C in a vacuum oven for 24 hours) in order to determine the non-solubilized dry mass. Solubility is defined as the percentage of dry mass of the film that is solubilized in distilled water under standardized conditions and is calculated as follows:

$$Water\ solubility\ (\%) = \frac{dry\ mass_{initial} - dry\ mass_{final}}{dry\ mass_{initial}}\ x\ 100 \quad (4)$$

Mechanical Properties

Tensile tests were performed using a universal testing machine (Instron testing machine, model 3345, Instron Corp., USA), provided with a load cell of 100 N. The geometry of the samples was rectangular (6 x 60 mm), the distance between the pneumatic clamps was 20 mm and the speed of vertical movement of the superior clamp was 50 mm/min. Experimental determinations were made from nine replicates.

From the data of force (F, N) versus displacement (D, mm), the stress ($\sigma = F/A$, where A is the sample section; MPa); and the deformation ($\varepsilon = D/L_0$, where L_0 is the initial length of the samples) parameters were calculated. The curves stress (σ, MPa) versus deformation (ε) were drawn and the stress at break (σ_r) and deformation at break (ε_r) were determined. The Elastic Modulus (Ec, MPa) was evaluated from the initial zone of the curve of true stress ($\sigma_T = \sigma\ (1+\varepsilon)$) versus true deformation ($\varepsilon_T = Ln\ [L/L_0]$; where ($L = D + L_0$), using the following exponential equation (Chillo and Del Nobile, 2008):

$$\sigma_T(\epsilon_T) = E_c\ \epsilon_T\ exp\ (-\epsilon_T\ K) \quad (5)$$

where K is a fit constant of the model.

Water Vapor Permeability (WVP)

The water vapor permeability of the films was determined gravimetrically, at 25°C, adapting the procedure recommended by the ASTM E96-00 (2000). To perform the permeability test, acrylic cells were used with the following dimensions: 4.4 cm internal diameter, 8.4 cm external diameter, resulting an exposed area of 15,205 cm^2. The depth of the cells was 3.5 cm and the films were placed between the main body of the cell and its lid. The cells containing $CaCl_2$ (Anedra, Argentina) inside, and maintaining a 10 mm of head space between the desiccant and the film, had an internal partial water vapor pressure ≈ 0 Pa. The tightness of the closing of the cells, was assured by applying vacuum grease to the rubber sheets adhered to the lid and main body of the cells, as well as by the adjustment of four equidistant screws. The cells were placed in humidity and temperature-controlled chamber (Ibertest, Spain) set to 25ºC and 70% R.H. (partial water vapor pressure ≈ 2288 Pa). After approximately 12 h, water vapor transmission rate was attained and, from that moment on, changes in weight of the cell (to the nearest 0.1 mg) were recorded daily over a 3-day period. The weight variation versus time data, were adjustment to a linear trend and the water vapor transmission rate (WVTR) was calculated according to equation:

$$WVTR = \frac{G}{t\,x\,A} \tag{6}$$

where G is the change in weight of the cell in grams, t is the time elapsed in h and A is the area of exposed film in m^2.

The WVP was obtained using the equations:

$$P' = \frac{WVTR}{\Delta p} \quad WVP = P' x\, e \tag{7}$$

where P′ is the permeance, Δp is the difference in water vapor pressure in the chamber and e is the thickness of the material. The thickness of the films was determined using a digital micrometer (Mitutoyo, Japan).

Antimicrobial Functionality of Edible Films

Culture Media and Strains

The microorganisms used in this study were: *Zygosaccharomyces bailii* (NRRL 7256), *Pseudomonas fluorescens* (ATCC 49838) and *Lactobacillus plantarum* (ATCC 8014). Sabouraud broth (Biokar, France) was used for the growth of *Z. bailii*, Mueller-Hinton broth (Biokar, France) was used for *P. fluorescens* and MRS broth (Biokar, France) was used for *L. plantarum*. For plate counting, the corresponding agars were used, incubating 5 days at 25ºC in the case of yeast or 72 h at 37ºC in the case of bacteria.

Preparation of Inoculum

For the preparation of inoculum, two aliquots of the reference microorganism were taken from a stock strains, using a loop in sterile conditions. The aliquots were transferred to a tube with 10 mL of the corresponding broth. These pre-cultures were incubated 24 h in a chamber at 25°C for yeast and 18-20 h at 37°C for bacteria.

Diffusion Assay in Agar

For the diffusion test, 15 mL of each of the agars necessary for the growth of the microorganisms tested were dispensed on Petri dishes. On each plate containing the agar, 1 mL of the corresponding inoculum was placed and left to dry under a laminar flow chamber for 20 min. Subsequently, three (3) discs of 10 mm diameter from each of the studied systems were put in contact with the inoculated agar and stored for 48 hours at 7°C. Then, the dishes were incubated at 25°C, for yeast or at 37°C, for bacteria, for 24 h. The antimicrobial action of the films was determined by observing the existence of clear zones in the contact zone, as well as around the discs, which expressed the inhibition exerted by the antimicrobials.

Statistical Analysis

Data analysis and linear regressions were performed with the software Statgraphics Centurion XV, V 2.15.06 (StatPoint Inc., U.S.A) for Windows®. The experimental results were reported as the average and standard deviation of at least two replicates. The significant differences between the means were determined by one-way analysis of variance (ANOVA) followed by a *post hoc* test (*t* Student or a LSD Fisher). A 95% confidence level was applied to all statistical analyses.

RESULTS AND DISCUSSION

Influence of the Emulsification Speed on the Physical Properties of the Films

In a first step, the influence of the emulsification speed (6500 rpm or 21500 rpm) on the physical properties of the films containing 0.1% w/w was analyzed.

Physical Characterization

X-Ray Crystallography

Figure 3 shows the X-ray diffraction patterns of studied films. It was determined that the patterns did not exhibit the sharp peaks characteristic of native starch. In the present work, the crystallinity analysis revealed a structure predominantly amorphous in both films, those that were subjected to low emulsification speed (LS films, 6500 rpm) and those made at high shearing rate (HS films, 21500 rpm). It is concluded that the crystallinity of the films would not be influenced by the emulsification speed used but would depend on the composition of the system (starch, HPMC, glycerol, potassium sorbate and carvacrol) and the filmmaking process that involve the starch gelatinization. It has been reported that there are four main types of diffraction patterns of native starches: A, B, C and V (Liu,

2005). Flores and Gerschenson (2007) studied starch films with and without potassium sorbate and different preparation methods and observed that films without potassium sorbate showed a higher crystallinity, which was evidenced in the pattern of X-ray diffraction by presenting greater number of sharp peaks, and a B-V-type crystal structure probably due to the presence of glycerol. However, the films with potassium sorbate did not present sharp peaks since their plasticizing behavior and the consequent inhibition of the crystallization development during retrogradation. The sorbate interaction with the biopolymeric chains would make their alignment difficult, as well as the preservative could interfere in the packaging of amylose. X-ray profiles reported by Flores and Gerschenson (2007) in the presence of sorbate are analogous to those observed in this work. On the other hand, Gerschenson and Alzate (2018) reported an amorphous character for edible films elaborated with starch, HPMC, glycerol and potassium sorbate concentrations similar to those used in this research.

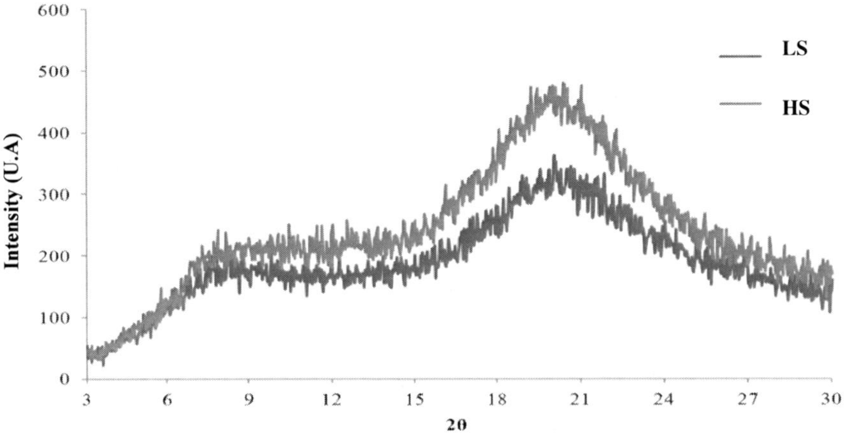

Figure 3. X-ray diffraction patter for edible films elaborated at low shear (LS) and high shear (HS) emulsion speed.

Color Determination

Table 2 summarizes the color parameters (L*, a*, b*, YI, DE and CI) of the LS (low shear, 6500 rpm) and HS (high shear, 21500 rpm) films. It was observed, in general, that the color parameters studied showed significant differences between both samples, as follow:

- Parameter L*: the HS sample presented a value slightly higher than LS sample, being both values close to 100 (maximum brightness), which is desirable since it implies that the films allowed to visualize the white background against which they were supported during the measurement and, therefore, it is inferred that the visual characteristics of a food that has been coated with these films, shall remain unchanged.

- Parameter a*: both systems presented negative magnitudes and small module. This corresponds to a slightly green component that is not visually appreciable. The a* module for HS films was smaller than for LS films.
- Parameter b*: in both systems this parameter presented values of 3.5 and 4, specifying a slightly yellow color. HS films had a slightly lower value for this parameter.
- Parameter YI: in line with b*, the HS films presented a lower value of YI.
- Parameter ΔE: The value of ΔE is used to study the similarity of color with respect to the pattern (white plate). The smallest value (2.7) corresponded to HS films, showing that these films were the closest to the standard value. In addition, ΔE values higher than 2, indicate that the color of films might be perceived by the consumers as different compared to the standard white.
- Parameter CI: The calculated color index indicates that the color of both films was found in the range between dark green (-20) and greenish-yellow (-2). These values are within the range of films based on proteins and polysaccharides (Murillo-Martínez and Vernon-Carter, 2011).

Table 2. Color parameters of edible films elaborated at low shear (LS) and high shear (HS) emulsion speed

System	Color Parameters					
	L*	a*	b*	YI	ΔE	CI
LS	88.9 ± 0.3	-1.48 ± 0.05	4.0 ± 0.2	7.0 ± 0.3	3.4 ± 0.3	-4.2 ± 0.3[a]
HS	89.5 ± 0.3	-1.32 ± 0.03	3.5 ± 0.1	6.1 ± 0.2	2.7 ± 0.3	- 4.2± 0.2[a]

Equal letters in the same column indicate absence of significant differences ($p > 0.05$).

For a better understanding, a photograph of LS and HS films is shown in Figure 4.

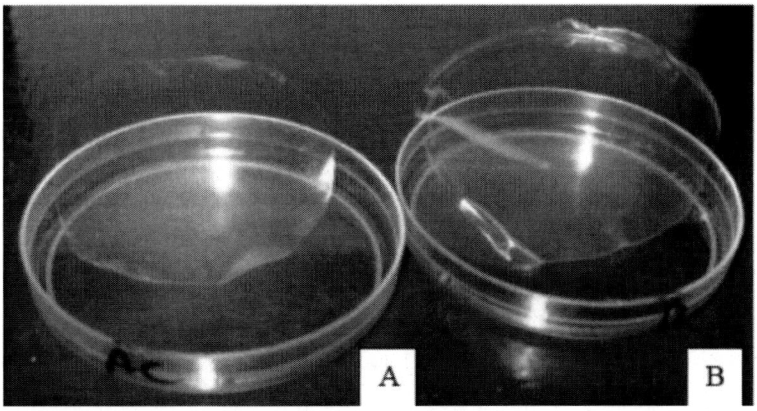

Figure 4. High shear film (A) and Low shear film (B).

Transparency and Opacity

Transparency is quantified as transmittance (percentage of intensity that passes through the sample). Therefore, a material presents high transparency when the transmittance is high enough to let the light through it easily. Table 3 shows the results for absorbance, transmittance and opacity of HS and LS films. It was observed that the HS system had an absorbance at 600 nm 136% higher than LS films. It is important to remark that, in the present work, edible films forming solutions were emulsified systems where the carvacrol droplets constituted the dispersed phase.

Table 3. Absorbance, transmittance and opacity of High Shear film (HS) and Low Shear (LS) film

Film	Absorbance (600 nm)	Transmittance (%)	Opacit (UA. nm)
LS	0.14	72.3	60
HS	0.33	46.6	136

Absence of letters in the same column indicate significant differences ($p < 0.05$) between samples.

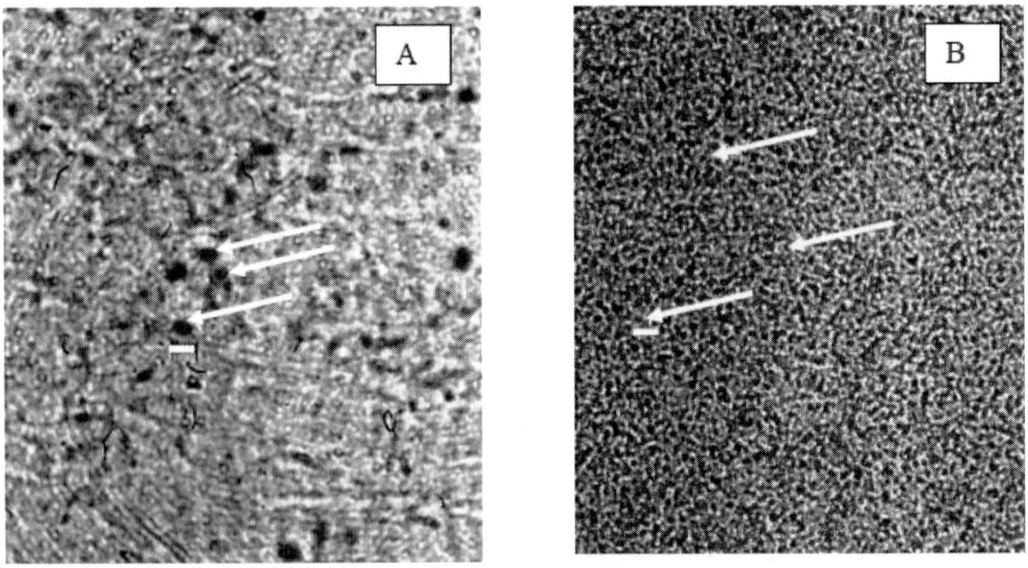

Figure 5. Optical microscopic observations of film-forming solutions. Panel A: low shear (LS) emulsification. Panel B: high shear (HS) emulsification. A bar of 50 μm length is included in both panels. Magnification: 100X. Arrows point out some carvacrol droplests.

In Figure 5 panel A, it can be seen that the film forming solution emulsified at low shear (LS) presented, under the optical microscope, an oil droplet size of approximately 32 ± 6 μm, which trended to be separated and distributed in a slightly inhomogeneous way. In contrast, in HS film forming solution (Figure 5, panel B) the droplet size of the dispersed phase was approximately 14 ± 2 μm with much denser and uniform droplets distribution.

Figure 6 (panels A and B) shows the absorbance spectrum between 400 and 800 nm for the studied films. The HS system presented greater absorbance in the entire range than the LS system and both films showed a downward trend of absorbance as the wavelengths increased.

It would be concluded that the forming solutions with smaller droplet size, (HS) would result in films that scatter more light, i.e., have less transmission at 600 nm and more opacity (Table 3). Murillo-Martínez and Vernon-Carter (2011) studied films of high opacity conformed by double emulsions based on low methoxylation pectins and whey protein isolate or sodium carboxymethylcellulose and whey protein isolate. The authors concluded that the opacity in both films was probably due to the morphology of the double emulsion, whose oil droplets had a relatively large size, which in turn contained multiple water droplets dispersed inside, causing a high degree of reflection of the spectrophotometer light beam.

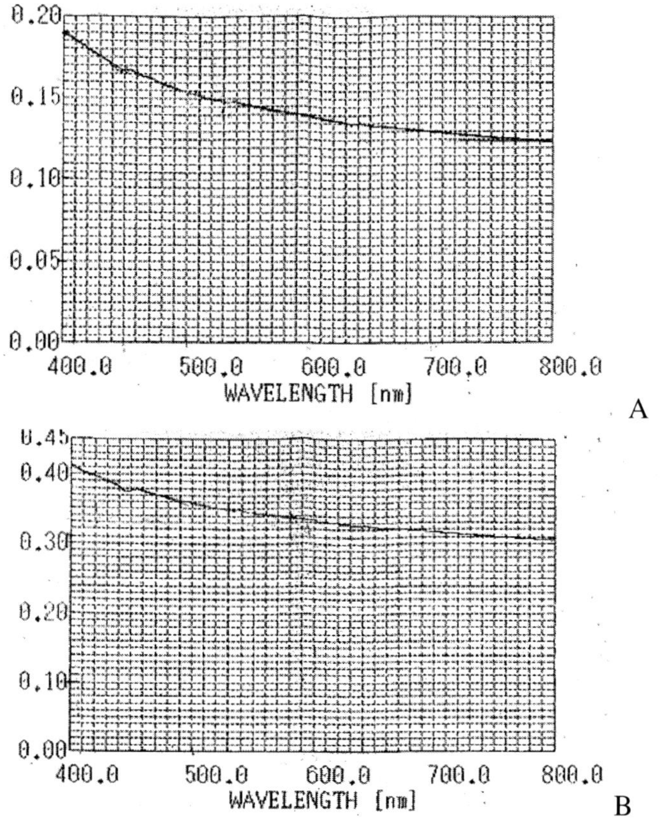

Figure 6. Absorbance spectrum for A) low shear (LS) film and B) high shear (HS) film.

The transmittance value obtained from the films to which the lower shear speed was applied, LS, was similar to that reported for surimi-based films (70.8%) and lower than that reported for low density polyethylene (86.9%) and for polyvinylidene chloride (90%) (Shiku and Tanaka, 2004). Moreover, Tejinder (2003) reported opacity values for films based on β-glucan extracts from barley and oats, similar to those obtained in this work: β-glucan from oats dissolved in water at 4% w/w had an opacity value of 63 UA.nm, just above the value of the LS film. In those formulated with barley glucans at 2% w/w in water, values of 140 UA.nm were obtained, comparable with the opacity value presented by HS films.

Water Solubility

An important feature in the application of edible films in foods is the film solubility in water. The solubility value modulates the film suitability to be applied in a food with a higher or lower percentage of humidity or the convenience to expose the film to atmospheres of high humidity. A film with a high percentage of solubility will see its stability compromised if it is applied in high water content food or if the environment where it will be stored has a high relative humidity. However, a high solubility will be desirable if the film was intended to be consumed together with the food or solubilized during cooking. It has been observed that the presence of antimicrobials, such as potassium sorbate, in starch films leads to a less organize matrix structure, which results in an increased solubility, irrespective of the drying method used. Flores and Gerschenson (2007) determined that films without antimicrobial had solubility values of around 20%.

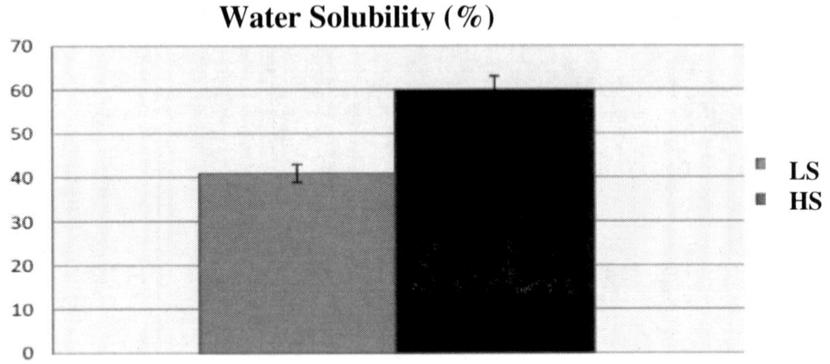

Figure 7. Solubility for low shear (LS) and high shear (HS) emulsified systems.

The values were 30% in films containing potassium sorbate. Figure 7 shows that the LS film had solubility around (40 ± 2)%, being higher than the previously mentioned values. However, HS films showed a significant increase in their solubility, (60 ± 3)%. It could be proposed that the rise in shear speed decreases the oil drop size and this determined a larger interfacial area between the polymer network and the carvacrol, affecting the structure of the polymer matrix, which would generate an increase in film solubility. In a study carried out by Espinel and Gerschenson (2014) with films formulated with combinations of starch, HPMC, potassium sorbate and glycerol, it was observed that the increase in the proportion of HPMC and glycerol and the decrease in the proportion of starch, increased solubility.

The values reported in this study were around 48% for films with similar contents of starch, HPMC and glycerol to those in the present work.

Mechanical Properties

In order to study the effect produced by the emulsification speed on the mechanical properties of the films, quasi-static tests were carried out in tensile mode and the stress (MPa) versus strain curves were obtained. The HS films presented an average value of stress at break and Elastic Modulus greater than those corresponding to LS films. The recorded strain at break does not show significant differences between films (Table 4). Murillo-Martinez and Vernon-Carter (2011) studied films conformed by double emulsions based on low methoxylation pectins and whey protein isolate (LMP-WPI) or sodium carboxymethylcellulose and whey protein isolate (CMC-WPI). They were able to conclude that the differences in mechanical properties found between the two types of film, were because of the size of the droplets in the emulsion and the interactions that take place between the biopolymer molecules that form the film structure. Thus, the LMP-WPI film formed by relatively small emulsion droplets with a less ordered and crosslinked matrix, showed higher tensile strength, higher Young's modulus and lower elongation than the CMC-WPI film with larger droplet size. Other studies performed by Nussinovitch (2003) showed that in gelled emulsions based on agar, the increase of the drop size decreased the strength of the gel evaluated by compression tests. The results obtained in the present work could be attributed to the smaller droplet size of the HS films due to the effect of the shear applied to the forming solution.

Table 4. Stress at break, strain at break and Elastic modulus of LS and HS films

Film	Strain at break	Stress at break (MPa)	Elastic Modulus (MPa)
LS	0.68 ± 0.05[a]	2.1 ± 0.2	12 ± 3
HS	0.59 ± 0.04[a]	3.5 ± 0.4	25 ± 6

Equal letters in the same column indicate absence of significant differences ($p > 0.05$).

Final Considerations on Process Conditions

From the analysis of the tests carried out under different process conditions, precisely different emulsification speeds, it can be highlighted that: both LS and HS films were structurally amorphous, the color of the films was a greenish yellow tone and high luminosity, however the HS film presented a lower degree of yellowish and green color, which could generate greater consumer acceptance. HS film had higher solubility in water and higher tensile stress than LS film, while deformation showed no significant differences between films.

Then, giving greater relevance to the mechanical and color properties, the HS procedure was chosen to continue with the experimental work. In the next section it will be discussed the impact of carvacrol addition at a level of 0.5% (w/w) on the physical and antimicrobial properties of the films.

Antimicrobial Activity of Edible Films Containing Potassium Sorbate and Carvacrol

Given the recognized action of carvacrol as an antifungal and antibacterial agent (Chavan and Tupe, 2014; Kurek and Debeaufort, 2013), the study of the antimicrobial activity of films containing potassium sorbate 0.3% (w/w) and potassium sorbate 0.3% (w/w) combined with carvacrol 0.5% (w/w) was performed using the yeast *Z. bailii* and the bacteria *L. plantarum* and *P. fluorescens* as microorganisms representative of the food spoilage.

Agar Diffusion Test

Table 5 shows the results of the halo test for films made with starch and added with 0.5% (w/w) of carvacrol.

Table 5. Agar diffusion test of films based on starch and added with potassium sorbate and carvacrol

Film	Inhibition zone	Contact Area		
		Z. bailii	*L. plantarum*	*P. fluorescens*
Control	No	High growth	High growth	High growth
Potassium Sorbate	No	Low growth	Low growth	Low growth
Potassium Sorbate - 0,5% (w/w) carvacrol	No	No growth	No growth	No growth

It can be observed that the control system, allowed the growth of microorganisms, since it did not possess any antimicrobial agent in its formulation. The film with potassium sorbate did not exert considerable inhibitory effect, except for the yeast *Z. bailii* due to its antifungal action. The incorporation of carvacrol to formulation, improved the effectiveness of the evaluated films since it was observed a decrease of the growth in the system containing 0.2% (w/w) of carvacrol and absence of growth in the system containing 0.5% (w/w) of carvacrol, both in the yeast and in the bacteria. Figures 8 to 10 show the images of the diffusion test results.

It has been reported that carvacrol supported in cassava starch-HPMC films at levels of 0.01 to 1.0% (w/w), presented a very good inhibitory capacity against *Z. bailii*, according to the inhibition zone trial and that the increase in the amount of carvacrol in the films increased the size of the halos observed (Alzate and Gerschenson, 2017). Manohar and Preuss (2001) attributed the protective activity of carvacrol against *Candida albicans* to the inhibition of the germinal tubes formation, necessary for the development of yeast mycelium. On the other hand, Rojas-Grau and McHugh (2006) worked with apple puree-based films with oregano essential oil (0 - 0.1% w/w) and tested the antimicrobial activity against *E. coli* O157:H7. These authors reported inhibition zones of 1.4 mm diameter for the maximum essential oil concentration and justified these results by the characteristics of cell wall structure and membrane composition of Gram-negative bacteria, which conditioned the interaction with lipophilic essential oils components.

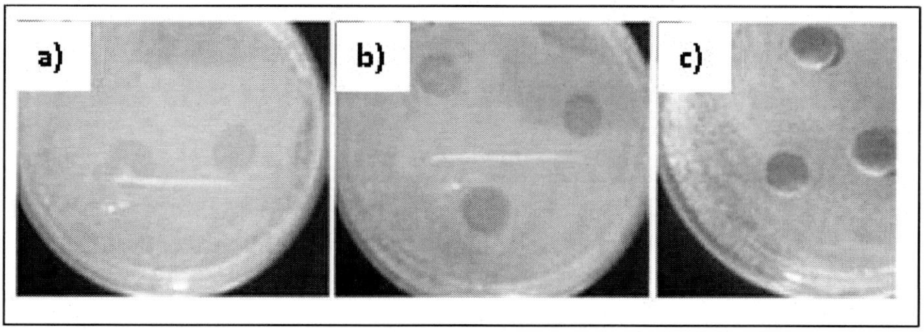

Figure 8. Inhibition zones against *Z. bailii*: a) control (without antimicrobials), b) 0.3% (w/w) potassium sorbate and c) 0.3% (w/w) potassium sorbate and 0.5% (w/w) of carvacrol.

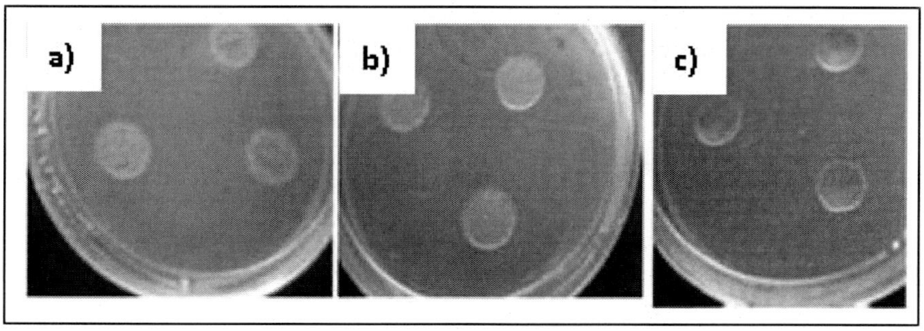

Figure 9. Inhibition zones against *L. plantarum:* a) control (without antimicrobials), b) 0.3% (w/w) potassium sorbate and c) 0.3% (w/w) potassium sorbate and 0.5% (w/w) of carvacrol.

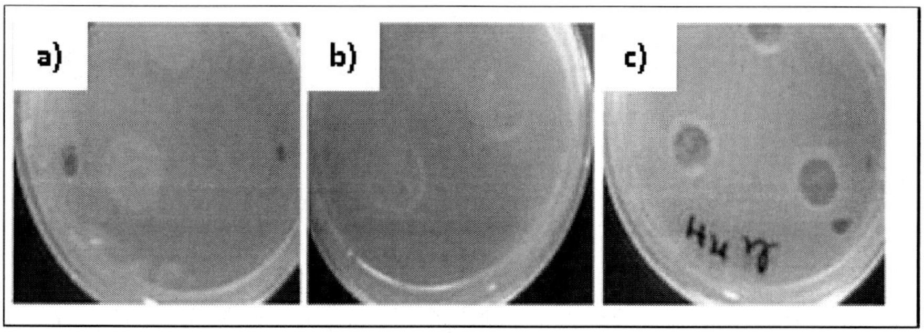

Figure 10. Inhibition zones against *P. fluorescens:* a) control (without antimicrobials), b) 0.3% (w/w) potassium sorbate and c) 0.3% (w/w) potassium sorbate and 0.5% (w/w) of carvacrol.

Physical Characterization of Edible Films Containing Potassium Sorbate and Carvacrol

It is necessary to consider that the inclusion of carvacrol at a level of 0.5% (w/w) could modify the physical properties of films containing sorbates, therefore it was necessary to evaluate these properties for new formulation. The effect of the presence of 0.5% carvacrol (w/w) on the WVP, color, solubility in water and mechanical properties of the films is shown in Table 6. These results were compared with films containing only potassium sorbate.

It was observed that, in general, the color parameters of films were not affected by the incorporation of carvacrol. Du and Friedman (2008) reported that b* parameter decreased with increasing concentration of carvacrol in films based on apple polysaccharides. In this study, the same trend was observed in b* and YI, but without significant differences.

Table 6. Physical properties of films based on cassava starch, HPMC and containing potassium sorbate or potassium sorbate/carvacrol

Property		Film	
		Potassium Sorbate	Potassium Sorbate/Carvacrol
Color	*L**	90.4 ± 0.3^{a}	90.7 ± 0.4^{a}
	*a**	-1.28 ± 0.06^{b}	-1.44 ± 0.03^{b}
	*b**	4.9 ± 0.3^{d}	4.6 ± 0.1^{d}
	YI	8.8 ± 0.6^{f}	8.2 ± 0.2^{f}
Mechanical properties	Ec (MPa)	3.7 ± 0.7	1.7 ± 0.1
	σ_r (MPa)	1.2 ± 0.1	0.80 ± 0.03
	ε_r (%)	74 ± 7	54 ± 8
Solubility	(%)	38 ± 9^{j}	31 ± 3^{j}
WVP x 10^9	g/Pa m s	1.07 ± 0.05^{l}	1.2 ± 0.1^{l}

Equal letters in the same row indicate absence of significant differences ($p > 0.05$). Ec (Elastic modulus); ε_r (strain at break); σ_r (stress at break).

Regarding mechanical parameters, it was determined that the incorporation of carvacrol significantly reduced the mechanical resistance, since Ec and σ_r values decreased, compared to formulations with potassium sorbate only. Du and Friedman (2008) studied the mechanical properties of films made from apple puree and containing carvacrol in a concentration range of 0.5 to 1.5% (w/w). These authors reported that the increase in the carvacrol amount did not produce significant changes in the stress at low oil levels, while for higher concentrations they observed a decrease from 1.9 to 1.6 MPa. On the other hand, ε_r showed a significant decrease when carvacrol was added. It should be noted that the carvacrol films were obtained through an emulsification process in order to homogeneously distribute the main component of the essential oil of oregano. Arrieta and Jiménez (2013), reported that the presence of carvacrol in the formulation of sodium or calcium caseinate films and glycerol, improved the ductile properties of these matrices.

Regarding solubility, a tendency to decrease was observed when the carvacrol was present in the formulation, which would be determined by its hydrophobic character; however, this difference was not statistically significant ($p > 0.05$).

No significant differences were observed for WVP results, being the average value for these systems $(1.13 \pm 0.05) \times 10^{-9}$ g/Pa m s.

CONCLUSION

The carvacrol, one of the components of oregano essential oil, was successfully used to formulate antimicrobial edible films based on cassava starch and HPMC plasticized with glycerol and added with potassium sorbate. The films developed in this research showed adequate physical and microbiological properties.

In order to evaluate the effect of the process variable (emulsification speed) on the film physical properties, two rates were tested: 6500 rpm (LS film) or 21500 rpm (HS film). The results showed that the crystallinity was not influenced by the emulsification rate, resulting in predominantly amorphous structures. Both films had a slightly greenish-yellow tonality and high luminosity but the HS film presented less color than the LS one. Therefore, the color of a food coated by this film would not be significantly altered. The water solubility increased with emulsification rate while the tensile stress was higher in HS films and the strain did not show significant differences in comparison with LS films.

When films were added with 0.5% (w/w) carvacrol and using the HS procedure, the antimicrobial activity was tested through the diffusion assay.

It was verified that the addition of carvacrol significantly improved the antimicrobial action of the films against *Lactobacillus plantarum, Pseudomonas fluorescens* and *Zygosaccharomyces bailii* in relation with the protective action of films containing only potassium sorbate.

The mechanical properties decreased with respect to those films that did not contain the component of the essential oil of oregano.

The results presented in this research reveal that the developed films have potential to be used as an antimicrobial stress factor or as active packaging material, contributing to the preservation of food quality and safety. This makes it possible to enrich the existing information base and contributes to improve the process of selecting appropriate formulations and processes in accordance with the requirements of the final application.

ACKNOWLEDGMENTS

The authors thank the financial assistance from UBA (UBACYT 2011-2014/726, 2014-2017/550BA), CONICET of Argentina (PIP 2010-2012/531, 2013-2015/507),

National Agency of Scientific and Technological Promotion of Argentina (PICT-2012-0183, PICT 2015-2109).

REFERENCES

Aguilera, J. and Stanley, D. (1999). *Microstructural principles of food processing and engineering. An Aspen Food Engineering Series Book*. Second edition.

Alzate, P., Miramont, S., Flores, S. and Gerschenson, L. N. (2017), Effect of the potassium sorbate and carvacrol addition on the properties and antimicrobial activity of tapioca starch – Hydroxypropyl methylcellulose edible films. *Starch - Stärke*, 69: 1600261.

Arismendi, C., Chillo, S., Conte, A., Del Nobile, M., Flores, S. and Gerschenson, L. (2013). Optimization of physical properties of xanthan gum/tapioca starch edible matrices containing potassium sorbate and evaluation of its antimicrobial effectiveness. *LWT - Food Science and Technology*, 53: 290 – 296.

Arrieta, M., Peltzer, M., Garrigós, M. and Jiménez, A. (2013). Structure and mechanical properties of sodium and calcium caseinate edible active films with carvacrol. *Journal of Food Engineering*, 114: 486–494.

Arrieta, M., Peltzer, M., López, J., Garrigós, M., Valentec, A. and Jiménez, A. (2014). Functional properties of sodium and calcium caseinate antimicrobial active films containing carvacrol. *Journal of Food Engineering*, 121: 94–101.

Barzegar, H., Hossein Azizi, M., Barzegar, M. and Hamidi-Esfahani, Z. (2014). Effect of potassium sorbate on antimicrobial and physical properties of starch–clay nanocomposite films. *Carbohydrate Polymers*, 110: 26–31.

Bertuzzi, M.A., Castro Vidaurre, E.F., Armada, M. and Gottifredi, J.C. (2007). Water vapor permeability of edible starch based films. *Journal of Food Engineering*, 80: 972–978.

Campos, C., Alzamora, S. and Gerschenson, L. (2000). Inhibitory action of potassium sorbate degradation products against Staphylococcus aureus growth in laboratory media. *International Journal of Food Microbiology*, 54: 117–122.

Carrillo, L. and Audisio, M.C. (2007). *Manual of Microbiology of Foods*. San Salvador de Jujuy. 1-191.

Chang, Y., Cheah, P. and Seow, C. (2000). Plasticizing-antiplasticizing effects of water on physical properties of tapioca starch films in the glassy state. *J. Food Sci.* 65(3): 445-451.

Chavan, P. and Tupe, S. (2014). Antifungal activity and mechanism of action of carvacrol and thymol against vineyard and wine spoilage yeasts. *Food Control*, 46: 115 – 120.

Chillo, S., Flores, S., Mastromatteo, M., Conte, A., Gerschenson, L. and Del Nobile M. (2008). Influence of glycerol and chitosan on tapioca starch-based edible film properties. *Journal of Food Engineering*, 88: 159–168.

Chiumarelli, M. and Hubinger, M. (2012). Stability, solubility, mechanical and barrier properties of cassavastarch - Carnauba wax edible coatings to preserve fresh-cut apples *Food Hydrocolloids*, 28: 59 – 67.

Chiumarelli, M. and Hubinger, M. (2014). Evaluation of edible films and coatings formulated with cassava starch, glycerol, carnauba wax and stearic acid. Food Hydrocolloids, 38: 20 -27.

Coffey, D., Bell, A. and Henderson, A. (1995). Cellulose and cellulose derivatives. In Stephen, A.M.[ed.], *Food Polysaccharides and their applications*, 123-153. Marcel Dekker, NY, USA.

De Vriesa, M., Vaughan, E., Kleerebezem, M. and De Vos, W. (2006). Lactobacillus plantarum—survival, functional and potential probiotic properties in the human intestinal tract. *International Dairy Journal*, 16: 1018–1028.

Du, W.X., Olsen, C.W., Avena-Bustillos, R., Mchugh, T., Levin, C. and Friedman, M. (2008). Storage stability and antibacterial activity against *Escherichia coli* O157:H7 of carvacrol in edible apple films made by two different casting methods. *J. Agric. Food Chem*, 56: 3082–3088

Espinel Villacrés, R., Flores, S. and Gerschenson, L. (2014). Biopolymeric antimicrobial films: Study of the influence of hydroxypropyl methylcellulose, tapioca starch and glycerol contents on physical properties. *Materials Science and Engineering C*, 36: 108–117.

Espinel, R., (2009). Innovations in the development of antimicrobial edible films based on biopolymers and oregano. Thesis presented to qualify for the title of Master in Food Science and Technology of Food Industrialization of the University of Buenos Aires.

Famá, L., Goyanes, S. and Gerschenson, L. (2007). Influence of storage time at room temperature on the physicochemical properties of cassava starch films. *Carbohydrate Polymers*, 70: 265–273.

Fanelli, B. (2009). *Starch.* Universidad Nacional de Quilmes. Available in: http://psceni.blog.unq.edu.ar/modules/docmanager/view_file.php?curent_file=78&curent_dir=26

Fang, Y., Tung, M. A., Britt, I. J., Yada, S. and Dalgleish, D. G. (2002). Tensile and barrier properties of edible films made from whey proteins. *Journal of Food Science*, 67, 188-193.

Fernández Cervera, M., Karjalainen, M., Airaksinen, S., Rantanen, J., Krogars, K., Heinämäki, J., Iraizoz Colarte, A. and Yliruusi, J. (2004). Physical stability and moisture sorption of aqueous chitosan–amylose starch films plasticized with polyols. *Eur J of Pharm Biopharm*. 58: 69–76

Fialova, J., Chumchalova, J., Mikova, K. and Hrusova, I. (2008). Effect of food preservatives on the growth of spoilage lactobacilli isolated from mayonnaise-based sauces. *Food Control*, 19: 706–713.

Flores, S., Conte, A., Campos, C., Gerschenson, L. and Del Nobile, M. (2007). Mass transport properties of tapioca-based active edible films. *Journal of Food Engineering*, 81: 580–586.

Flores, S., Costa, D., Yamashita, F., Gerschenson, L. and Grossman, M.V. (2010). Mixture design for evaluation of potassium sorbate and xanthan gum effect on properties of tapioca starch films obtained by extrusion. *Materials Science and Engineering C*, 30: 196–202.

Flores, S., Fama, L., Rojas, A., Goyanes, S. and Gerschenson, L. (2007). Physical properties of tapioca-starch edible films: Influence of filmmaking and potassium sorbate. *Food Research International* 40: 257–265.

García-García, R.M. and Palou-García, E. (2008). Mechanisms of antimicrobial action of thymol and carvacrol on microorganisms of interest in food. *Selected Topics of Food Engineering*, 2 -2: 41 – 51.

Gerez, C.L., Torres, M.J., Font de Valdez, G. and Rollán, G. (2013). Control of spoilage fungi by lactic acid bacteria. *Biological Control*, 64: 231–237.

Gerschenson, L., Rojas, A.M. *and* Flores, S.K. Films & Coatings: Migration of ingredients. (2016). In *Edible Films and Coatings: Fundamentals and Applications*. Editores: Montero, M.P.; Gómez-Guillén; M.C.; López-Caballero, M.E. y Barbosa-Cánovas, G.V. CRC Press, Taylor & Francis Group, Boca Raton, Florida. Copyright 2016. ISBN: 978-1-48-221831-2.

Hewage, S. and Vithanarachchi, S. M. (2008). Preparation and characterization of biodegradable polymer films from cowpea (*Vigna unguiculata*) protein isolate. Department of Chemistry, Faculty of Science, University of Colombo.

Higueras, L., López-Carballo, G., Gavara, R. and Hernández-Muñoz, P. (2015). Incorporation of hydroxypropyl-β-cyclodextrins into chitosan films to tailor loading capacity for active aroma compound carvacrol. *Food Hydrocolloids*, 43: 603-611.

Homayouni, H., Kavoosi, G. and Nassiri, S. (2017). Physicochemical, antioxidant and antibacterial properties of dispersion made from tapioca and gelatinized tapioca starch incorporated with carvacrol. *LWT – Food Science and Technology*, 77: 503 – 509.

Iturriaga, L., Olabarrieta, I. and Martínez de Marañón, I. (2012). Antimicrobial assays of natural extracts and their inhibitory effect against *Listeria innocua* and fish spoilage bacteria, after incorporation into biopolymer edible films. *International Journal of Food Microbiology*, 158: 58–64.

Jakobsen, M. and Narvhus, J. (1996). Yeasts and their possible beneficial and negative effects on the quality of dairy products. *Ht. Dairy Journal*, 6: 755-768.

Kralj, I., Plavec, J., Smole, S. and Zupancic-Kralj, L. (2001). Characterization of sorbate geometrical isomers. *Journal of Chromatography* A, 905: 359–366.

Kurek, M., Moundanga, S., Favier, C., Galic, K. and Debeaufort, F. (2013). Antimicrobial efficiency of carvacrol vapour related to mass partition coefficient when incorporated in chitosan based films aimed for active packaging. *Food Control*, 32: 168 - 175.

Laxmikant, B., Borah, P. and Deka, S. (2014). Antimicrobial and enzymatic antibrowning film used as coating for bamboo shoot quality improvement. *Carbohydrate Polymers*, 103: 213–220.

Lebert, I., Robles-Olvera, V. and Lebert, A. (2000). Application of polynomial models to predict growth of mixed cultures of Pseudomonas spp. and Listeria in meat. *International Journal of Food Microbiology*, 61: 27–39.

Murillo-Martinez, M. M., Pedroza-Islas, R., Lobato-Calleros, C., Martinez-Ferez, A. and Vernon-Carter, E. J. (2010), Designing W1/O/W2 double emulsions stabylizaed by protein-polysaccharide complexes for producing edible films: Rheological, mechanical and water vapour properties. *Food hydrocolloids,* 25: 577-585.

Nussinovitch, A. (2003). Hydrocolloids in the production of special textures. In: *Watersoluble Polymer Applications in Foods*. Blackwell Publishing, Malden, MA, USA. Chapter 9, 203-204.

Ollé, C., Jagus, R. and Gerschenson, L. (2014). Natamycin efficiency for controlling yeast growth in models systems and on cheese surfaces. *Food Control*, 35: 101 – 108.

Ozdemir, M. and Floros, J. (2008). Optimization of edible whey protein films containing preservatives for water vapor permeability, water solubility and sensory characteristics. *Journal of Food Engineering*, 86: 215–224.

Peressini, D., Bravin, B., Lapasin, R., Rizzotti, C. and Sensidoni, A. (2003). Starch–methylcellulose based edible films: rheological properties of film-forming dispersions. *Journal of Food Engineering*, 59: 25–32.

Phan, T. D., Debeaufort, F., Luu, D., Voilley, A. (2005). Functional properties of edible agar-based and starch-based films for food quality preservation. *J. Agric. Food Chem.*, 53, 973–981.

Prakash Marana, J., Sivakumarb, V., Sridharc, R. and Thirugnanasambandhamd, K. (2013). Development of model for barrier and optical properties of tapioca starch based edible films. *Carbohydrate Polymers*, 92: 1335–1347.

Sothornvit R. and Krochta, J. M. (2005). Plasticizers in edible films and coatings. Chapter 23. *Innovations in Food Packaging*. 403 – 428

Sarkar, N. and Walker, L.C. (1995). Hydration-dehydration properties of methylcellulose and hydroxypropylmethylcellulose. *Carbohydrate Polymers*, 27, 177-185.

Shiku, Y., Hamaguchi, P., Benjakul, S., Visessanguan, W., Tanaka, M. (2004). Effect of Surimi Quality on Properties of Edible Films Based on Alaska Pollack. *Food Chemistry*, 86: 493–499.

Souza, E.L., Stamford, T.L., Lima, E.O. and Trajano, V.N. (2007). Effectiveness of Origanum vulgare L. essential oil to inhibit the growth of food spoiling yeasts. *Food Control*, 18: 409–413.

Tongdeesoontorn, W., Mauer, L. J., Wongruong, S., Sriburi, P. and Rachtanapun, P. (2011). Effect of carboxymethyl cellulose concentration on physical properties of biodegradable cassava starch-based films. *Chemistry Central Journal*, 1: 1186 – 1752.

Trezza, T. A. and Krochta, J. M. (2000). Color stability of edible coatings during prolonged storage. *Journal of Food Science*, 65(1), 1166-1169.

Tunç, S. and Duman, O. (2011). Preparation of active antimicrobial methyl cellulose/carvacrol/montmorillonite nanocomposite films and investigation of carvacrol release. *LWT - Food Science and Technology*, 44: 465 - 472.

Vásconez, M., Flores, S., Campos, C., Alvarado, J. and Gerschenson, L. (2009). Antimicrobial activity and physical properties of chitosan–tapioca starch based edible films and coatings. *Food Research International*, 42: 762–769

Ventura, S., De Barros, R., Sintra, T., Soares, C., Lima, A. and Coutinho, J. (2012). Simple screening method to identify toxic/non-toxic ionic liquids: Agar diffusion test adaptation. *Ecotoxicology and Environmental Safety*, 83: 55–62.

Wu, D. and Sun, D.W. (2013). Colour measurements by computer vision for food quality control: A review. *Trends in Food Science & Technology*, 29: 5-20.

In: Oregano: Properties, Uses and Health Benefits
Editor: Gema Nieto Martínez
ISBN: 978-1-53616-284-4

Chapter 4

IMPROVING FOOD SHELF LIFE WITH OREGANO EXTRACT AND ESSENTIAL OIL

José M. Lorenzo[1,*], Paulo E. S. Munekata[1], Mladen Brnčić[2], Suzana Rimac Brnčić[2], Fabienne Remize[3] and Francisco J. Barba[4]

[1]Meat Technological Center of Galicia, Ourense, Spain
[2]Department of Food Engineering, University of Zagreb, Zagreb, Croatia
[3]UMR QualiSud, Université de La Réunion, CIRAD, Université Montpellier, Montpellier SupAgro, Université d'Avignon, Sainte Clotilde, France
[4]Preventive Medicine and Public Health, Food Science, Toxicology and Forensic Medicine Department, Universitat de València, València, Spain

ABSTRACT

Oregano is one of the main seasonings used worldwide in the preparation of dishes at both household and industrial level because of its unique sensory properties. Moreover, the composition of oregano leaves has been associated with a preservative effect in food matrixes. The investigation of oregano composition revealed that products of secondary metabolism in plant tissues, mainly essential oils (e.g., terpenes) and phenolic compounds are the main classes of compounds to exert such an effect in food. Consequently, several studies explored the impact of oregano components in food. Some approaches have been developed in order to prevent food quality loss such as addition of oregano as an ingredient in the product formulation, soaking food matrix into a solution with oregano active compounds, production of nanoparticles, inclusion into films and into food package material. It is worth mentioning that the antimicrobial potential of oregano has been reported in meat, meat products, fish, fish products, vegetables, bread, oils, salad dressing and fruits. This chapter discusses the use of oregano extracts in food matrixes, which also

* Corresponding Author's E-mail: jmlorenzo@ceteca.net.

includes technologies, antimicrobial mechanisms, and the relation between food matrix characteristics and enhancement of shelf life.

Keywords: *Origanum vulgare*, microbial stability, oxidation, sensory attributes, films, shelf life, meat products, fresh food, modified atmosphere

INTRODUCTION

The concept of food quality is composed of multi-variable aspects such as microbiological, physico-chemical, nutritional, and sensory characteristics of a particular food. However, food quality is also associated with subjective aspects of consumer's life and experience, the personal relationship with food and a particular product, the context and the moment of purchase and the location where consumer buys a particular food (Cardello, 1995). In the context of fresh vegetables, the perception of freshness and general appearance are key characteristics related to the moment of purchase (Rico et al., 2007). Likewise, meat and meat products quality are also influenced by consumer's perception of several attributes such as color, level of visible fat, price, type of cut and general aspect (Grunert, Bredahl, and Brunsø, 2004).

In addition, the perception of post-purchase characteristics of food are the main factors that influence further purchases. In this context the food elaboration, sensory characteristics (e.g., taste, flavor, and texture), convenience and the general experience with a particular food can lead to further purchases (Grunert, Bredahl, and Brunsø, 2004). The combination of both pre and post-purchase factors must be considered in the context of food quality. Conversely, exploring and understanding the factors and changes in food characteristics during quality decay are crucial to improve current minimally-processed and processed foods towards consumer's expectations and needs. The main current trends driving food development are health, environmental-friendly products and search of authenticity. Therefore, the use of natural sources of preservative compounds have been receiving great attention from researchers and food industries (Carocho et al., 2014). Tamaño letra

Oregano (*Origanum* L.) is an herb traditionally used as seasoning in food preparation. The Mediterranean region is the location with the greater diversity of this aromatic spice, where more of 60-70 species and hybrids can be found (Aboukhalid et al., 2017). The geographical distribution of the plant also influenced the local culinary traditions, leading to use into local foods, which are part of the local heritage, such as observed for Italian culinary (Cappellini and Parsons, 2014). The characterization of oregano composition and further exploration of active components revealed that such a spice can be used to improve the quality and preserve food (Figure 1), by delay of microbial spoilage and decrease of oxidative reactions (Tajkarimi, Ibrahim, and Cliver, 2010; Rodriguez-Garcia et al., 2016).

The present chapter deals with the use of oregano, by means of its preservative components, to improve the shelf life of fresh, minimally-processed and processed food.

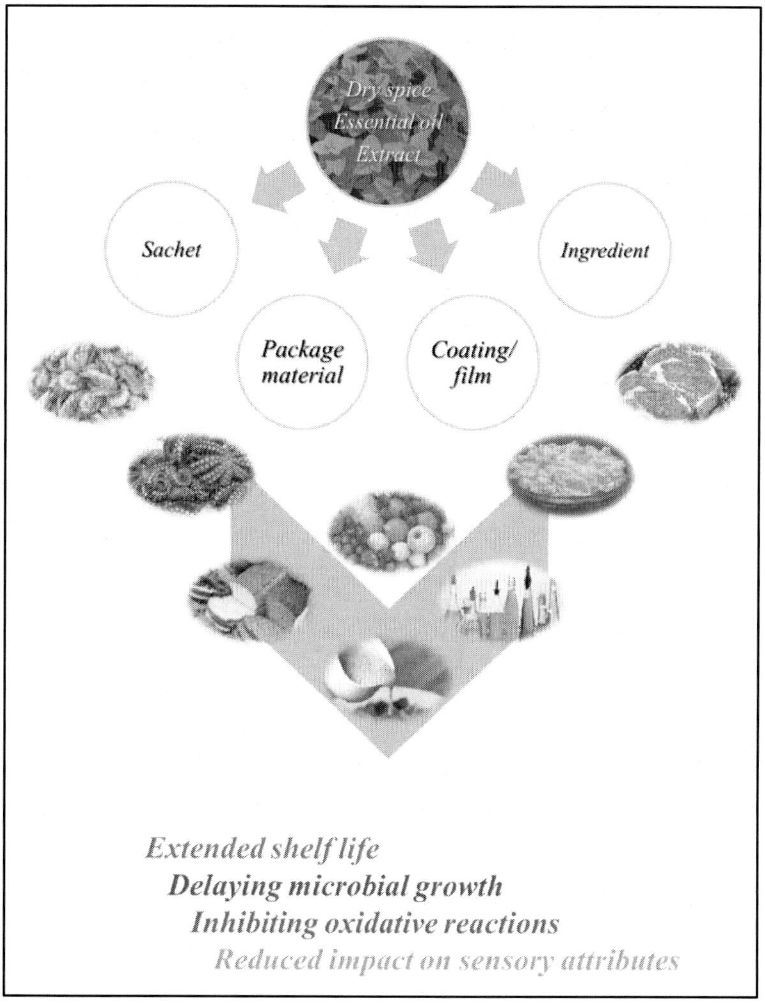

Figure 1. Schematic representation of oregano preservative components effect on food stability during storage.

PRESERVATIVE COMPONENTS AND TECHNOLOGIES OF USE

Oregano is a rich source of compounds with potential application in food industry. Extracts and fractions of oregano components have been explored over the last decades in order to improve the shelf life of fresh, minimally-processed and processed food. Essential oils and phenolic compounds are considered as the main preservative agents responsible of oregano protective effect in food. The essential oil of oregano is composed of several hydrophobic compounds such as carvacrol and thymol followed by *p*-pymene, terpinen-4-

ol, sabinene, *trans*-sabinene hydrate, and γ-terpinene (Table 1). The phenolic composition of oregano tissues revealed that rosmarinic acid is the major compound, followed by other phenolic acids (caffeic, protocatechuic acid) and flavonoids (Table 1). These compounds are related to antimicrobial and antioxidant activities, which in turn can delay the loss of quality during storage and consequently improve the shelf life of several products.

Table 1. Main compounds in oregano essential oil and phenolic fraction

Main compounds	Other compounds	Reference
Essential oils		
trans-sabinene hydrate (17.9-28.2 g/100 g) and thymol (12.1-18.6 g/100 g)	terpinen-4-ol (6.2-9.5 g/100 g), γ-terpinene (g/100 g), orto-cymene (5.1-6.3 g/100 g), and sabinene (3.6-4.5 g/100 g)	(Asensio, Grosso, and Juliani, 2015)
terpineol (E) beta (55.5 g/100 g)	terpinen-4-ol (15.9 g/100 g) and thymol (12.9 g/100 g)	(Olmedo, Nepote, and Grosso, 2013)
carvacrol (47.2% area)	β-caryophyllene (9.6% area), β-bisabolene (5.2% area), and thymoquinone (3.3% area)	(Damašius et al., 2009)
carvacrol (0-30.2% area) and terpinen-4-ol (8.5-21.6% area)	*trans*-sabinene hidrate (0-23.9% area), γ-terpinene (7.3-11.8% area), and *p*-cymene (0-14.6% area)	(Asensio et al., 2014)
carvacrol (81.8% area)	thymol (4.1% area), *p*-cymene (3.3% area), and γ-terpinene (2.3% area)	(Jouki et al., 2014)
carvacrol (47.8% area)	thymol (21.4% area), γ-terpinene (13.4% area), and *p*-cymene (8.5% area)	(Van Haute et al., 2016)
carvacrol (71.2% area)	*p*-cymene (4.4% area), thymol (4.3% area), and linalool (3.1% area)	(Carrión-Granda et al., 2016)
thymol (32% area)	4-terpineol (12% area), α-terpinene (10% area), carvacrol (6% area) and *trans*-sabinene hidrate (6% area)	(Hashemi et al., 2017)
carvacrol (68.5% area)	thymoquinone (12.1% area) and *p*-cymene (7.8% area)	(Gutierrez, Barry-Ryan, and Bourke, 2008)
Phenolic compounds		
rosmarinic acid (4.8-8.9 mg/g dw)	coumaric acid (0.9-3.9 mg/g dw) and quercetin (1.04-3.24 mg/g dw)	(Chun et al., 2005)
rosmarinic acid (173-1271 mg/100 g plant extract)	caffeic acid (traces)	(Exarchou et al., 2002)
rosmarinic acid (2562.7 mg/100 g dw)	caffeoyl derivatives (1324.2 mg/100 g dw), *p*-coumaric acid (214.8 mg/100 g dw) and other phenolic acids (208.5 mg GAE/100 g dw)	(Shan et al., 2005)
rosmarinic acid (52.2 μg/g dw)	caffeic (10.6 μg/g dw) and protocatechuic acid (9.9 μg/g dw)	(Vallverdú-Queralt et al., 2014)

dw: dry weight; GAE: gallic acid equivalent.

In order to successfully apply these compounds into food matrix, several researchers explored strategies to prepare oregano preservative compounds for food use (Figure 1). The direct use of oregano either as ingredient or on the surface (e.g., direct application, dipping into solution, and marinating) of food is the simplest technology to preserve food. This strategy originates from the traditional use of oregano, added as ingredient in the elaboration of food. From those, scientific advances in the characterization of oregano composition and their role in the protective effect of oregano on food were made. Although adding oregano into food can be consider a simplistic approach, more complex strategies to improve the preservation of food rely on the same concept.

A relevant example of a complex strategy is food coating with oregano preservative components in a film. The preservative component is incorporated to the film matrix that is further used to wrap food and so-called active packaging. The main advantage of this strategy is the progressive release of preservative components during shelf life, which balances the growth and activity of microorganisms (Appendini and Hotchkiss, 2002). Another application which ressembles to the use of films for active packaging, is direct coating of food. For that purpose, a solution containing both coating material and preservative components is directly applied onto the surface of food (by brushing, dipping, or spraying) prior to solidification of coating. In this approach, the preservative compounds are continuously released during the storage period (Aloui and Khwaldia, 2016).

Another way to improve shelf life is to put in the packaging together with the food to preserve a sachet containing the preservative components. In this concept the progressive release of preservatives from a carrier matrix trough a permeable outer layer is expected. The sachet remains in constant contact with food (Otoni et al., 2016).

Lastly, oregano preservative extracts can be directly incorporated into package material. The concept of diffusion is analogous to that of sachets: the preservative compounds are incorporated troughout the surface of a package material. Additional layers can be applied to slow down the release flux. The immobilization instead of incorporation of preservative compounds onto the package material is another possible alternative but in both cases, the contact with food is necessary (Bastarrachea, Dhawan, and Sablani 2011). In further sections, the use of each one of these strategies is discussed regarding selected food categories.

USE IN FOOD PRESERVATION

Meat and Meat Products

The use of oregano, and particularly essential oil of oregano, in meat and meat products has shown promising results to improve shelf life and, in some cases, displayed equivalent capacity to replace synthetic preservatives (Table 2). It has been mainly investigated to limit the development of spoilage microorganisms. For instance, a study characterized the antimicrobial potential of oregano essential oil (0.25%) on raw chicken breast meat. *Brochothrix thermosphacta*, *Enterobacteriaceae*, lactic acid bacteria (LAB), *Pseudomonas* spp., total plate count (TPC), and yeasts andmoulds (Y&M) growth were inhibited during refrigerated storage, whereas sensory acceptance was identical to that of control samples (Petrou et al., 2012). The authors also reported that combining oregano essential oil with chitosan prevented the reduction of sensory acceptance of taste and odor observed for control samples. In another study, the incorporation of essential oil in the range of 0.5-2.0% in a film or in coating material showed positive results to prevent fresh meat deterioration. The development of *Enterobacteriaceae*, LAB, psychrotrophic bacteria, TPC, and Y&M was inhibited in comparison to uncoated chicken breast meat (Chaleshtori and Chaleshtori, 2017) over 6 days of refrigerated storage. The protective of oregano essential oil during storage was also reported for fresh foal meat (Lorenzo, Batlle, and Gómez, 2014). In this study, an active film containing oregano essential oil (2%) was combined with modified atmosphere. This film inhibited the growth of total aerobic bacteria, *Pseudomonas* spp., *Enterobacteriaceae*, Y&M. The protective effect was also observed on lipid oxidation and sensory properties, particularly by improving the stability of red color and by reducing the discoloration and off odor formation.

The interest in oregano preservative effects was not limited to fresh meat but also investigated for processed meat products. In the same way as for meat, the use of oregano extract as preservative into raw sheep patties supported its technological function (Fernandes et al., 2016). During the refrigerated storage (under modified atmosphere) up to 20 days, both lipid and protein oxidation were inhibited along with the loss of red color, and deterioration of sensory properties. In addition, the authors concluded that oregano extract (1000 ppm) could be considered as a potential alternative to the synthetic antioxidant butylated hydroxytoluene (BHT). In a further study, the same oregano extract was evaluated as potential preservative for frozen stored raw lamb burgers. A protective effect against deterioration was also reported by the authors regarding the lipid and protein oxidation, and the loss of red color (Fernandes et al., 2017).

The protective effect of oregano extract (at 6630.98 and 8038.20 mg/kg) was also observed during storage of sheep sausages at ambient temperature (Fernandes et al., 2018). The experiment with this matrix characterized the protective effect on lipids and proteins, the preservation of red color and reduced the formation of volatile compounds associated with lipid oxidation. Under these storage conditions, sausages containing the oregano extract could be stored up to 135 days. Moreover, the authors also highlighted the potential of the extract to replace the synthetic antioxidant sodium erythorbate.

In another approach, the use of oregano essential oil (in combination with orange dietary fiber) as preservative improved the microbial stability of bologna sausages during refrigerated storage. Lower aerobic bacteria and LAB counts were observed throughout 24 days of storage. Moreover, the observations were enhanced by combining oregano essential oil and orange dietary fiber with packaging technology, particularly with modified atmosphere and vacuum packaging (Viuda-Martos et al., 2010).

Interestingly, oregano essential oil (0.4%) was associated with improved shelf life of vacuum packaged sliced cooked ham in a recent study (Menezes et al., 2018).

Table 2. Preservative effect of oregano on storage stability of meat and meat products

Food	Strategic use	Study conditions	Preservative effect	Reference
Fresh chicken breast meat	Adding essential oil (0.25%) onto the surface after dipping in chitosan solution	21 days at 4°C; MA (70% NO_2 and 30% CO_2)	Inhibition of total aerobic bacteria *Enterobacteriaceae*, LAB, *Pseudomonas* spp., *Brochothrix thermosphacta*, Y&M growth, lipid oxidation and redness loss; no impact on sensory acceptance; *shelf life: 15 days*	(Petrou et al., 2012)
Fresh chicken breast meat	Coating with chitosan-essential oil (0.5, 1 and 2%)	9 days at 4°C	Inhibition of *Enterobacteriaceae*, LAB, psychrotrophic, total aerobic bacteria, and Y&M growth	(Chaleshtori and Chaleshtori, 2017)
Fresh foal meat	Wrapping with oregano essential oil film (2%)	14 days at 2°C; MA (80% O_2 and 20% CO_2)	Inhibition of total aerobic, *Pseudomonas* spp., *Enterobacteriaceae*, Y&M growth, lipid oxidation; preservation of red color and reduced discoloration and off odor	(Lorenzo, Batlle, and Gómez, 2014)
Raw sheep burgers	As ingredient (lyophilized extract, 1000 ppm)	20 days at 4°C; MA (80% O_2 and 20% CO_2)	Inhibition of lipid oxidation and protein oxidation, loss of red color, and sensory properties deterioration; *shelf life: 10 days, 4°C*	(Fernandes et al., 2016)
Raw lamb burger	As ingredient (aqueous extract, 24 mL/kg)	120 days at -18°C	Inhibition of lipid and protein oxidation, and loss of red color; *shelf life: 120 days, -18°C*	(Fernandes et al., 2017)
Sheep sausage	As ingredient (aqueous extract, 500 mg/kg)	135 days at 20°C VP	Inhibition of lipid and protein oxidation, loss of red color, and formation of volatile compounds; similar effect to commercial antioxidant	(Fernandes et al., 2018)
Bologna sausage	As ingredient (essential oil, 0.02%) with orange dietary fiber (1%)	24 days at 4°C, MA (80% N_2 and 20% CO_2), VP or air pouches	Inhibition of total aerobic bacteria and LAB, lipid oxidation; MA packaging and VP improved the inhibitory effects	(Viuda-Martos et al., 2010)
Cooked sliced ham	Appling essential oil (0.4%) onto the surface	45 days at 6°C, 18 days at 12 and 15°C, and 6 days at 20 and 25°C VP	Inhibition of LAB counts for refrigerated samples (at 6 and 12°C); *shelf life: >45 days at 6°C*	(Menezes et al., 2018)
Chicken pâté	As ingredient (essential oil nano-emulsion, 12 g/kg)	8 days at 4°C	Partial inhibition of *Escherichia coli* and *Staphylococcus aureus* growth	(Moraes-lovison et al., 2017)
Paínho sausage	Coating with WPC and essential oil solution (1%)	126 days at 4°C; VP	Inhibition of total aerobic bacteria and color fading; *shelf life: 104 days, 4°C*	(Catarino et al., 2017)
Alheira sausage	Coating with WPC and essential oil solution (1%)	106 days at 4°C; VP	Inhibition of total aerobic bacteria and lipid oxidation; *shelf life: 98 days, 4°C*	(Catarino et al., 2017)

MA: modified atmosphere; VP: vacuum packaged; LAB: lactic acid bacteria; WPC: whey protein concentrate; Y&M: yeasts and moulds.

The evaluation of the temperature effect on the growth of LAB indicated that the inhibitory effect was reduced as the temperature increased from 6 to 15°C for samples added of essential oil. The authors also observed that shelf life was drastically reduced from >45 to 12-14 days by this increase of temperature. All together these data support the role of oregano essential oil as food preservative and indicate the necessity to prevent temperature abuse in this kind of products.

The use of a nanoemulsion containing oregano oil (12 g/kg) was evaluated as natural preservative during 8 days of refrigerated storage of chicken pâté. The nanoemulsion inhibited the growth of *Escherichia coli* and *Staphylococcus aureus*, particularly on the last days of refrigerated storage (Moraes-lovison et al., 2017). Conversely, the use of oregano (particularly essential oil) can also induce the development of spoilage bacteria leading to low quality products. This effect was reported in an experiment with cooked chicken patties that combined oregano and thyme essential oil in an edible film and observed a reduction on shelf life of 5 days (Soni et al., 2018). A similar outcome regarding the psychrotrophic growth (0.02 and 0.1% of oregano extract) was reported for raw beef patties stored for 24 days at 2°C (Sánchez-Escalante et al., 2003).

Finally, regarding dry-cured and fermented sausages, the use of oregano as preservative improved the shelf life of two traditional Portuguese sausages: *Paínho* and *Alheira* (Catarino et al., 2017). According to the authors, coating both kind of sausages with 1% oregano essential oil (composed of whey protein, glycerol and ethanol) at the end of processing (prior to vacuum packaging) prevented the growth of aerobic bacteria during storage. The shelf life of *Paínho* sausage was improved by 20 days to 98 days and that of *Alheira* sausage was increased by 15 days to 104 days. Moreoever, while color fading was particularly inhibited in *Paínho*, the development of lipid oxidation was reduced in *Alheira* sausage.

Fish and Seafood

Due to the fast deterioration of fish and seafoods, appropriate technologies and strategies are required to preserve quality, safety and sensory properties. The role of oregano as preservative in this category of food is similar to that observed for meat and meat products by preventing the growth of spoilage microorganisms (Table 3). Regarding oregano use on fresh fish fillets, oregano (by dipping into an 0.05% essential oil solution) can inhibit the growth of *Photobacterium phosphoreum* in fresh cod (*Gadus morhua*) fillets and extend the shelf life at 2°C from 21 to 26 days. The combination of oregano essential oil with modified atmosphere (60% CO_2 and 40% N_2) used to improve storage time in this study was also associated with a reduced trimethylamine formation, improving thus the quality of fillets (Mejlholm and Dalgaard, 2002). An important deteriorative indicator in fish and seafood is the production of nitrogenous compounds, which is linked to the activity of spoilage microorganisms and endogenous enzymes (Goulas and Kontominas 2007; Mejlholm and Dalgaard 2002). For instance, the effect of oregano essential oil on the production of nitrogenous compounds was investigated during refrigerated storage of fresh Sea bream (*Sparus aurata*) fillets packaged under modified atmosphere. Both total volatile basic nitrogen and trimethylamine nitrogen contents were reduced in the presence of oregano oil in a concentration-dependent manner for 33 days. Moreover, lipid oxidation and sensory (odor, flesh texture, and flesh color) decay were markedly delayed (Goulas and Kontominas, 2007).

A comparative study about the use of modified atmosphere supported the efficacy of its combination with oregano essential oil to preserve the quality of fresh Swordfish (*Xiphias gladius*) fillets (Giatrakou et al., 2008). The authors observed that 0.1% oregano essential oil could inhibit the growth of total aerobic bacteria during aerobic refrigerated storage (over 4 days) while the combination of modified atmosphere (50% CO_2, 45% N_2 and 5% O_2) and oregano oil increased the shelf life by 8 days. The growth rate of *Enterobacteriaceae*, *Pseudomonas* and H_2S-producing bacteria was also decreased by 0.1% oregano essential oil under both aerobic and modified atmosphere packaging. Another important result indicated in this study was the reduction of odor and taste decay during storage. However, oregano essential oil did not prevent the production of lipid oxidation products and the growth of LAB.

A similar outcome was reported for fresh rainbow trout (*Onchorynchus mykiss*) fillets treated with oregano essential oil packaged with an O_2 absorber. The growth of *Enterobacteriaceae*, H_2S-producing bacteria, LAB, *Pseudomonas* spp., and TVC was inhibited during 21 days of refrigerated storage, which improved the shelf life to 13-14 days. As observed on other studies, the development of oxidative reactions was also inhibited, as well as the formation of volatile nitrogenous compounds. Interestingly, the authors evaluated the association between variables and obtained a positive correlation between H_2S-producing bacterial counts and odor and between lipid oxidation indexes and taste (Mexis, Chouliara, and Kontominas 2009). Another efficient strategy to prevent the deterioration of fresh rainbow trout fillets thanks to oregano essential oil activity was its association with quince seed mucilage film. The use of this film inhibited the growth of total aerobic, psychrophilic, LAB and H_2S-producing bacteria during refrigerated storage. The authors observed that oregano essential oil concentration was one of the main factors to successfully improve trout fillets deterioration, wherein 2% film was the most efficient in comparison to 1 and 1.5% films. The development of lipid oxidative reactions and the production of nitrogenous compounds were also reduced by the active film. In addition, the decay of sensory attributes (color, odor, texture, and overall acceptance) of wrapped trout fillets was delayed (Jouki et al., 2014).

Table 3. Preservative effect of oregano on stability of fish and seafood during storage

Food	Strategic use	Study conditions	Preservative effect	Reference
Fresh cod fillets	Dipping into oregano oil solution (0.05%)	26 days at 2°C; MA (60% CO_2 and 40% N_2)	Inhibition of *Photobacterium phosphoreum* growth and trimethylamine formation; *shelf life: 21-26 days*	(Mejlholm and Dalgaard, 2002)
Fresh sea bream fillets	Adding essential oil (0.4 and 0.8%) and salt	33 days at 4°C; MA (40% CO_2, 30% O_2 and 30% N_2)	Inhibition of nitrogenous compounds production and lipid oxidation; preservation of sensory properties; *shelf life: 15-16 days*	(Goulas and Kontominas, 2007)
Fresh Swordfish fillets	Adding essential oil (0.1%)	18 days at 4°C; aerobic and MA (50% CO_2, 45% N_2 and 5% O_2)	Inhibition of total aerobic bacteria (both packaging systems), *Enterobacteriaceae*, *Pseudomonas* and H_2S-producing bacteria growth, and nitrogenous compounds; reduced the sensory decay of odor and taste; *shelf life: increased by 4 (aerobic packaging) and 8 (MA packaging) days, 4°C*	(Giatrakou et al., 2008)
Fresh rainbow trout fillets	Adding essential oil (0.4%) and O_2 absorber	21 days at 4°C	Inhibition of *Enterobacteriaceae*, H_2S-producing bacteria, LAB, *Pseudomonas* spp., and total aerobic bacteria growth; delaying sensory decay; inhibiting lipid oxidation and the production of nitrogenous compounds; *shelf life: 13-14 days, 4°C*	(Mexis, Chouliara, and Kontominas, 2009)
Fresh rainbow trout fillets	Wrapping with quince seed mucilage and essential oil film (1, 1.5, or 2%)	18 days at 4°C	Inhibition of total aerobic, psychrophilic, LAB and H_2S-producing bacteria growth, lipid oxidation and nitrogenous compounds production; reduced sensory decay of color, odor, texture, and overall acceptance; *shelf life: 15-18 days, 4°C*	(Jouki et al., 2014)
Fresh asian sea bass fish	Adding essential oil (0.05%)	33 days at 0-2°C	Inhibition of total aerobic bacteria; delaying of sensory properties deterioration; partial inhibition of nitrogenous compounds production; *shelf life: 33 days, 0-2°C*	(Harpaz et al., 2003)
Fresh trout fillets	Adding essential oil (0.2 and 0.4%)	18 days at 4°C; VP	Inhibition of *Enterobacteriaceae*, H_2S-producing bacteria, LAB, *Pseudomonas* spp., and total aerobic microorganism' growth, nitrogenous compounds production; delayed sensory properties decay; *shelf life: 11-12 days, 4°C*	(Frangos et al., 2010)
Fresh grass carp fillets	Wrapping with gelatin-chitosan and essential oil film (4%)	12 days at 4°C	Inhibition of total aerobic bacteria growth and nitrogenous compound production	(Wu et al., 2014)

Food	Strategic use	Study conditions	Preservative effect	Reference
Fresh salmon fillets	Marinating with oregano oil (1%)	6 days at 4°C	Partial inhibition of total aerobic psychrotrophic bacteria growth	(Van Haute et al., 2016)
Fresh octopus tentacles	Adding essential oil (0.2 and 0.4%)	24 days at 4°C; VP	Inhibition of *Enterobacteriaceae*, H_2S-producing bacteria, LAB, *Pseudomonas* spp., and total aerobic bacteria growth and nitrogenous compounds production; *shelf life: 17-23 days, 4°C*	(Atrea et al., 2009)
Fresh scampi	Marinating with oregano essential oil (1%)	6 days at 4°C	Partial inhibition of total aerobic psychrotrophic and LAB growth	(Van Haute et al., 2016)
Pre-fried squid rings	Coating with multi-component mixture (essential oil 0.010, 0.025, and 0.050%)	14 days at 4°C MA (70% N_2, 25% CO_2 and 5% O_2)	Inhibition of total aerobic bacteria; partial inhibition of *Enterobacteriaceae*, total anaerobic, and psychrotrophic microorganism growth, and lipid oxidation	(Sanjuás-Rey et al., 2012)
Cooked shrimp	Wrapping with chitosan and essential oil film (0.5%)	12 days at 4°C, MA (40% CO_2 and 60% N_2)	Inhibition of psychrotrophic and total aerobic microorganism growth; partial inhibition of *Enterobacteriaceae* and LAB	(Carrión-Granda et al., 2016)
Cooked shrimp	Dipping into essential oil-water emulsion (0.5%)	12 days at 4°C MA (40% CO_2 and 60% N_2)	Inhibition of total aerobic bacteria and *Enterobacteriaceae* microorganism growth; partial inhibition of psychrotrophic and LAB growth	(Carrión-Granda et al., 2016)

MA: modified atmosphere; VP: vacuum packaged; LAB: lactic acid bacteria.

Likewise, oregano essential oil (0.05%) was used on packaged Asian sea bass fish (*Lates calcarifer*). A general impact on growth of aerobic bacteria during storage was reported on both fish surface and flesh. According to the authors, the sensory properties were also influenced by oregano treatment, which delayed the decay of freshness perception (Harpaz et al., 2003). Similarly, the storage of fresh trout fillets was improved by oregano essential oil. Microbial growth (*Enterobacteriaceae*, H_2S-producing bacteria, LAB, *Pseudomonas* spp., and TPC) was inhibited as well as the decay of sensory properties (odor, taste, and overall acceptability), resulting in an increase of the time of storage to 11-12 days, particularly for 0.2% oregano oil treatment. It worths mentioning that fillets with 0.4% oregano oil received a low sensory score by consumer while the highest scores were attributed to 0.2% oregano oil treatment throughout the storage time (Frangos et al., 2010).

Regarding the development of films with incorporated oregano essential oil, an experiment with a gelatin-chitosan film added of oregano essential oil improved the shelf life of Fresh grass carp (*Hypophthalmichthys molitrix*) fillets. During the storage, the growth of aerobic bacteria of fish samples wrapped with the active film was inhibited, which yielded a product with lower aerobic bacteria counts. The authors also indicated that wrapped samples displayed a lower content of nitrogenous compounds than control sample (unwrapped) and parafilm packaged fillets (Wu et al., 2014). Although oregano essential oil partially prevented the growth of aerobic psychrotrophy bacteria up to 3 days in fresh salmon (*Salmo salar*) fillets, no influence in the development of LAB and Y&M was observed. In this study, salmon fillets were marinated with oregano oil and other ingredients (NaCl, sodium lactate, lactic acid, and Tween 80) for 2 min (Van Haute et al., 2016).

In a similar way, the shelf life of seafood can be improved by oregano. For example, an experiment with oregano essential oil and fresh octopus (*Octopus vulgaris*) tentacles revealed that *Enterobacteriaceae*, H_2S-producing bacteria, LAB, *Pseudomonas* spp., and total aerobic microorganism were inhibited. Moreover, the inhibitory effect was influenced by the concentration of oregano essential wherein higher concentration (0.4 vs 0.2% of oregano essential oil) led to higher inhibitory effects of spoilage microorganism during storage (24 days at 4°C, vacuum packaged). In addition, the production of nitrogenous compounds (total volatile basic nitrogen and trimethylamine nitrogen content) was also reduced throughout storage time, in a concentration-dependent manner. Although a desirable and pleasant odor was perceived by panelists on oregano treated samples, the authors commented that non-significant differences were obtained among treatments for odor during storage. Oregano essential oil treatments improved the shelf life to 17-23 days (Atrea et al., 2009). However, oregano oil (as ingredient in the marinating step) partially prevented the growth of spoilage microorganism in fresh scampi (*Penaeus monodon*) during refrigerated storage. While total aerobic psychrotrophic and LAB growths were partially inhibited, no effect on Y&M was reported (Van Haute et al., 2016).

The storage stability of ready-to-eat or partially prepared seafood can also be enhanced by oregano. This outcome was reported for cooked shrimps (*Penaeus vannamei*) subjected to either essential oil-water emulsion or coated with essential oil-chitosan film. The use of essential oil emulsion inhibited the growth of total aerobic bacteria and *Enterobacteriaceae* microorganism, while chitosan coating affected the growth of psychrotrophic and total aerobic bacteria. Both strategies led to a partial inhibition of LAB during storage. Likewise, the use of oregano essential oil in a coating mixture (wheat flour, cold water and essential oil) inhibited the growth of total aerobic bacteria during storage (14 days at 4°C) of cooked shrimp. However, the coating mixture partially affected the development of *Enterobacteriaceae*, total anaerobic, and psychrotrophic microorganism growth, and lipid oxidation (Carrión-Granda et al., 2016).

Fruits, Vegetables and Bread

The preservative effect of oregano was also reported for fresh or fresh-cut vegetables and fruits (Table 4). An experiment with fresh lamb's lettuce revealed that using oregano essential oil solution (250 mg/L, with 1% ethanol) during washing/decontamination step resulted in the same microbial counts than those observed with chlorine (120 mg/L), from the day of washing to 8 days at 6°C. Mesophilic aerobic bacteria, LAB and yeasts were equally affected by both treatments. Moreover, the combination of oregano essential oil with either thyme oil or carvacol did not modified the growth of the monitored microorganisms, compared to chlorine (Siroli et al., 2015). The storage of fresh-cut iceberg lettuce with a sachet containing oregano essential oil microparticles displayed promising results. The growth of yeast and molds was significantly reduced, particularly with 3/5 to 5/5 (w/w) oil/polyvinyl alcohol protportions used in the sachet, during 5 days at 20°C. An interesting aspect explored in this study was the effect of a high relative humidity (85%), which improved the release of oregano essential oil from sachet to lettuce. However, the growth of mesophilic aerobic bacteria was not affected by the sachet at any concentration of oregano oil (Chang et al., 2017).

Table 4. Preservative effect of oregano on storage stability of bread and food of vegetable origin

Food	Strategic use	Study conditions	Preservative effect	Reference
Vegetables				
Fresh lamb's lettuce	Washing with oregano essential oil solution (250 mg/L)	8 days at 6°C; MA (artificial ordinary atmosphere)	Similar effect on total aerobic bacteria, LAB and yeasts as observed for control sanitizing solution (120 mg/L chlorine)	(Siroli et al., 2015)
Fresh-cut iceberg lettuce	Packaging with essential oil sachet (1/5-5/5 oil/PVA)	5 days at 20°C	Inhibition of Y&M growth	(Chang et al., 2017)
Fresh cut apricot	Coating with essential oil film (1-6%)	8 days at 4°C	Inhibition of Y&M growth; higher scores for odor and overall acceptability on the last day of storage;	(Hashemi et al., 2017)
Fresh apple pieces	Coating with essential oil solution (0.1 and 0.5%)	21 days at 4°C	Inhibition of psychrophilic, Y&M;	(Rojas-Graü et al., 2007)
Fresh strawberries	Coating with essential oil solution (0.2%)	14 days at 4°C	Reducing the percentages of fruits showing decay	(Vu et al., 2011)
Fresh Cherry tomatoes	Package containing essential oil (5.5%)	10 days at 21°C	Reducing the percentage of fruits showing decay	(Lafuente, Nerin, and Batlle, 2010)
Bread				
Sliced bread	Nano-emulsion with essential oil (4%)	15 days at room temperature	Inhibition of Y&M growth	(Otoni et al., 2014)
Sliced bread	Coating with methylcellulose and essential oil (4%) film	15 days at room temperature	Inhibition of Y&M growth	(Otoni et al., 2014)
Sliced bread	Packaging with essential oil sachet (0.04, 0.08, and 0.12%)	15 days at room temperature	No effect	(Passarinho et al., 2014)

MA: modified atmosphere; LAB: lactic acid bacteria; PVA: polyvinyl alcohol.

Oregano essential oil has been considered for its effect on foodborne pathogens. When compared to other essential oils, it showed a lower afficacy than tea tree (*Melaleuca alternifolia*) or rosemary (*Rosmarinus officinalis*) oils (Alvarez, Ponce, and Moreira, 2013). In another study, the antimicrobial effect of oregano essential oil (20 discs with 10 μl/disc) was demonstrated on both pathogen (*E. coli* O157:H7, *Salmonella* Typhimurium, *Listeria monocytogenes*, *S. aureus*, and *Bacillus cereus*) and spoilage microorganisms. To preserve fresh cabbage, the oil was applied by the disc volatilization method, which is similar to sachet technology, and combined with modified atmosphere (100% CO_2) packaging (Hyun et al., 2015).

Regarding the use of oregano as preservative in fruits, a film incorporated with oregano essential oil (1-6%) inhibited the growth of Y&M of fresh-cut apricot during 8 days at 4°C. The effect was concentration-dependent, wherein higher oregano essential oil concentration led to higher inhibition levels. In addition, the evaluation of odor and overall acceptability after 8 days revealed that apricots coated with oregano film received higher scores than control samples, in a concentration-dependent manner. However, no significant inhibitory effect on mesophilic bacteria was indicated by authors (Hashemi et al., 2017). A similar study was carried with fresh apple pieces indicating that oregano essential oil (0.1 and 0.5%) film prevented the growth of psychrophilic and Y&M in a concentration-dependent manner. The experiment was carried out for 21 days at 4°C and also indicated that ethylene production (a trigger of climacteric fruit ripening) was reduced with oregano essential oil film throughout storage time. However, the authors mentioned that sensory properties of apple coated with oregano essential oil received low scores by panelists, particularly for overall acceptance (Rojas-Graü et al., 2007).

The shelf life of strawberries was also improved by coating these fruits with oregano essential oil (0.2%). The authors observed that the percentage of fruits showing decay was reduced in comparison to non-coated fruits during 14 days of storage at 4°C (Vu et al., 2011). Likewise, cherry tomatoes were protected by packaging containers composed of oregano essential oil active paper. The percentage of tomatoes showing showing decay during 10 days of storage at 21°C was significantly reduced in comparison to control (Lafuente, Nerin, and Batlle, 2010).

The use of oregano essential oil was assayed to inhibit the growth of foodborne pathogens in ready-to-eat fruits and vegetables. In their study, Harich et al. (2018) used successfully two essential oil preparations sprayed on cranberries, pre-fried potatoes or fresh-cut red peppers to inhibit the development of *E. coli* O157:H7, *Salmonella* Tiphymurium and *L. monocytogenes*. However, the most efficient strategy seems to be a combination of treatments, as performed on ready-to-eat carrots, treated with essential oil, nisin and irradiation.

Although poorly explored, improving the shelf life of bakery products is another relevant example of oregano preservative effect. An interesting example explored the application of either nano-emulsion or methylcellulose film containing oregano essential oil to extend the shelf life of sliced bread. Both strategies were equally effective to prevent the growth of Y&M between 10th and 15th day of storage at room temperature (Otoni et al., 2014). Conversely, the use of sachets incorporated with oregano essential oil (0.04, 0.08, and 0.12%) did not show clear results regarding the inhibition of Y&M (Passarinho et al., 2014).

However, for fruits as well as for bakery products, a special attention has to be paid to sensory characteristics, possibly modified by the use of oregano extracts.

Cheese

Oregano can be an interesting preservative in dairy industry, particularly in the production of cheese (Table 5). The use of oregano essential oil (0.2 g/100 g) in flavored cream cheese improved the microbial stability by inhibiting the growth of total aerobic bacteria during 35 days at 5°C. Moreover, lipid oxidation was delayed by oregano essential oil and except for the characteristic aroma of oregano, sensory attributes of cream cheese were similar to conventional product (Olmedo, Nepote, and Grosso, 2013).

In another study about the impact of oregano origin (Compacto, Cordobes, Criollo, Mendocino; Argentine) on stability over storage of ricotta cheese, the inhibition of total aerobic bacteria during 30 days at 23°C was reported, regardless the origin of oregano. However, sensory attributes were affected in all cheese samples elaborated with oregano essential oil (0.05%) (Asensio et al., 2014). A complementary experiment with the same essential oil in cottage cheese indicated that the natural compounds delayed the production of lipid oxidative products during 30 days at 40°C. The authors also indicated that production of organic acids was also inhibited by adding oregano essential oil, particularly for oregano obtained from Cordobes and Criollo region (Asensio, Grosso, and Juliani, 2015).

Table 5. Preservative effect of oregano on storage stability of cheese

Food	Strategic use	Study conditions	Preservative effect	Reference
Flavored cream cheese	As ingredient (essential oil, 0.2%)	35 days at 5°C	Inhibition of total aerobic bacteria; improved oxidative stability	(Olmedo, Nepote, and Grosso, 2013)
Ricotta cheese	As ingredient (essential oil, 0.05%)	30 days at 23°C	Inhibition of total aerobic bacteria	(Asensio et al., 2014)
Cottage cheese	As ingredient (essential oil, 0.05%)	30 days at 40°C	Inhibition of lipid oxidation and production of organic acids	(Asensio, Grosso, and Juliani, 2015)
Low-fat cheese	Coating with essential oil nano-emulsion (1.5-2.5%)	15 days at 4°C	Inhibition of Y&M growth; partial inhibition of psychrophilic bacteria growth; preservation of color	(Artiga-Artigas, Acevedo-Fani, and Martín-Belloso, 2017)

MA: modified atmosphere; LAB: lactic acid bacteria; PVA: polyvinyl alcohol.

The potential application of oregano essential oil in a coating matrix to improve storage stability of cheese was explored. Oregano essential oil nano-emulsion (1.5, 2.0, and 2.5%) coating a low-fat cheese delayed the growth of Y&M and psychrophilic bacteria during 5 days at 4°C. While the 2.5% treatment delayed the growth of psychrophilic bacteria for 5 days and inhibited the growth of Y&M throughout storage time, 1.5% and 2.0% treatments did not display the same protective effect. It's worth mentioning that cheese color was equally preserved by all treatments with oregano essential oil (Artiga-Artigas, Acevedo-Fani, and Martín-Belloso, 2017).

Salad Dressing and Oils

Oils of animal or plant origin are important sources of nutrients in modern diets. In order to prevent loss of quality during storage, particularly due to oxidative reactions on lipid fraction, oregano (either as a dry spice, a concentrated extracted or essential oil) has been explored to delay, at some extent, the progression of oxidation reactions. It is important mentioning, the unsaturated fatty acids in fish oil are oxidized during storage leading to important alteration regarding the formation of derived products (Table 6).

In this context, ground oregano was used to prevent the formation of peroxides of Mackerel (*Scomber scombrus*) oil for at least 30 days at 40°C (Tsimidou, Papavergou, and Boskou, 1995). A similar outcome was reported for oregano essential oil added to extra-virgin olive oil stored for 28 days at room temperature and exposed to lightness or darkness wherein both primary and secondary lipid oxidation production were reduced. In addition, the formation of free fatty acids, usually from triglycerides, was inhibited during storage at room temperature. However, this study revealed that storage at 60°C (in darkness) did not prevent the chemical deterioration of olive oil, which was similar to those of control oil without antioxidant. However, the generation of free fatty acids was inhibited in samples stored at 60°C (Asensio, Nepote, and Grosso, 2011). Differently, the study about the protective effect of oregano concentrated extract towards the oxidative stability of Menhaden oil indicated that nutritionally relevant long chain omega-3 fatty acids DHA and EPA were slightly protected. Both DHA and EPA contents were reduced to 16 and 18% of its initial concentration (Bhale et al., 2007).

Another relevant food matrix to explore the protective effect of oregano is salad dressing, which is an oil-in-water emulsified product mainly composed of oil, water, a thickening agent, herbs and spices. As observed for oils from animal and plant origin, the effect of oregano is controversial. A study explored three strategies to incorporate oregano active components into a salad dressing: (i) by direct incorporation of a concentrated extract into the salad dressing (0.06% of oil content), (ii) by mixing the extract in olive oil (3%) and (iii) by elaborating liposomes (by ultrasonification and microfluidization techniques) prior to salad dressing preparation. The authors indicated that storage in darkness at both room temperature and at 60°C delayed the formation of hydroperoxides in salad dressings for the first two strategies. However, when salad dressing was exposed to light during storage, no protective effect was observed. Linoleic acid content and production of hydroperoxides and hexanal were similar to that observed for control (without antioxidant) during storage. The third strategy (liposomes with concentrated extract) prevented the formation of hexanal after 30 days at 40°C but hydroperoxide generation was not influenced (Abdalla and Roozen, 2001). A protective effect of oregano, as a dry spice, was also observed in a mayonnaise-based salad composed of mayonnaise (63% soybean oil), tuna, maize, peas, bell pepper, and onion. In this matrix, oregano prevented the formation of volatile compounds associated with lipids (2-pentenal and pentanal) during 57 days at 2°C. The use of 1% oregano dry spice lso induced the formation of hydroperoxides during storage (Sørensen, Nielsen, and Jacobsen, 2010).

Table 6. Preservative effect of oregano on storage stability of salad dressing and oils

Food	Strategic use	Study conditions	Preservative effect	Reference
Mackerel oil	Adding as dry spicy (0.5%)	Up to 50 days at 40°C	Inhibition of peroxide formation	(Tsimidou, Papavergou, and Boskou, 1995)
Extra-Virgin Olive Oil	Adding essential oil (0.05%)	28 days at room temperature or 60°C, in darkness or exposed to light	Inhibition of and primary and secondary oxidation products and free fatty acid formation in darkness and exposed to light; minimal protective effect during storage at 60°C	(Asensio, Nepote, and Grosso, 2011)
Menhaden Oil	Adding concentrated extract (1, 2.5, and 5%)	5 days at 60°C	Low protective effect of DHA and EPA from oxidation	(Bhale et al., 2007)
Salad dressing	As ingredient (concentrated extract, 0.06% in oil content) or in olive oil (concentrated extract, 3%)	6 months at room temperature in darkness, 30 days at 40°C in darkness and 12 weeks at room temperature (exposed to light	Inhibition of hydroperoxide formation for samples storage in darkness; non-protective effect on hydroperoxide and hexanal formation, degradation of linoleic acid exposed to light	(Abdalla and Roozen, 2001)
	As ingredient in liposomes produced by ultrasonification and microfluidisation technique (concentrated extract, 3%)	30 days at 40°C (dark)	Inhibition of hexanal formation for both liposome production technique; non-protective effect on hydroperoxides formation	(Abdalla and Roozen, 2001)
Mayonnaise-based salad	As ingredient (dry spice, 1%)	57 days at 2°C (dark)	Inhibition of 2-pentenal and pentanal formation; induction of peroxide production	(Sørensen, Nielsen, and Jacobsen, 2010)

MA: modified atmosphere; LAB: lactic acid bacteria.

CONCLUSION

The preservative components of oregano are of great value for food industry and researchers in order to improve the stability and shelf life of fresh, minimally-processed and processed food. The use of essential oils, mainly thymol and carvacrol, is directly associated with protective effects against the growth of spoilage microorganisms and the evolution of oxidative reactions. Phenolic compounds also play an important role in the preservation of food. However, the protective effect is dependent on the food matrix, the technology to apply preservative agents and storage conditions. Understanding the interactions between these factors is essential to achieve successful shelf life improvement. Oregano active components can enhance the storage time of several foods, but additional technologies may be required to prevent premature quality decay. A relevant consideration about the influence of such factors is the use of modified atmosphere in meat and meat products storage and the prevention against high temperature in edible oils.

However, the impact of oregano, either by essential oil, concentrated extract or dried spice, on the sensory properties of food may reduce the acceptance of food. It is important to prevent deleterious effects of oregano active components on the sensory attributes of food. Some studies reported that oregano characteristic flavor/aroma or spice flavor/aroma led to significant reduction of product acceptance and sensory attributes. This scenario highlights the importance of proper characterization of sensory attributes in the use of oregano preservative components in food. In this sense, the most promising approch to explore the preservative effect of oregano active components is to apply a coating layer or wrapping with a film, which can limit quality decay and reduce the impact on sensory attributes of food.

The development of further studies is suggested to overcome current hurdles as low level of information in some food matrix, such as baked food, fruits and vegetables; explore the possible advantages/disadvantages of emerging processing technologies (particularly the non-thermal technologies) and preserve the natural nutritional value of food; explore the potential contribution on functional food (in order to improve the stability of natural or intentionally added functional component); and finally evaluate the economical relevance of oregano preservative components in the processing cost and product final price.

ACKNOWLEDGMENTS

Paulo E. S. Munekata acknowledges postdoctoral fellowship support from Ministry of Economy and Competitiveness (MINECO, Spain) "Juan de la Cierva" program (FJCI-2016-29486). José M. Lorenzo and Paulo E. S. Munekata are members of the MARCARNE network, funded by CYTED (ref.116RT0503).

REFERENCES

Abdalla, Ahmed E, and Jacques P Roozen. 2001. "The Effects of Stabilised Extracts of Sage and Oregano on the Oxidation of Salad Dressings." *European Food Research and Technology* 212: 551–60. https://doi.org/10.1007/s002170100288.

Aboukhalid, Kaoutar, Nathalie Machon, Josie Lambourdière, Jawad Abdelkrim, Mohamed Bakha, Ahmed Douaik, Grazyna Korbecka-Glinka, et al. 2017. "Analysis of Genetic Diversity and Population Structure of the Endangered Origanum Compactum from Morocco, Using SSR Markers: Implication for Conservation." *Biological Conservation* 212: 172–82. https://doi.org/10.1016/j.biocon.2017.05.030.

Aloui, Hajer, and Khaoula Khwaldia. 2016. "Natural Antimicrobial Edible Coatings for Microbial Safety and Food Quality Enhancement." *Comprehensive Reviews in Food Science and Food Safety* 15: 1080–1103. https://doi.org/10.1111/1541-4337.12226.

Alvarez, María V, Alejandra G Ponce, and R Moreira. 2013. "Antimicrobial Efficiency of Chitosan Coating Enriched with Bioactive Compounds to Improve the Safety of Fresh Cut Broccoli." *LWT - Food Science and Technology* 50 (1): 78–87. https://doi.org/10.1016/j.lwt.2012.06.021.

Appendini, Paola, and Joseph H Hotchkiss. 2002. "Review of Antimicrobial Food Packaging." *Innovative Food Science & Emerging Technologies* 3: 113–26.

Artiga-Artigas, María, Alejandra Acevedo-Fani, and Olga Martín-Belloso. 2017. "Improving the Shelf Life of Low-Fat Cut Cheese Using Nanoemulsion-Based Edible Coatings Containing Oregano Essential Oil and Mandarin Fiber." *Food Control* 76: 1–12. https://doi.org/10.1016/j.foodcont.2017.01.001.

Asensio, Claudia M, Nelson R Grosso, and H Rodolfo Juliani. 2015. "Quality Preservation of Organic Cottage Cheese Using Oregano Essential Oils." *LWT - Food Science and Technology* 60 (2): 664–71. https://doi.org/10.1016/j.lwt.2014.10.054.

Asensio, Claudia M, Valeria Nepote, and Nelson R Grosso. 2011. "Chemical Stability of Extra-Virgin Olive Oil Added with Oregano Essential Oil." *Journal of Food Science* 76 (7): S445–50. https://doi.org/10.1111/j.1750-3841.2011.02332.x.

Asensio, Claudia M, Mercedes Oliva, Mirta S Demo, and Nelson R Grosso. 2014. "Sensory and Bio-Chemical Preservation of Ricotta Cheese Using Natural Products." *International Journal of Food Science and Technology* 49: 2692–2702. https://doi.org/10.1111/ijfs.12604.

Atrea, I, Aikaterini Papavergou, Ioannis Amvrosiadis, and Ioannis N. Savvaidis. 2009. "Combined Effect of Vacuum-Packaging and Oregano Essential Oil on the Shelf-Life of Mediterranean Octopus (Octopus Vulgaris) from the Aegean Sea Stored at 4°C." *Food Microbiology* 26 (2): 166–72. https://doi.org/10.1016/j.fm.2008.10.005.

Bastarrachea, Luis, Sumeet Dhawan, and Shyam S Sablani. 2011. "Engineering Properties of Polymeric-Based Antimicrobial Films for Food Packaging." *Food Engineering Reviews* 3 (2): 79–93. https://doi.org/10.1007/s12393-011-9034-8.

Bhale, S D B, Z Xu, W Prinyawiwatkul, J M King, and J S G Odber. 2007. "Oregano and Rosemary Extracts Inhibit Oxidation of Long-Chain n-3 Fatty Acids in Menhaden Oil." *Journal of Food Science* 72 (9): 504–8. https://doi.org/10.1111/j.1750-3841.2007.00569.x.

Cappellini, Benedetta, and Elizabeth Parsons. 2014. "Constructing the Culinary Consumer: Transformative and Reflective Processes in Italian Cookbooks." *Consumption Markets & Culture* 17 (1): 71–99. https://doi.org/10.1080/10253866.2012.701893.

Cardello, Armand V. 1995. "Food Quallty: Relativity, Context and Consumer Expectations." *Food Quality and Preference* 6 (3): 163–70.

Carocho, Márcio, Maria Filomena Barreiro, Patricia Morales, and Isabel C F R Ferreira. 2014. "Adding Molecules to Food, Pros and Cons: A Review on Synthetic and Natural Food Additives." *Comprehensive Reviews in Food Science and Food Safety* 13: 377–99. https://doi.org/10.1111/1541-4337.12065.

Carrión-Granda, Ximena, Idoya Fernández-Pan, Isabel Jaime, Jordi Rovira, and Juan I Maté. 2016. "Improvement of the Microbiological Quality of Ready-to-Eat Peeled Shrimps (Penaeus Vannamei) by the Use of Chitosan Coatings." *International Journal of Food Microbiology* 232: 144–49. https://doi.org/10.1016/j.ijfoodmicro.2016.05.029.

Catarino, Marcelo D, Jorge M Alves-Silva, Rui P Fernandes, Maria J Gonçalves, Lígia R Salgueiro, Marta F Henriques, and Susana M Cardoso. 2017. "Development and Performance of Whey Protein Active Coatings with Origanum Virens Essential Oils in the Quality and Shelf Life Improvement of Processed Meat Products." *Food Control* 80: 273–80. https://doi.org/10.1016/j.foodcont.2017.03.054.

Chaleshtori, Farhad S, and Reza S Chaleshtori. 2017. "Antimicrobial Activity of Chitosan Incorporated with Lemon and Oregano Essential Oils on Broiler Breast Meat during Refrigerated Storage." *Nutrition & Food Science* 47 (3): 306–17. https://doi.org/10.1108/NFS-08-2016-0123.

Chang, Yoonjee, Inyoung Choi, Ah Reum Cho, and Jaejoon Han. 2017. "Reduction of Dickeya Chrysanthemi on Fresh-Cut Iceberg Lettuce Using Antimicrobial Sachet Containing Microencapsulated Oregano Essential Oil." *LWT - Food Science and Technology* 82: 361–68. https://doi.org/10.1016/j.lwt.2017.04.043.

Chun, Sung-Sook, Dhiraj A Vattem, Yuan-Tong Lin, and Kalidas Shetty. 2005. "Phenolic Antioxidants from Clonal Oregano (Origanum Vulgare) with Antimicrobial Activity against Helicobacter Pylori." *Process Biochemistry* 40: 809–16. https://doi.org/10.1016/j.procbio.2004.02.018.

Damašius, Jonas, Petras Rimantas Venskutonis, Jordi Rovira, Javier González, Lucia González, and Rimantė Vinauskienė. 2009. "Characterisation of Oregano Water Extracts and Their Effect on the Quality Characteristics of Cooked Pork." *International Journal of Food Science and Technology* 44: 394–401. https://doi.org/10.1111/j.1365-2621.2008.01781.x.

Exarchou, Vassiliki, Nikolaos Nenadis, María Tsimidou, Ioannis P. Gerothanassis, Anastassios Troganis, and Dimitrios Boskou. 2002. "Antioxidant Activities and Phenolic Composition of Extracts from Greek Oregano, Greek Sage, and Summer Savory." *Journal of Agricultural and Food Chemistry*, 5294–99. https://doi.org/10.1021/jf020408a.

Fernandes, Rafaella De P P, Marco A Trindade, Jose M Lorenzo, and Marize P De Melo. 2018. "Assessment of the Stability of Sheep Sausages with the Addition of Different Concentrations of Origanum Vulgare Extract during Storage." *Meat Science* 137: 244–57. https://doi.org/10.1016/j.meatsci.2017.11.018.

Fernandes, Rafaella De P P, Marco A Trindade, Jose M Lorenzo, Paulo E S Munekata, and Mariza P. De Melo. 2016. "Effects of Oregano Extract on Oxidative, Microbiological and Sensory Stability of Sheep Burgers Packed in Modified Atmosphere." *Food Control* 63: 65–75. https://doi.org/10.1016/j.foodcont.2015.11.027.

Fernandes, Rafaella De P P, Marco A Trindade, Fernando G Tonin, Silvana M P Pugine, Cesar G Lima, Jose M Lorenzo, and Marize P De Melo. 2017. "Evaluation of Oxidative Stability of Lamb Burger with Origanum Vulgare Extract." *Food Chemistry* 233: 101–9. https://doi.org/10.1016/j.foodchem.2017.04.100.

Frangos, L, Nikoletta Pyrgotou, Vasiliki I Giatrakou, Athina G Ntzimani, and Ioannis N Savvaidis. 2010. "Combined Effects of Salting, Oregano Oil and Vacuum-Packaging on the Shelf-Life of Refrigerated Trout Fillets." *Food Microbiology* 27 (1): 115–21. https://doi.org/10.1016/j.fm.2009.09.002.

Giatrakou, Vasiliki I, Sonia Kykkidou, Aikaterini Papavergou, Michael G Kontominas, and Ioannis N Savvaidis. 2008. "Potential of Oregano Essential Oil and MAP to Extend the Shelf Life of Fresh Swordfish: A Comparative Study with Ice Storage." *Journal of Food Science* 73 (4): 167–73. https://doi.org/10.1111/j.1750-3841.2008.00729.x.

Goulas, Antonios E, and Michael G Kontominas. 2007. "Effect of Light Salting, Modified Atmosphere Packaging and Oregano Essential Oil on the Shelf-Life of Sea Bream (Sparus Aurata): Biochemical and Sensory Attributes." *Food Chemistry* 100: 287–96. https://doi.org/10.1016/j.foodchem.2005.09.045.

Grunert, Klaus G, Lone Bredahl, and Karen Brunsø. 2004. "Consumer Perception of Meat Quality and Implications for Product Development in the Meat Sector - a Review." *Meat Science* 66: 259–72. https://doi.org/10.1016/S0309-1740(03)00130-X.

Gutierrez, Jorge A, Catherine Barry-Ryan, and Paula Bourke. 2008. "The Antimicrobial Efficacy of Plant Essential Oil Combinations and Interactions with Food Ingredients." *International Journal of Food Microbiology* 124: 91–97. https://doi.org/10.1016/j.ijfoodmicro.2008.02.028.

Harich, Mehdi, Behnoush Maherani, Stephane Salmieri, and Monique Lacroix. 2018. "Evaluation of Antibacterial Activity of Two Natural Bio-Preservatives Formulations on Freshness and Sensory Quality of Ready to Eat (RTE) Foods." *Food Control* 85: 29–41. https://doi.org/10.1016/j.foodcont.2017.09.018.

Harpaz, Sheenan, Larisa Glatman, Vladimir Drabkin, and Alexander G Gelman. 2003. "Effects of Herbal Essential Oils Used to Extend the Shelf Life of Freshwater-Reared Asian Sea Bass Fish (Lates Calcarifer)." *Journal of Food Protection* 66 (3): 410–17.

Hashemi, Seyed M Bagher, Amin Mousavi Khaneghah, Maryam Ghaderi Ghahfarrokhi, and Eş Ismail. 2017. "Basil-Seed Gum Containing Origanum Vulgare Subsp. Viride Essential Oil as Edible Coating for Fresh Cut Apricots." *Postharvest Biology and Technology* 125: 26–34. https://doi.org/10.1016/j.postharvbio.2016.11.003.

Haute, Sam Van, Katleen Raes, Paul Van Der Meeren, and Imca A. Sampers. 2016. "The Effect of Cinnamon, Oregano and Thyme Essential Oils in Marinade on the Microbial Shelf Life of Fish and Meat Products." *Food Control* 68: 30–39. https://doi.org/10.1016/j.foodcont.2016.03.025.

Hyun, Jeong-Eun, Young-Min Bae, Jae-Hyun Yoon, and Sun-Young Lee. 2015. "Preservative Effectiveness of Essential Oils in Vapor Phase Combined with Modified Atmosphere Packaging against Spoilage Bacteria on Fresh Cabbage." *Food Control* 51: 307–13. https://doi.org/10.1016/j.foodcont.2014.11.030.

Jouki, Mohammad, Farideh T Yazdi, Seyed Ali Mortazavi, Arash Koocheki, and Naimeh Khazaei. 2014. "Effect of Quince Seed Mucilage Edible Films Incorporated with Oregano or Thyme Essential Oil on Shelf Life Extension of Refrigerated Rainbow Trout Fillets." *International Journal of Food Microbiology* 174: 88–97. https://doi.org/10.1016/j.ijfoodmicro.2014.01.001.

Lafuente, Angel Rodriguez, Cristina Nerin, and Ramon Batlle. 2010. "Active Paraffin-Based Paper Packaging for Extending the Shelf Life of Cherry Tomatoes." *Journal of Agricultural and Food Chemistry* 58: 6780–86. https://doi.org/10.1021/jf100728n.

Lorenzo, José M, Ramón Batlle, and María Gómez. 2014. "Extension of the Shelf-Life of Foal Meat with Two Antioxidant Active Packaging Systems." *LWT - Food Science and Technology* 59 (1): 181–88. https://doi.org/10.1016/j.lwt.2014.04.061.

Mejlholm, Ole, and Paw Dalgaard. 2002. "Antimicrobial Effect of Essential Oils on the Seafood Spoilage Micro-Organism Photobacterium Phosphoreum in Liquid Media and Fish Products." *Letters in Applied Microbiology* 34: 27–31. https://doi.org/10.1046/j.1472-765X.2002.01033.x.

Menezes, Natielle M C., Wiaslan F Martins, Daniel A Longhi, and Gláucia M F Aragão. 2018. "Modeling the Effect of Oregano Essential Oil on Shelf-Life Extension of Vacuum-Packed Cooked Sliced Ham." *Meat Science* 139: 113–19.

Mexis, Stamatios F, Eirini Chouliara, and Michael G Kontominas. 2009. "Combined Effect of an Oxygen Absorber and Oregano Essential Oil on Shelf Life Extension of Rainbow Trout Fillets Stored at 4°C." *Food Microbiology* 26 (6): 598–605. https://doi.org/10.1016/j.fm.2009.04.002.

Moraes-lovison, Marília, Luís F P Marostegan, Marina S Peres, Isabela F Menezes, Marluci Ghiraldi, Rodney A F Rodrigues, Andrezza M Fernandes, and Samantha C Pinho. 2017. "Nanoemulsions Encapsulating Oregano Essential Oil: Production,

Stability, Antibacterial Activity and Incorporation in Chicken pâTé." *LWT - Food Science and Technology* 77: 233–40.

Olmedo, Rubén H, Valeria Nepote, and Nelson R Grosso. 2013. "Preservation of Sensory and Chemical Properties in Flavoured Cheese Prepared with Cream Cheese Base Using Oregano and Rosemary Essential Oils." *LWT - Food Science and Technology* 53 (2): 409–17. https://doi.org/10.1016/j.lwt.2013.04.007.

Otoni, Caio G, Paula J P Espitia, Roberto J Avena-bustillos, and Tara H Mchugh. 2016. "Trends in Antimicrobial Food Packaging Systems: Emitting Sachets and Absorbent Pads." *Food Research International* 83: 60–73. https://doi.org/10.1016/j.foodres.2016.02.018.

Otoni, Caio G, Silvania F O Pontes, Eber A A Medeiros, and Nilda F F Soares. 2014. "Edible Films from Methylcellulose and Nanoemulsions of Clove Bud (Syzygium Aromaticum) and Oregano (Origanum Vulgare) Essential Oils as Shelf Life Extenders for Sliced Bread." *Journal of Agricultural and Food Chemistry* 62 (22): 5214–19. https://doi.org/10.1021/jf501055f.

Passarinho, Amanda Tafuri Paniago, Natália Fialho Dias, Geany Peruch Camilloto, Renato Souza Cruz, Caio Gomide Otoni, Allan Robledo Fialho Moraes, and Nilda Fátima Ferreira Soares. 2014. "Sliced Bread Preservation Through Oregano Essential Oil-Containing Sachet." *Journal of Food Process Engineering* 37: 53–62. https://doi.org/10.1111/jfpe.12059.

Petrou, Stavros, Maria I. Tsiraki, Vasiliki I. Giatrakou, and Ioannis N. Savvaidis. 2012. "Chitosan Dipping or Oregano Oil Treatments, Singly or Combined on Modified Atmosphere Packaged Chicken Breast Meat." *International Journal of Food Microbiology* 156 (3): 264–71. https://doi.org/10.1016/j.ijfoodmicro.2012.04.002.

Rico, Daniel, Ana B Martín-Diana, José M Barat, and Catherine Barry-Ryan. 2007. "Extending and Measuring the Quality of Fresh-Cut Fruit and Vegetables: A Review." *Trends in Food Science & Technology* 18: 373–86. https://doi.org/10.1016/j.tifs.2007.03.011.

Rodriguez-Garcia, Isela, Brenda A Silva-Espinoza, Luis A Ortega-Ramírez, Juan M Leyva, Mohammed W Siddiqui, Manuel R Cruz-Valenzuela, Gustavo A González-Águilar, and Jesús F Ayala-Zavala. 2016. "Oregano Essential Oil as an Antimicrobial and Antioxidant Additive in Food Products." *Critical Reviews in FoodScience and Nutrition* 56: 1717–27. https://doi.org/10.1080/10408398.2013.800832.

Rojas-Graü, Maria A, Rosa M Raybaudi-Massilia, Robert C Soliva-fortuny, Roberto J Avena-Bustillos, Tara H McHugh, and Olga Martín-Belloso. 2007. "Apple Puree-Alginate Edible Coating as Carrier of Antimicrobial Agents to Prolong Shelf-Life of Fresh-Cut Apples." *Postharvest Biology and Technology* 45: 254–64. https://doi.org/10.1016/j.postharvbio.2007.01.017.

Sánchez-Escalante, Armida, Djamel Djenane, Gastón Torrescano, José A. Beltrán, and Pedro Roncalés. 2003. "Antioxidant Action of Borage, Rosemary, Oregano, and

Ascorbic Acid in Beef Patties Packaged in Modified Atmosphere." *Journal of Food Science* 68 (1): 339–44.

Sanjuás-Rey, Minia, Parastoo Pourashour, Jorge Barros-Velázquez, and Santiago P. Aubourg. 2012. "Effect of Oregano and Thyme Essential Oils on the Microbiological and Chemical Quality of Refrigerated (4°C) Ready-to-Eat Squid Rings." *International Journal of Food Science and Technology* 47: 1439–47. https://doi.org/10.1111/j.1365-2621.2012.02991.x.

Shan, Bin, Yizhong Z Cai, Mei Sun, and Harold Corke. 2005. "Antioxidant Capacity of 26 Spice Extracts and Characterization of Their Phenolic Constituents." *Journal of Agricultural and Food Chemistry* 53: 7749–59. https://doi.org/10.1021/jf051513y.

Siroli, Lorenzo, Francesca Patrignani, Diana I Serrazanetti, Silvia Tappi, Pietro Rocculi, Fausto Gardini, and Rosalba Lanciotti. 2015. "Natural Antimicrobials to Prolong the Shelf-Life of Minimally Processed Lamb's Lettuce." *Postharvest Biology and Technology* 103: 35–44. https://doi.org/10.1016/j.postharvbio.2015.02.016.

Soni, Arvind, Kandeepan Gurunathan, Sanjod K. Mendiratta, Suman Talukder, Rohit K. Jaiswal, and Heena Sharma. 2018. "Effect of Essential Oils Incorporated Edible Film on Quality and Storage Stability of Chicken Patties at Refrigeration Temperature (4 ± 1°C)." *Journal of Food Science and Technology* 55 (9): 3538–46. https://doi.org/10.1007/s13197-018-3279-7.

Sørensen, Ann-dorit Moltke, Nina Skall Nielsen, and Charlotte Jacobsen. 2010. "Oxidative Stability of Fish Oil-Enriched Mayonnaise-Based Salads." *European Journal of Lipid Science and Technology*, 476–87. https://doi.org/10.1002/ejlt.200900180.

Tajkarimi, Mehrdad M, Salam A Ibrahim, and Dean O Cliver. 2010. "Antimicrobial Herb and Spice Compounds in Food." *Food Control* 21 (9): 1199–1218. https://doi.org/10.1016/j.foodcont.2010.02.003.

Tsimidou, María, Ekaterini J Papavergou, and Dimitrios G Boskou. 1995. "Evaluation of Oregano Antioxidant Activity in Mackerel Oil." *Food Research International* 28 (4): 431–33.

Vallverdú-Queralt, Anna, Jorge Regueiro, Miriam Martínez-Huélamo, José F R Alvarenga, Leonel N Leal, and Rosa M Lamuela-Raventos. 2014. "A Comprehensive Study on the Phenolic Profile of Widely Used Culinary Herbs and Spices: Rosemary, Thyme, Oregano, Cinnamon, Cumin and Bay." *Food Chemistry* 154: 299–307. https://doi.org/10.1016/j.foodchem.2013.12.106.

Viuda-Martos, Manuel, Yolanda Ruíz-Navajas, Juana Fernández-López, and José A. Pérez-Alvarez. 2010. "Effect of Orange Dietary Fibre, Oregano Essential Oil and Packaging Conditions on Shelf-Life of Bologna Sausages." *Food Control* 21 (4): 436–43. https://doi.org/10.1016/j.foodcont.2009.07.004.

Vu, Khanh D, Robert G Hollingsworth, E Leroux, Stéphane Salmieri, and M Lacroix. 2011. "Development of Edible Bioactive Coating Based on Modified Chitosan for

Increasing the Shelf Life of Strawberries." *Food Research International* 44: 198–203. https://doi.org/10.1016/j.foodres.2010.10.037.

Wu, Jiulin, Shangying Ge, Hui Liu, Shuang Wang, Shanfei Chen, Jianhua Wang, Jianhua Li, and Qiqing Zhang. 2014. "Properties and Antimicrobial Activity of Silver Carp (Hypophthalmichthys Molitrix) Skin Gelatin-Chitosan Films Incorporated with Oregano Essential Oil for Fish Preservation." *Food Packaging and Shelf Life* 2 (1): 7–16. https://doi.org/10.1016/j.fpsl.2014.04.004.

In: Oregano: Properties, Uses and Health Benefits
Editor: Gema Nieto Martínez
ISBN: 978-1-53616-284-4

Chapter 5

OREGANO: HEALTH BENEFITS AND ITS USE AS FUNCTIONAL INGREDIENT IN MEAT PRODUCTS

Lorena Martínez, Gaspar Ros and Gema Nieto*
Department of Food Technology, Nutrition and Food Science,
University of Murcia, Murcia, Spain

ABSTRACT

Oregano (*Origanum vulgare*) is a perennial herb used as condiment, that mainly grows in the Mediterranean region. However, different varieties of oregano also grow around Europe, Asia and Latinoamerica, each one with distinctive compounds that has been tested in order to know their possible health benefits. This aromatic spice is rich in antioxidant compounds such as monoterpens as carvacol, flavonoids as epicatechine, epigallocatechine, catequin, rutin, kaempferol, and luteonin, and phenolic acids as rosmarinic. Due to its molecular structure, its regular consumption has reported several beneficial effects such as antioxidant, anti-inflammatory, anticancer, and antimicrobial. For these reasons, the use of oregano extract is a good strategy to use in meat products to replace synthetics additives. Additionally, this extract has a pleasant odour and flavour, so it could be used in order to improve the organoleptic quality of the meat products when it is added as ingredient. The present review exposes the health benefits provided by oregano consumption and the latest research about its use on meat, together new trends about its application as ingredient in functional meat products will be expossed.

Keywords: oregano, health, antioxidant, antimicrobial, antiinflammatory, functional, meat

---

* Corresponding Author's E-mail: gnieto@um.es.

INTRODUCTION

The use of natural ingredients obtained from fruits, vegetables, spices and herbs to keep the shelf life of meat and meat products has reported similar preservative properties compared to some synthetic additives without any damage to health after continued consumption (Ribeiro et al. 2019; Jian & Xiong, 2016; Ahmad, Don Bosco & Ahmad, 2014). Natural antioxidants prevent oxidation by different ways such as scavenging initiating radicals of oxidation chain, breaking oxidation chain reaction, decomposing peroxides or other secondary oxidation products, binding metal ions, and decreasing oxygen concentration.

Culinary herbs have been used in cuisine as food, flavorings, functional ingredients or even for medicinal purposes for centuries. One of the most commonly commercialized is the oregano, which is a perennial herb that includes at least 61 species of 17 genera belonging to six families. The *Lamiaceae* family is considered the most important group that contains the genus *Origanum* and involves Turkish and Greek types. The *Verbenaceae* family (genus *Lanata* and *Lippia*) is used for production of oregano herbs. While *Rubiaceae, Scrophulariaceae, Apiaceae*, and *Asteraceae* families have showed less importance. Generally, consumption of herb species classified as oregano has reported potential health benefits attributed to the phytochemicals and bioactive compounds that are present in their composition, such as phenolic acids and flavonoids with known antioxidant, anti-inflammatory and anti-cancer properties that are going to be exposed in the present review.

For this reason, oregano use as meat preservative would be an excellent functional ingredient to avoid food degradation in different matrix. For example, regular consumption of meat and meat products (two times per week or 500 – 600 g per week) has been described as necessary for a balanced diet due to it is an important source of high-quality proteins (20 – 25%), minerals (Fe – hemo form –, Mg, K, Zn, P and Se) and vitamins (A, thiamine, riboflavin, niacin, retinol, B6, folic acid, B12, D and K). However, manufactured meat products are usually rich in saturated fatty acids, synthetic additives, and other carcinogen compounds formed during their storage from lipid and protein oxidation or during their cooking from Maillard reaction. This kind of compounds are responsible for the statements of World Health Organization (WHO) in 2015, who classified processed meat as carcinogen (Group I) and red meat as possible carcinogen (Group 2A) (IARC, 2015).

In this way, the continued consumption of several synthetic preservatives as sulfites (E-220 to 228), nitrites (E-249 and E-250), BHT (Butyl hydroxytoluene, E-321) and BHA (Butylated hydroxyanisole, E-320) have reported a directly correlation with the chronic disease development such as asthma, hyperactivity or cancer (Soubra et al. 2007). Furthermore, lipid peroxidation produces reactive species (ROS) responsible for rancid flavour like hydroxyl radical, superoxide anion, ferryl and perferryl species, lipid peroxyl radical and secondary products such as Malondialdehyde (MDA) and 4-Hydroxynonenal

(4-HNE). This reaction occurs through the radical chain reaction mechanism and some factors can accelerate this process, such as oxygen presence, polyunsaturated fatty acids concentration, the deficit of natural antioxidants, high concentration of prooxidants agents, or free radical presence of salt added (NaCl) (Chang & Pan, 2008; Clough, 2014).

In addition, protein oxidation also has an important influence on meat quality produced by a covalent modification of protein structure induced by ROS or secondary oxidative stress products, which results in thiol groups loss, carbonyl formation, and reactions with aldehydes or ketones able to produce complexes between proteins and proteins, proteins and carbonyls, or proteins and lipids (Nieto et al. 2013). Moreover, this modification is also induced by hydroxyl radical (*OH) in presence of ROS or metals as Fe or Cu, which cause modifications of amino acids and increase the concentration of proteolytic enzymes and protein polymerization. These reactions modify the texture and toughens of the meat by the production of soluble aggregates that decrease the organoleptic quality and increase free radical generation which also has an impact on human health and safety product (Xiong, 2000; Xiong et al. 2010; Estévez, 2011).

The objective of this paper is to review the latest literature about oregano consumption benefits, its extraction, its used as natural preservative, and its application in meat and meat products with special emphasis on new trends and future perspectives in meat industry.

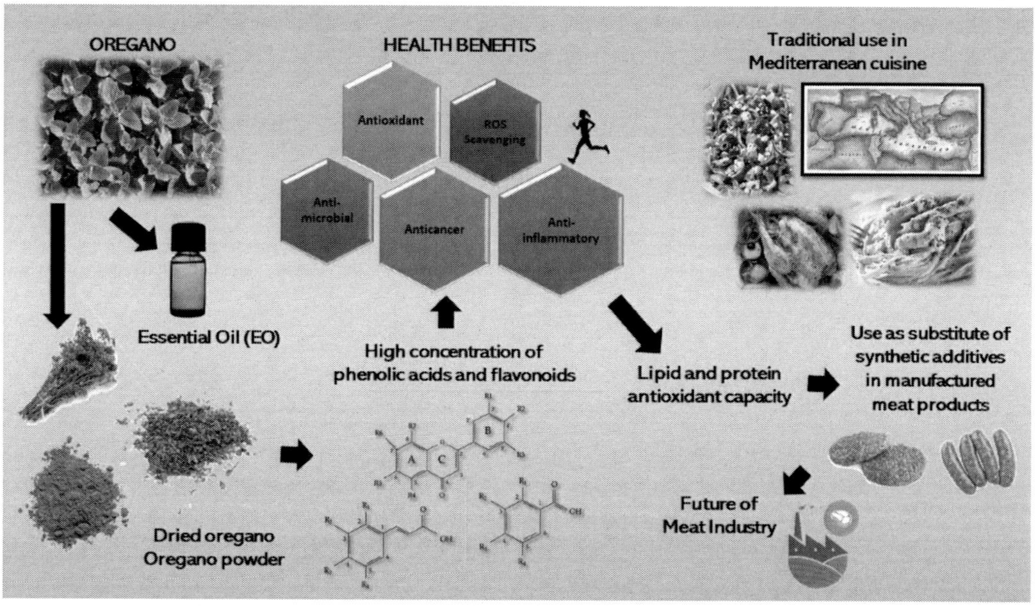

Figure 1. Schematic representation of oregano health benefits and its use a substitute of synthetic additives in meat products.

Oregano Composition

The chemical composition of oregano is divided in two groups: essential oils, such as thymol or *trans*-Sabinene hydrate, with hydrophobic properties, and phenolic compounds, such as phenolic acids (rosmarinic acid) and flavonoids (kaempferol, catechin or epocatechin, among others), with hydrophilic properties. Actually, phenolic compounds are responsible of characteristic flavour of this herb and the USDA database established the total phenolic content of this herb at 3789 mg GAE per 100 g product (Haytowitz & Bhagwat, 2010). This fact can be compared with current values obtained by us in once of our last study of 1439.7 mg GAE per 100 g oregano (water as solvent) (Figure 2) or 5500 mg GAE per 100 g oregano (70% methanol as solvent) showed by Skendi, Irakli & Chatzopoulou (2017). Previous reports from different oregano species have shown as the most common flavonoids found in oregano are flavones, flavonols, flavanones and flavanols.

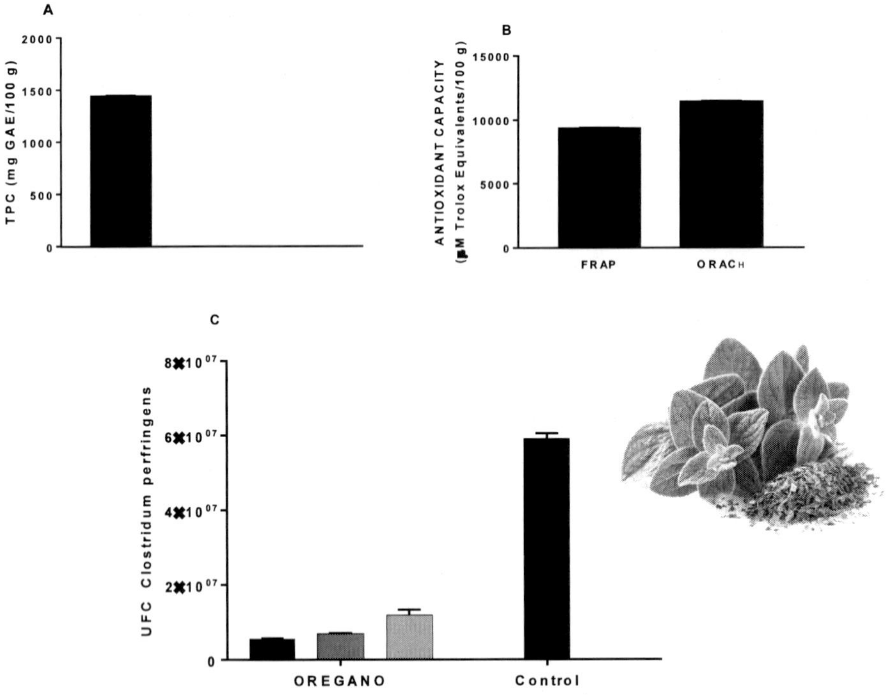

Figure 2. Total phenolic content (A), antioxidant (B) and antimicrobial activity *in vitro* against Clostridium perfringens (C) of Oreganum vulgare L. (1000, 500, 250 ppm). Control is the total normal growth of *C. perfringens* without any external agent.

Therefore, the most abundant phenolic acids are hydroxycinnamic, hydroxybenzoic acid, and their derivatives, while carvacrol (monoterpen), rosmarinic acid, apigenin, luteolin, catechin, and scutellarein are the major compounds identified (Figure 3) (Leyva et al. 2016; Gonçalves et al. 2017). In addition, it should be taken into account that the concentration of phenolic compounds in oregano depends on several factors like geographical localization, cultivar, weather, daylight, temperature, soil conditions, harvesting time, water availability, among others (Croteau, Kutchan & Lewis, 2015).

Similarly, the flavonoid and phenolic acids profile of each oregano specie can vary also depending on the oregano chemotypes within the same species of this herb, as it was reported by Gutiérrez-Grijalva et al. (2017) who developed an exhaustive review among the latest studies about flavonoid and phenolic acid contents from oregano and its essential oil. However, Skendi, Irakli & Chatzopoulou (2017) analysed the phenolic content in *Origanum vulgare ssp hirtum* L. from Greece and obtained 24 different compouds (phenolic acids and their derivatives, flavonoids and monoterpenes) detected by HPLC-DAD being carvacrol, rosmarinic acid, naringenin, rutin, caffeic acid, kaempferol, luteolin, epicatechin and epigallocatechine the most abundant compounds. Likewise, oregano essential oil is also rich in sesquiterpenoids, diterpenoids, triterpenoids, and cymyl-, sabinyl-, acyclic-, and bornyl- compounds, being *trans*-sabinene hydrate the most abundant compound in essential oils of four oregano-types from Argentina (Asensio et al. 2015).

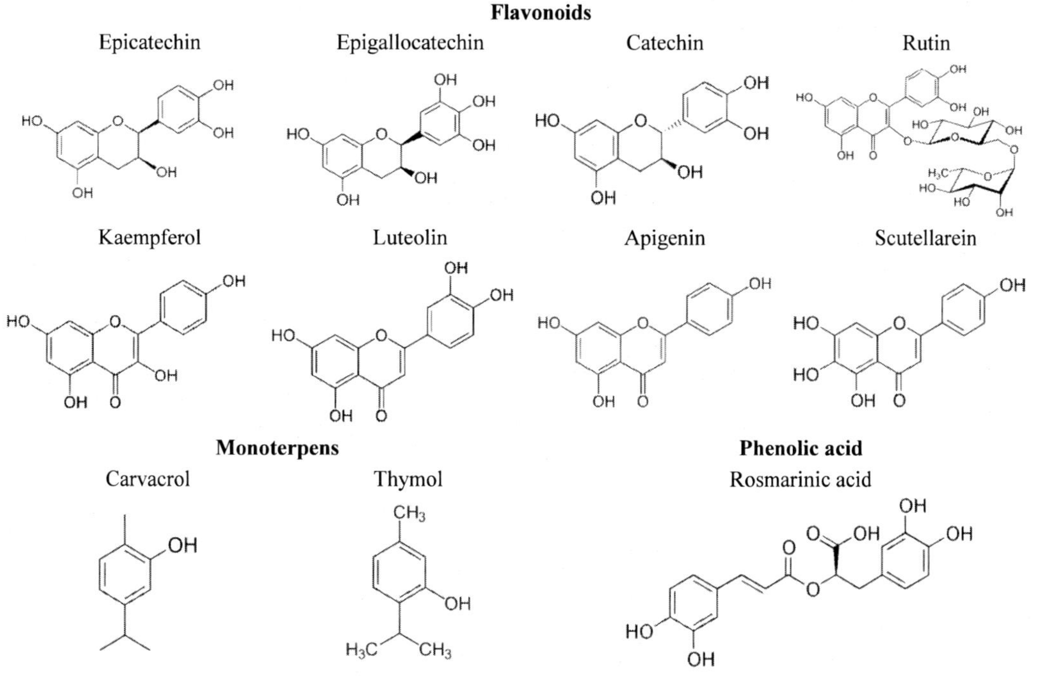

Figure 3. Principal phenolic compounds found in oregano.

Moreover, different results have been also obtained depending on the different solvent extraction used (water, methanol at different concentrations, buffers, acetone, ethyl acetate, hexane, etc.), which is not surprising knowing that there are so many species of oregano with different profiles of bioactive constituents and, consequently, beneficial effects.

Health Benefits

Oregano herb has been used for medicinal purposes since the ancient Greek and Roman, when its leaves were applied as antiseptic and to treat skin sores and aching muscles. Oregano has been also used in traditional medicines in order to treat illness such as asthma, cramping or digestion disorders. Currently, in some parts of Greece, an oregano infusion is still used as a traditional remedy against colds or to maitain general health (Shan et al. 2005). Oregano extracts, essential oils and individual compounds from this herb have demonstrated antioxidant, antiinflamatory, anticancer, and antimicrobial actions, which may contribute to the capacity to avoid human infections or to protect the cardiovascular and nervous systems by blood glucose and lipid modulation., which are going to be exposed in this section.

Oxidant balance in the human body helps to maintain the cell membrane integrity and functionality so, an imbalance is linked to impaired cell functions, cell death, impaired immunity and DNA damage which could conduct to cancer (Knight, 2000). For this reason, there is a correlation between increased dietary intake of antioxidants and a lower incidence of morbidity and mortality (epidemiological evidence showed by Desvasagayam et al. 2004). The antioxidant mechanisms of essential oils and phenolic compounds are based on its ability to donate a hydrogen, to quench free radicals by donation of an electron and its ability to delocalize the unpaired electron within the aromatic structure of the phenolic constituents (Fernández-Pachón et al. 2008).

Health benefits showed by application and consumption of oregano are showed in Table 1. Firstly, antioxidant capacity of oregano lies in the concentration of phenol and cathecol groups in the molecular structure of its principal monoterpens, flavonoids and phenolic acids compounds, able to scavenge free radicals through the oxidation of their hydroxyl group (·OH) before the formation of stable phenoxyl radicals (Rodríguez-García et al. 2015). Values of 11436 or 9355 μM Trolox Equivalents per 100 g were obtained by measurement of the hydrophilic oxygen radical absorbance capacity ($ORAC_H$) and ferric ion reducing antioxidant power assay (FRAP), respectively, in a current study presented by our group (Figure 2), where it was also showed the scavenging capacity against some radicals, DPPH and ABTS. However, in this research, water was the solvent used and oregano composition is divided in hydrophilic and hydrophobic compounds, which can explain higher values showed by other researchers using polar solvents as methanol (Lagouri & Alexandri, 2013; Yan et al. 2016; Skendi, Irakli & Charzopoulou, 2017). Due to the high quantity in phenolic compounds cited above, oregano has demonstrated radical scavenging action, supression of lipid peroxidation, inhibition of nitric oxide activity, and protection of DNA induced oxidant damage (Aherne, Kerry, O'Brien, 2007; Tsai et al. 2007; Zheng & Wang, 2001). This fact could explain also the antioxidative properties that oregano has reported as preservative in different food matrix, for example, meat and meat products. Currently, Gutiérrez-Grijalva et al. (2019) showed celular antioxidant capacity of polyphenols from oregano extracts with hypoglycemic and hypolipidemic properties by measurement of α-Glucosidase and α-Amylase inhibition assays.

On the other hand, oregano has shown an excellent antimicrobial activity against different bacteria, such as *Escherichia coli, Listeria monocytogenes, Bacillus enteritidis, Shigabacillus, Salmonella,* or *Staphylococcus aureus* (Rodríguez-García, 2015; Adame-Gallegos, Andrade-Ochoa & Nevarez-Moorillon, 2016). Oregano essential oil has proven to be the best antimicrobial agent compared to other species such as thyme, rosemary or sage (Rodríguez-García et al. 2015). In a similar way, in our last work, oregano was also the best antimicrobial agent against *Clostridium perfringens* in comparison with other water soluble extracts obtained from citrics, acerola or leafy green vegetables rich in nitrates such as, beet, lettuce, arugula, spinach, chard, celery, and watercress. Obtained results of this study showed as 250 ppm oregano inhibited in 80% the bacterial growth, 500 ppm in 90%, and 1000 ppm in 92% regarding to the Control (Figure 2). In parallel, Dutra et al. (2019) have also demonstrated the effectivenes of oregano (*Origanum vulgare*) essential oil against *Alicyclobacillus* spp., which was due to the high concentration of carvacrol (59.6%). This compound is responsible of great part of the antioxidant and antimicrobial properties of oregano, as it has also been cited above. In the same way, antiviral activity of mexican oregano essential oil (*Lippia graveolens)* was shown against animal and human viruses, such as acyclovirresistant herpes simplex virus type 1 (ACVR-HHV-1), acyclovir-sensitive HHV-1, human respiratory syncytial virus (HRSV), bovine herpesvirus type 2 (BoHV-2), and bovine viral diarrhoea virus (BVDV) (Pilau et al. 2011).

Furthermore, oregano has also reported to have antiinflammatory properties. Inflammation is a biological response of the human body against a damage, infections and external agents that results in the production of inflammatory mediators as cytokines, prostaglandins, enzymes, nitric oxide, and reactive oxygen species (ROS). When these substances are overproduced, they migh produce pathologic processed related to chronic diseases (cardiovascular diseases, arthritis, cancer, etc.). For example, carvacrol and thymol, monoterpenes obtained from oregano species reduced significantly ROS and NO levels in macrophage cells stimulated by lipopolysaccharide (LPS) (Leyva-López et al. 2016). Lima et al. (2013) also studied the antiinflammatory power of carvacrol, which reduced proinflammatory mediator levels (IL-1β, PGE_2, COX-2) while antiinflammatory cytokines (IL-10) were increased. This fact could also explain the biological activity of oregano essential oil to reduced the risk to suffer atherosclerosis and other cardiovascular diseases result of a huge inflammatory response (Alves-Silva et al. 2016; Dantas et al. 2015). Parallelly, anti-inflammatory and anticancer activities of oregano essential oil have also proven in a human skin disease model by Han & Parker (2017). In this model, oregano essential oil presence inhibited several inflammatory biomarkers, which provides evidences of the influence of oregano in human dermal fibroblasts.

Table 1. Health benefits of oregano consumption as *in vtro* as *in vivo*

Health benefit	Form/Specie	Dose used	Model	Main effects	Reference
Antioxidant	Extracts from *Origanum majoricum* and *Origanum vulgare*	75 mM	*In vitro* ORAC, Total phenolic content, HPLC	Oregano showed one of the highest antioxidant capacity due to the higher concentration in phenolic compounds, measured by HPLC	Zheng & Wang (2001)
Antioxidant	Extract from *Origanum vulgare*	100, 250, and 500 µm	*In vitro* Human colon cancer cell line (Caco-2) exposed to hydrogen peroxide	Affected cell viability in a dose-dependent manner. Protected against DNA damage induced by H_2O_2, which was related with the concentration of phenolic compounds	Aherne, Kerry & O'Brien (2007)
Anti-inflammatory	Dried *Origanum vulgare*	60 µL	*In vitro* Total phenolic content, DPPH RAW 264.7 macrophage cell line stimulated by lipopolysaccharide (LPS) to measure nitric oxide (NO)	NO supressive activity was showed by oregano, but not antioxidant activity regarding to the rest of analyzed extract (clove, thyme, basil, cinnamon, tarragon, and rosemary)	Tsai et al. (2007)
Antioxidant and antimicrobial	Essential oil/ *Origanum majorana* and *Origanum vulgare*	From 0.5 to 500.0 µg/mL for antioxidant capacity, 10 µL for antimicrobial, and from 0 to 0.50 mg/mL for anticancer	*In vitro:* Antioxidant: DPPH and linolenic acid system. Antimicrobial: *Staphylococcus aureus, Bacillus cereus, B. subtilis, Pseudomonas aeruginosa, Salmonella poona, Escherichia coli,* and *ampicillin-resistant E. coli.* Anticancer: Human breast cancer cell line MCF-7	Antioxidant power to quench DPPH and in the linolenic acid system. Antibacterial capacity against all the studied strains. Cytotoxic potential, which produced apoptosis of human breast cells	Hussain et al. (2011)
Antiviral	Essential oil/ *Lippia graveolens*	6400 µg/ml in MEM (minimum essential medium)	*In vitro* Cell lines: Mardin-Darby bovine kidney (MDBK) cells, MA104 cells, and HEp-2 cells Viral strains: ACVR-HHV-1, HRSV, BoHV-1 Cooper, BoHV-5 607, BoHV-2, HHV-1 and RV	Oregano essential oil inhibited acyclovirresistant herpes simplex virus type 1 (ACVR-HHV-1), acyclovir-sensitive HHV-1, human respiratory syncytial virus (HRSV), bovine herpesvirus type 2 (BoHV-2), and bovine viral diarrhoea virus (BVDV). Carvacrol alone exhibited high antiviral activity against Human Rotavirus (RV)	Pilau et al. (2011)

Health benefit	Form/Specie	Dose used	Model	Main effects	Reference
Anti-inflammatory	Carvacrol	50 and 100 mg/kg	*In vivo* Male Swiss rice (22-28 g)	Anti-inflammatory properties of carvacrol are dependent on its ability to reduce the production of inflammatory mediators, such as IL-1b and prostanoids.	Lima et al. (2013)
Antimutagenic	Essential oil/ *Origanum majorana*	64.0 mg/kg	*In vivo:* Male Wistar rats (150 ± 5 g)	Antigenotoxic and anticytotoxic potential of orégano essential oil against prallethrin-induced genotoxic and cytotoxic effects in rat bone marrow cells were showed	Mossa et al. (2013)
Anticancer	Essential oil/ *Origanum vulgare*	From 10 to 500 mg/mL	*In vitro* Human breast adenocarcinoma (MCF-7), and human colon adenocarcinoma (HT-29) cell lines	Induced a high cytotoxicity effect in HT-29, however it was less effective in the MCF-7 cell line, which was related with concentration of major compounds, such as 4-terpineol.	Begnini et al. (2014)
	Ethanol extract/ *Origanum marjorana*	40, 80 and 120 µg/mL	*In vitro* Cancer cell line of fibrosarcoma: HT-1080	Ethanol extract has shown significant cytotoxicity in fibrosarcoma cell line and toxicity against normal human lymphocytes	Rao, Timsine & Nadumane (2014)
Cardiovascular protection	Carvacrol	1, 5, 10, and 20 mg/kg	*In vivo* Male Wistar rats (250-300 g)	Vasorelaxant effect on isolated rat superior mesenteric artery rings, probably by inhibiting calcium influx, but also by store and receptor operated channels inhibition, which was correlated with the inhibition of transiente receptor potential	Dantas et al. (2015)
Antioxidant, antimicrobial, and anticancer	Essential oils from *Origanum dictamnus, Origanum microphyllum* and *Origanum libanoticum*	Antioxidant: 1 mL Antimicrobial: 25 and 50 mg/mL Antiproliferative: 100 mg/mL	*In vitro:* Antioxidant: DPPH and FRAP Antimicrobial: 10 Gram + and Gram - bacteria Antiproliferative: Human cancer cell lines: LoVo and HepG2	Antimicrobial and cytotoxic properties were showed. However, antioxidant capacity was higher measured by FRAP instead of applying DPPH method	Marrelli et al. (2015)
Anti-inflammatory	Methanol orégano extracts of *Lippia graveolens, Lippia palmeri* and *Hedeoma patens*	50 and 100 µg/mL for *Lippia graveolens,* 100 and 200 µg/mL for *Lippia palmeri,* and 200 and 400 µg/mL for *Hedeoma patens*	*In vitro* RAW 264.7 macrophage cell line stimulated by lipopolysaccharide (LPS) to measure nitric oxide (NO) and reactive oxygen species (ROS), and evaluation of cyclooxygenase activity (COX-1, COX-2)	Inhibitory effect on ROS and NO production, mitochondrial activity in LPS-induced inflammation, and also against the activity of the cyclooxygenases COX-1 and COX-2.	Leyva et al. (2016)

Table 1. (Continued)

Health benefit	Form/Specie	Dose used	Model	Main effects	Reference
Anti-inflammatory, tissue remodeling, immunomodulatory, and anticancer	Essential oil/ *Origanum vulgare*	0.0037% (v/v)	*In vitro* Human neonatal fibroblasts cell line stimulated with a mix of interleukin-1β, tumor necrosis factor-α, interferon-γ, basic fibroblast growth factor, epidermal growth factor, and platelet-derived growth factor	Inhibited the levels of many inflammatory and tissue remodeling biomarkers, including MCP-1, VCAM-1, ICAM-1, IP-10, ITAC, IP-10, MIG, collagen I, collagen III, M-CSF, EGRF, MMP-1, PAI-1, TIMP1, and TIMP2, which demonstrated its potential anti-inflammatory and anticâncer activity	Han & Parker (2017)
Anticancer	Essential oil/ *Origanum vulgare*	10, 25 and 50 μg/mL	*In vitro* Human cancer cell lines (AGS)	Inhibited lipogenesis pathway by downregulating transcripts and proteins such as ACC, FASN, SREPB1 (fatty acid biosynthesis) and HMGCR (cholesterol biosynthesis). In addition, it leads to the activation of BAX (anti-apoptotic protein) and downregulation of BCL2 (proapoptotic proteins) and resulted in apoptosis of AGS cancer cells	Balusamy et al. (2018)
Cellular antioxidant	Oregano powder obtained from: *Hedeoma patens, Lippia graveolens* and *Lippia palmeri*	25, 50, 100, and 200 μg dried extract/mL	*In vitro* Human colorectal adenocarcinoma cell line (Caco-2) with α-glucosidase from *Saccharomyces cerevisiae* and α-amylase from porcine pancreas	Oregano species were able to inhibit enzymes involved in carbohydrate and lipid metabolism. Digestion process increased bioactivity of oregano species polyphenol-rich extracts due to their biotransformation as evidenced by the increased inhibitory rate of α-amylase and pancreatic lipase	Gutiérrez-Grijalva et al. (2019)

In this way, antiproliferative effects of oregano essential oil have been demonstrated in the hepatocarcinoma cell line (HepG2), human breast adenocarninoma (MCF-7), and human colon adenocarcinoma (HT-29) in 50% (Marrelli et al. 2015; Begnini et al. 2014). In addition, essential oils from oregano has been classified as dietary inhibitors of mutagenesis and carcinogenesis (Mossa et al. 2013). Hussain et al. (2011) showed an 80% inhibitory effect on cancer cell viability in human breast (MCF-7) and prostate (LNCaP) cancer cell lines. This effect can be related to the oregano composition and its antioxidant capacity, which might contribute to reduce the lipid peroxidation (Mossa et al. 2013). In addition, in fibrosarcoma cancer cell line HT-1080, *Origanum majorana* ethanol extract has shown cytotoxicity, but also against human lymphocytes, which demonstrates its anticancer potential (Rao, Timsina & Nadumane, 2014). Balusamy et al. (2018) have also shown the anti-proliferative activity of oregano essential oil application through lipogenesis inhibition and apoptosis in human stomach cancer cell lines (AGS).

Role Oregano Consumption in Diet

It is generally known that several factors of Mediterranean diet have been linked with a lower risk of inflammation diseases and cancer. In particular, oregano has been widely used in Mediterranean cuisine providing its distinctive flavour, well known as "Italian taste," to enhance the organoleptic characteristics of a variety of foods, such as pizza, pasta, bread, fish, vegetables, legumes, bread, and sauces.

Actually, the spices average consumption in Spain in 2017 was 1.28 kg/person/year (MAPA, 2018). Knowing that oregano is one of the spices commonly consumed, it can be said that this herb is generally present in Spanish diet, unless other data from Europe have not been found. In the same way, oregano essential oil is also present in Spanish diet. Regarding to the National inform of food consumption in Spain in 2017 (MAPA, 2018), consumption of seed oil was 0.34 L/person/year, including grape seed, rice, hazelnut, walnut, sesame, peanuts, sweet almonds, oregano, linseed, wheat germ and coconut.

Oregano Used as a Functional Ingredient in Meat Products

The use of oregano, both as essential oil and extract, endogenously applied as dietary antioxidant or, exogenously applied as a direct food additive to prevent the oxidation of foods has been effective in several animal models and different food systems, storage time, and conditions. Firstly, Zou et al. (2017) showed that a dietary supplementation of 25 ppm oregano essential oil combined with 200 ppm vitamin E in pigs after a 28-day feeding trial, can alleviate stress, improve intestinal morphology, and increase meat quality after the transportation of pigs. These results indicated that the endogenous incorporation of oregano was beneficial to improve the pork meat quality.

Table 2. Oregano used as a functional ingredient in manufactured meat products

Extract form	Specie	Dose used	Meat product	Storage conditions	Main effects	Reference
Essential oils	*Origanum vulgare*	1% in milk-protein based edible film	Beef slices inoculated with *Pseudomonas* spp. and *E. Coli* O157:H7.	7 days at 4°C	Reduced lipid oxidation; antimicrobial activity against *Pseudomonas* spp. and *E. Coli* O157:H7.	Oussalah et al. (2004)
		1 - 2% in chitosan based edible film	Bologna slices inoculated with *Listeria monocytogenes* and *E. Coli* O157:H7	5 days at 10°C	Antimicrobial activity against *Listeria monocytogenes* and *E. Coli* O157:H7.	Zivanovic, Chi & Draughon (2005)
		3%	Ground porcine/bovine meat	12 days at 4°C	Reduced lipid oxidation	Fasseas et al. (2007)
		0.1% - 1%	Fresh chicken breast	MAP 30% CO_2/70% N_2 and MAP 70% CO_2/30% N_2 25 days at 4°C	Reduced lipid oxidation (0.1%); colour maintenance; and microbiological control (TVC, *Pseudomonas* spp., lactic acid bacteria, yeast, *Brochothrix thermosphacta* and *Enterobacteriaceae).*	Chouliara et al. (2007)
		0.02%	Bologna sausages	24 days RT	Reduced lipid oxidation and colour maintenance	Viuda-Martos et al. (2010)
		0.6 - 0.9%	Minced sheep meat inoculated with *Salmonella enteritidis.*	12 days at 4 or 10°C.	Antimicrobial activity against *Salmonella enteritidis*; good sensory acceptance	Govaris et al. (2010)
	Origanum heracleoticum	5%	Ground beef patties coated with isolated soy protein films incorporated essential oils	12 days at 4°C	Antimicrobial activity against *Escherichia coli, E. coli* O157:H7, *Staphylococcus aureus, Pseudomonas aeruginosa,* but not against *Lactobacillus plantarum.*	Emiroğlu et al. 2010
	Origanum vulgare	0.1% - 0.3%	Chicken liver meat	20 days at 4°C	Reduced lipid oxidation	Hasapidou & Savaidis (2011)
	Origanum majorana	200 ppm	Beef patties	3 months at -18°C	Reduced lipid oxidation; improved sensory quality	Mohamed & Mansour (2012)
	Origanum vulgare	0.05 - 0.4%	Pork patties	12 days MAP 70% O_2/20% CO_2/10% N_2 or Anaerobic conditions at 4°C.	Reduced protein oxidation	Nieto et al. (2013)
	Coridothymus capitatus (485.6 g/kg carvacrol)	5, 10, 20, and 30 g/kg	Chicken breast under whey protein isolate film forming solutions that incorporated oregano essential oil	8 days at 4°C	Antimicrobial activity against *Enterobateriaceae,* lactic acid bacteria, and *Pseudomonas* spp.	Fernández-Pan, Mendoza & Maté (2013)
	Origanum vulgare	0.2%	Minced beef inoculated with *Listeria monocytogenes*	10 days at 3°C	Antimicrobial activity against *Listeria monocytogenes;* colour maintenance; good sensory acceptance	Hulankova, Borilova & Steinhauserova (2013)
		2%	Foal meat under antioxidant active packaging system that incorporated oregano essential oil	14 days MAP (80% O_2/20% CO_2) at 2°C	Antimicrobial activity against *Pseudomonas* spp., lactic acid bacteria, *Enterobacteriaceae,* moulds, and yeast. Reduced lipid and protein oxidation, preserved colour and sensorial properties	Lorenzo, Batlle & Gómez (2014)

Extract form	Specie	Dose used	Meat product	Storage conditions	Main effects	Reference
Essential oils	*Origanum vulgare*	1.5 – 2 ml	Dried beef meat inoculated with *Salmonella enteriditis* and *Escherichia coli*	6 h of drying at 55°C	Antimicrobial capacity against *Salmonella enteriditis* and *Escherichia coli* and good sensory acceptance	Hernández et al. (2016)
		2 – 4%	Pork fillets inoculated with *Listeria monocytogenes* and dipped in oregano essential oil.	15 days MAP 70% O_2/20% CO_2/10% N_2 at 4°C.	Antimicrobial activity against *Listeria monocytogenes* and *Pseudomonas*. Reduced lipid oxidation, reduced colour loss and good sensory acceptance in combination with chitosan.	Paparella et al. (2016)
		0.1%	Beef steaks in alginate-based edible coating with oregano essential oil	14 days at 2°C	Reduced weigh loss, lipid oxidation, preserved colour, and good sensory acceptance	Pelaes-Vital et al. (2016)
Extract		13.32, 17.79, 21.01 ppm	Lamb burgers	120 days at -18°C	Reduced lipid and protein oxidation; reduced colour loss; good sensory acceptance.	Fernandes et al. (2017)
Essential oils	*Origanum virens*	1%	Portuguese dry cured sausages (paínhos and alheiras) packed with whey protein active coatings with oregano essential oil	126 days for paínhos and 106 days for alheiras at 4°C	Antimicrobial activity, protected against colour loss, reduced lipid oxidation, and good sensory acceptance.	Catarino et al. (2017)
	Origanum vulgare	0.4%	Cooked sliced ham	Vacuum packed 45 days at 6°C 18 days at 12°C 12 days at 15°C 6 days at 20°C 3 days at 25°C	Antimicrobial activity. Increased shelf-life for 30 days more, compared to the control.	Costa-Menezes et al. (2018)
Extract		4964.51, 6630.98, 8038.20 ppm	Cooked sheep sausages	Vacuum packed 135 days RT	Reduced lipid and protein oxidation; reduced colour loss; good sensory acceptance.	Fernandes et al. (2018)
Essential oil		1%	Black wildebeest meat	9 days at 3°C	Reduced lipid oxidation; antimicrobial activity against TVC, lactic acid bacteria, and total coliforms; reduced colour loss.	Shange et al. (2019)

MAP: Modified Atmosphere Packaging; TVC: Total Viable Count; RT: Room Temperature.

On the other hand, some of the most current researchers about oregano used as an antioxidant ingredient in meat and meat products are summarized in Table 2. First of all, oregano essential oil has been extensively studied in different meat model systems and edible films used to preserve them. For example, Oussalah et al. (2004) reduced lipid oxidation and bacterial growth of *Pseudomonas* spp. and *E. Coli* O157:H7 in beef slices inoculated with these strains and covered with milk-protein based edible film that incorporated 1% oregano essential oil for 7 days under refrigerated storage. In the same way, Zivanovic, Chi & Draughon (2005) proved the antimicrobial activity of 1 – 2% oregano essential oil in chitosan edible film used to cover bologna slices inoculated with *Listeria monocytogenes* and *E. Coli* O157:H7 for 5 days at 10ºC. Both researchers demonstrated as oregano essential oil can also act as antimicrobial used directly in meat packaging, neither as ingredient nor through animal diet. In addition, using 3% oregano essential oil, Fasseas et al. (2007) managed to reduce lipid oxidation in ground porcine and bovine meat under refrigerated storage for 12 days. As well as, Chouliaria et al. (2007) also reduced lipid oxidation, bacterial growth (Total Viable Count (TVC), *Pseudomonas* spp., lactic acid bacteria, yeast, *Brochothrix thermosphacta* and *Enterobacteriaceae),* and maintained colour in fresh chicken breast with 0.1 - 1% oregano essential oil, modified atmosphere packaged (MAP) (30% CO_2/70% N_2 - 70% CO_2/30% N_2) for 25 days at 4ºC.

Parallelly, Viuda-Martos et al. (2010) reduced lipid oxidation and maintained colour of bologna sausages incorporated 0.02% oregano essential oil for 24 days at room temperature (RT). Moreover, antimicrobial activity against *Salmonella enteritidis* inoculated in minced sheep meat was showed by Govaris et al. (2010) for 12 days at 4ºC and 10ºC, using 0.6 - 0.9% of oregano essential oil. Hernández et al. (2016) studied the antimicrobial capacity of the application of 1.5 and 2 ml of oregano essential oil in dried beef meat against *Salmonella enteriditis* and *Escherichia coli* growth for 6 h of drying at 55ºC getting satisfactory results regarding to the microbial load and the general sensory attributes. Also lipid oxidation was reduced in chicken liver meat incorporated 0.1 - 0.3% oregano essential oil for 20 days under refrigerated storage (Hasapidou & Savaidis, 2011), while Mohamed & Mansour (2012) improved sensory acceptance of beef frozen patties with 200 ppm oregano essential oil.

Nevertheless, 0.05 - 0.4% oregano essential oil also reduced protein oxidation in pork patties for 12 days at 4ºC, both MAP 70% O_2/20% CO_2/10% N_2 or under anaerobic conditions, as Nieto et al. (2013) showed in their investigation. Hulankova, Borilova & Steinhauserova (2013) exhibited 0.2% oregano essential oil antimicrobial activity in miced beef inoculated with *Listeria monocytogenes* for 10 days at 3ºC, while colour and sensory quality were maintained. Also cooked sliced ham incorporated 0.4% oregano essential oil increased shelf-life for 30 days more in comparisson to the control at 6ºC. Finally, one of the last research in this field carried out by Shange et al. (2019) showed as lipid oxidation was reduced and bacterial growth was controlled using 1% oregano essential oil in black wildebeest meat storaged for 9 days at 3ºC. Apart from that, using oregano extract, lamb burgers incorporated 13.32, 17.79 and 21.01 ppm showed lipid and protein oxidation reduction and good sensory acceptance for 120 days at frozen storage conditions (Fernandes et al. 2017). In the same way, cooked sheep sausages incorporated 4964.51, 6630.98 and 8038.20 ppm obtained similar results as previously described for 135 days (Fernandes et al. 2018).

Additionally, oregano can preserve meat products by different incorporation ways. For example, as it has been cited above, Oussalah et al. (2004) and Zivanovic, Chi & Draughon (2005) studied the oregano essential oil incorporation in bioactive packaging systems. In the same way, Paparella et al. (2016) have also shown the antimicrobial capacity of 4% oregano essential oil in combination of chitosan based film, increasing from 12 to 18 days the shelf life of pork fillets compared to the control, under modified atmosphere packaging (MAP) (70% O_2/20% CO_2/10% N_2). Fernández-Pan, Mendoza & Maté (2013) applied an edible film base whey protein isolate and glycerol with oregano and clove essential oils. Obtained results showed a significant reduction of microbial growth on the surface of poultry. Moreover, antimicrobial capacity of soy protein edible films incorporated 5% oregano essential oil reported excellent results against *Escherichia coli, E. coli* O157:H7, *Staphylococcus aureus, Pseudomonas aeruginosa* and *Lactobacillus plantarum* growt in ground beef patties during 12 days of refrigerated storage (Emiroğlu et al. 2010). In the same research it was demonstrated the synergistic effect of the combination of oregano and thyme essential oils against bacterial growth. Nevertheless, lipid and protein oxidation were significantly reduced in fresh foal steaks by combining MAP (80 O_2/20 CO_2) with an active film containing 2% oregano essential oil (Lorenzo, Batlle & Gómez, 2014). This combination increased the shelf life maintaining the colour and decreasing the bacterial growth. Also Pelaes-Vital (2016) reduced weigh loss, lipid oxidation, preserved colour, and obtained good sensory acceptance in beef steaks packed using alginate-based edible coating with 0.1% oregano essential oil for 14 days stored at 2ºC. Currently, Catarino et al. (2017) developed a whey protein film as biopolymer matrix that incorporated 1% oregano extract in two traditional Portuguese meat products (painho and alheira), which presented lipid oxidation reduction. As it can be appreciated, the incorporation of oregano, both as essential oil or as extract in edible biodegradable films can also be an option to preserve meat products.

NEW TRENDS

Currently, there is a great opportunity for manufactured meat products to use natural antioxidants in their formulations to replace synthetic additives without quality loss. In addition, there are a lot of researchers to investigate the application of oregano by different ways in meat products, which it is important to modify the regulatory status regarding to new natural additives for their application. Additionally, with these kind of ingredients there is a possibility to influence in the colour, flavour, or aroma produced by their incorporation. For these reasons, researchers have currently been focused on the encapsulation of this extract and its directly incorporation to active packaging to prevent oreganoleptic organoleptic alterations on the quality of the product.

In addition, natural extracts as oregano, can be encapsulated and exogeously incorporated in manufactured products. For example, Almeida et al. (2013) created mocrospheres of different types of starch wrapping oregano essential oil using supercritical carbon dioxide (SC-CO_2), which can preserve its antioxidant and beneficial properties under mild operating conditions. Subsequently, microencapsulated Mexican oregano essential oils demonstrated to reduce the bacterial growth, lipid and oxymyoglobin oxidation of fresh pork meat maintaining the sensory quality after 15 days, whereas untreated meat samples were undesirable (Hernández-Hernández et al. 2017). Nevertheless, it must be taken into account that the application of this method could be really expensive but also innovative. So more researchers are needed in this field in order to find real conclusions about that.

Unless new methods to extract oregano bioactive compounds as well as different ways to apply these compounds to manufactured meat products, as it has been exposed in the present review, no one example of commercialization of these products has been found, apart from, of course, small commerces where butchers prepare their own product with natural ingredients, as oregano, in order to enhance flavour and odour of marinated and cured meat products. However, this fact is typical in traditional commerces of Spain, for example, but not used by big companies, whose products are usually bought by the major part of the population. Nevertheless, companies as the German Willy Benecke GMBH, the Chinese Shandong Bailong Chuandyuan BIO-TECH CO., LTD, and the Spanish Coralim ADITIVOS S.L. are experts in natural additives markets. In the same way, there are more companies focused in development, production, and distribution of free additives solutions used by Meat Industry, for example, the Murcian (Spain) Catalina Food Solutions S.L. Other multinational industries also focused in production of natural flavorings, have also aimed their view in Food Industry, such as the Spanish Indukern Food Division, which has developed the Blend-a-Kern CFX, CEX, and CII solutions for the elaboraion of manufactured meat products without E numbers, or the Israeli Frutarom Industries LTD., which specializes in the production and distributions of natural extracts obtained from herbs, fruits, and vegetables for flavor and fragances.

This kind of companies gives the posibility to Meat Industry to elaborate Clean Label meat products. For example, the North American Coleman Natural Foods LLC. is lauching a new clean label meat products line, such as beef burgers, chicken sausages, and maple-smoked bacon. Also the French ActiMeat® is on the look out for Clean Label and Organic products with the aim objective of develop natural, authentic and respectful with environment meat products. In the Spanish market, Domínguez Meat Products, SL. has developed the "Bo&San" line, which includes meat products free of additives and allergens, such as "Spanish cured "chorizo," bacon, roast ham, Celtic cured ham, and burgers, while Mafriseu S.A. produces traditional manufactured meat products, such as sausages, meat-balls, minced meat, Spanish "chorizo," burgers, "butifarra," paté, or "fuet," among others. Also Noel Alimentaria S. L. sells since several years ago roast ham and roast poultry breast free of additives.

As it has been previously exposed, these companies are pioneers in the field of Clean Label meat products elaboration, however, the specific use of oregano in their products has not been found, however, it is known that for the traditional recipe of Spanish "chorizo" is necessary the use of oregano in its formula, for example.

CONCLUSION

Beneficial effects of oregano consumption have been extensively investigated due to its antioxidant, antiinflammatory and antimicrobial power. For this reason, in last 20 years, researchers have focused on the elimination of preservatives and dyes by oregano incorporation in order to achieve "clean label" meat products. Fortunately, oregano could be incorporated to manufactured meat products through different ways to contribute health benefits by their consumption, since its characteristic flavour has been palatably accepted, as it has been described above. Therefore, it can be concluded that any studied ways, through animal diet, as an ingredient in their formula, through its application in new packaging systems or by encapsulation, are valid to obtain its health benefits and antioxidant properties on meat. Consequently, a great opportunity exists for meat processors to use natural antioxidants, like oregano, to replace synthethic additives while maintaining product quality.

REFERENCES

Adame-Gallegos, J. R., Andrade-Ochoa, S., Nevarez-Moorillon, G. V. (2016). Potential use of Mexicano regano essential oil against parasite, fungal and bacterial pathogens. *Journal of essential oil bearing plants, 19:* 553-567.

Aherne, S., Kerry, J., O'Brien, N. (2007). Effects of plant extracts on antioxidant status and oxidant-induced stress in Caco-2 cells. *Brithis Journal of Nutrition, 97:* 321-328.

Ahmad Shah, M., Don Bosco, S. J., Ahmad Mir, S. (2014). Plant extracts as natural antioxidants in meat and meat products. *Meat Science, 98(1):* 21-33.

Almeida, A. P., Rodríguez-Rojo, S., Serra, A. T., Vila-Real, H., Simplicio, A. L., Delgadilho, I., da Costa, S. B., da Costa, L. B., Nogueira, I. D., Duarte, C. M. M. (2013). Microencapsulation of oregano essential oil in starch-based materials using supercritical fluid technology. *Innovative food science & emerging technologies, 20:* 140-145.

Alves-Silva, J. M., Zuzarte, M., Marques, C., Salgueiro, L., Guirão, H. (2016). Protective effects of terpenes on the cardiovascular system: current advances and future perspectives. *Current medicinal chemistry, 23:* 4559-4600.

Asensio, C. M., Grosso, N. R., Juliani, H. R. (2015). Quality characters, chemical composition and biological activities of oregano (*Origanum* spp.) essential oils from central and southern Argentina. *Industrial crops and products, 63:* 203-213.

Balusamy, S. R., Perumalsamy, H., Huq, Md. A., Balasubramanian, B. (2018). Anti-proliferative activity of *Origanum vulgare* inhibited lipogenesis and induced mitocondrial mediated apoptosis in human stomach cancer cell lines. *Biomedicine & pharmacotherapy, 108:* 1835-1844.

Begnini, K. R., Nedel, F., Lund, R. G., Carvalho, P. H. D., Rodrigues, M. R. A., Beira, F. T. A., Del Pino, F. A. B. (2014). Composition and antiproliferative effect of essential oil of *Origanum vulgare* against tumor cell lines. *Journal of medicinal food, 17:* 1129-1133.

Catarino, M. D., Alves-Silva, J. M., Fernandes, R. P., Gonçalves, M. J., Salgueiro, L. R., Henriques, M. F., Cardoso, S. M. (2017). Development and performance of whey protein active coatings with *Origanum virens* essential oils in the quality and shelf life improvement of processed meat products. *Food control, 80:* 273-280.

Chang, T. W. & Pan, A. Y. (2008). Chapter 2: Cumulative Environmental Changes, Skewed Antigen Exposure and the Increase of Allergy. In: *Advances in Inmunology*, 98, 39-83.

Chouliara, E., Karatapanis, A., Savaidis, I. N., Kontominas, M. G. (2007). Combined effect of oregano essential oil and modified atmosphere packaging on shelf life extensión of fresh chicken breast meat, stored at 4 ºC. *Food microbiology, 24:* 607-617.

Clough, S. R. (2014). Sodium Sulfite. Reference Module in Biomedical Sciences. In: Encyclopedia of Toxicology (3ª Edition), 341-343.

Costa-Menezes, N. M., Figueiredo-Martins, W., Angelo-Longui, D., Falcão-de Aragão, G.M. (2018). Modeling the effect of oregano essential oil on shelf-life extensión of vacuum-packed cooked sliced ham. *Meat science, 139:* 113-119.

Croteau, R., Kutchan, I. M., Lewis, N. G. (2015). Natural products (secondary metabolites). In: Buchanan, B., Gruissem, W., Jones, R. (2015). Biochemistry & Molecular Biology of Plants. *Eds: American Society of Plants, Rockville, MD, USA:* 1250-1318.

Dantas, B. P. V., Alves, Q. L., de Assis, K. S., Ribeiro, T. P., de Almeida, M. M., de Vasconcelos, A. P., de Araújo, D. A. M., de Andrade Braga, V., de Medeiros, I. A., Alencar, J. L. et al. (2015). Participation of the trp channel in the cardiovascular effects induced by carvacrol in normotensive rat. *Vascular pharmacology, 67-69:* 48-58.

Desvasagayam, T. P. A., Tilka, J. C., Boloor, K. K., Sane, K. S., Ghaskadb, I., Lele, R. D. (2004). Free radicals and antioxidants in human health: current status and future prospects. *Journal of the Association of Physicians of India, 52:* 794-804.

Dutra, T. V., Castro, J. C., Menezes, J. L., Ramos, T. R., do Prado, I. N., Junior, M. M., Mikcha, J. M. G., de Abreu Filho, B. A. (2019). Bioactivity of oregano (*Origanum vulgare*) essential oil against *Alicyclobacillus* spp. *Industrial crops & products, 129:* 345-349.

Emiroğlu, Z. K., Yemiş, G. P., Coşkun, B. K, Candoğan, K. (2010). Antimicrobial activity of soy edible films incorporated with thyme and oregano essential oils on fresh ground beef patties. *Meat science, 86:* 283-288.

Estévez, M. (2011). Protein carbonyls in meat systems: a review. *Meat Science, 89(III),* 259-279. DOI: 10.1016/j.meatsci.2011.04.025.

Fasseas, M. K., Mountzouris, K. C., Tarantilis, P. A., Polissiou, M., Zervas, G. (2007). Antioxidant activity in meat treated with oregano and sage essential oils. *Food Chemistry, 106:* 1188-1194.

Fernandes, R. P. P., Trindade, M. A., Lorenzo, J. M., de Melo, M. P. (2018). Assessment of the stability of sheep sausages with the addition of different concentrations of *Origanum vulgare* extract during storage. *Meat science, 137:* 244-257.

Fernandes, R. P. P., Trindade, M. A., Tonin, F. G., Pugine, S. M. P., Lima, C. G., Lorenzo, J. M., de Melo, M. P. (2017). Evaluation of oxidative stability of lamb burger with *Origanum vulgare* extract. *Food chemistry, 233:* 101-109.

Fernández-Pachón, M. S., Villano, D., Troncoso, A. M., García-Parrilla, M. C. (2008). Antioxidant activity of phenolic compounds: from in vitro results to in vivo evidence. *Critical Reviews in Food Science and Nutrition, 48(VII):* 649-671.

Fernández-Pan, I., Mendoza, M., Maté, J. I. (2013). Whey protein isolate edible films with essential oils incorporated to improve the microbial quality of poultry. *Journal of the science of food and agriculture, 93(XII):* 2986-2994.

Gonçalves, S., Moreira, E., Grosso, C., Andrade, P. B., Valentão, P., Romano, A. (2017). Phenolic profile, antioxidant activity and enzyme inhibitory activities of extracts from aromatic plants used in mediterranean diet. *Journal of Food Science and Technology, 54:* 219–227.

Govaris, A., Solomakos, N., Pexara, A., Charzopoulou, P. S. (2010) The antimicrobial effect of oregano essential oil, nisin and their combination against *Salmonella enteritidis* in minced sheep meat during refrigerated storage. *International journal of food microbiology, 137:* 175-180.

Gutiérrez-Grijalva, E. P., Antunes-Ricardo, M., Acosta-Estrada, B. A., Gutiérrez-Uribe, J. A., Heredia, J. B. (2019). Cellular antioxidant activity and *in vitro* inhibition of α-glucosidase, αamylase and pancreatic lipase of oregano polyphenols under simulated gastrointestinal digestion. *Food research international, 116:* 676-686.

Gutiérrez-Grijalva, E. P., Picos-Salas, M. A., Leyva-López, N., Criollo-Mendoza, M. S., Vazquez-Olivo, G., Heredia, J. B. (2017). Flavonoids and phenolic acids from oregano: occurrence, biological activity and health benefits. Review. *Plants, 7(II).* DOI: 10.3390/plants7010002.

Han, X. & Parker, T. L. (2017). Anti-inflammatory, tissue remodeling, immunomodulatory, and anticancer activities of oregano (*Origanum vulgare*) essential oil in a human skin disease model. *Biochimie Open, 4:* 73-77.

Hasapidou, A. & Savaidis, I. N. (2011). The effects of modified atmosphere packaging, EDTA and oregano oil on the quality of chicken liver meat. *Food research international, 44(IX):* 2751-2756.

Haytowitz, D. B. & Bhagwat, S. (2010). USDA Database for the Oxygen Radical Absorbance Capacity (ORAC) of Selected Foods, Release 2. *U.S. Department of Agriculture (USDA), Maryland, USA.*

Hernández, H., Fraňková, A., Sýkora, T., Klouček, P., Kouřimska, L., Kučerová, I., Banout, J. (2016). The effect of oregano essential oil on microbial load and sensory attributes of dried meat. *Journal of science and food agricultura, 97:* 82-87.

Hernández-Hernández, E., Lira-Moreno, C. Y., Guerrero-Legarreta, I., Wild-Padua, G., Di Pierro, P., García-Almendárez, B. E., Regalado-González, G. (2017). Effect of nanoemulsified and microencapsulated Mexican oregano (*Lippia graveolens* Kunth) essential oil coatings on quality of fresh pork meat. *Food microbiology & safety, 82(VI):* 1423-1432.

Hulankova, R., Borilova, G., Steinhauserova, I. (2013). Combined antimicrobial effect of oregano essential oil and caprylic acid in miced beef. *Meat science, 95:* 190-194.

Hussain, A. I., Anwar, F., Rasheed, S., Nigam, P. S., Janneh, O., Sarker, S. D. (2011). Composition, antioxidant and chemotheraputic properties of the essential oils from two *Origanum* species growing in Pakistan. *Revista Brasileira de Farmacognosia – The Brazilian journal of pharmacognosy, 21:* 943-952.

Jian, J., & Xiong, Y. L. (2016). Natural antioxidants as food and feed additives to promote health benefits and quality of meat products: A review. *Meat Science, 120*: 107-117.

Knigh, J. A. (2000). Reviwe: Free radicals, antioxidants, and the immune system. *Annals of Clinical & Laboratory Science, 30(II):* 145-158.

Lagouri, V., Alexandri, G. (2013). Antioxidant properties of greek *O. dictamnus* and *R. officinalis* methanol and aqueous extracts – HPLC determination of phenolic acids. *International Journal of Food Properties, 16:* 549-562.

Leyva-López, N., Nair, V., Bang, W. Y., Cisneros-Zevallos, L., Heredia, J. B. (2016). Protective role of terpenes and polyphenols from three species of oregano (*Lippia graveolens, Lippia palmeri* and *Hedeoma patens*) on the suppression of lipopolysaccharide-induced inflammation in RAW 264.7 macrophage cells. *Journal of Ethnopharmacology, 187:* 302–312.

Lima, M. D. S., Quintans-Júnior, L. J., De Santana, W. A., Martins Kaneto, C., Pereira Soares, M. B., Villarreal, C. F. (2013). Anti-inflammatory effects of carvacrol: Evidence for a key role of interleukin-10. *European journal of pharmacology, 23:* 192-201.

Lorenzo, J.M., Batlle, R., Gómez, M. (2014). Extension of the shelf-life of foal meat with two antioxidant active packaging systems. *LWT-Food science and technology, 59(I):* 181-188.

MAPA – Ministerio de Agricultura, Pesca y Alimentación. (2018). Informe anual de consumo alimentario 2017. *Gobierno de España.*

Marrelli, M., Conforti, F., Formisano, C., Rigano, D., Arnold, N. A., Menichini, F., Senatore, F. (2015). Composition, antibacterial, antioxidant and antiproliferative activities of essential oils from three origanum species growing wild in Lebanon and Greece. *Natural producto research, 30:* 735-739.

Mohamed, H. M. H. & Mansour, H. A. (2012). Incorporating essential oils of marjoram and rosemary in the formulation of beef patties manufactured with mechanically deboned poultry meat to improve the lipid stability and sensory attributes. *LWT-Food science and technology, 45:* 79-87.

Mossa, A. T. H., Refaie, A. A., Ramadan, A., Bouajila, J. Antimutagenic effect of *Origanum majorana* L. essential oil against prallethrin-induced genotoxic damage in rat bone marrow cells. *Journal of medicinal food, 16:* 1101-1107.0.

Nieto, G., Jongberg, S., Andersen, M. L., Skibsted, L. H. (2013). Thiol oxidation and protein cross-link formation during chill storage of pork patties added essential oil of oregano, rosemary, or garlic. *Meat Science*, 95(II), 177-184.

Oussalah, M., Caillet, S., Salmiéri, S., Saucier, L., Lacroix, M. (2004). Antimicrobial and antioxidant effects of milk protein-based film containing essential oils for the preservation of whole beef muscle. *Journal of agricultural and food chemistry, 52(XVIII):* 5598-5605.

Paparella, A., Mazzarino, G., Chaves-López, C., Rossi, C., Sacchetti, G., Guerrieri, O., Serio, A. (2016). Chitosan boosts the antimicrobial activity of *Origanum vulgare* essential oil modified atmosphere packaged pork. *Food microbiology, 59:* 23-31.

Pelaes-Vital, A. C., Guerrero, A., Monteschio, J. de O., Velandia-Valero, M., Barbosa-Carvalho, C., de Abreu-Filho, B. A., Scaramal-Madrona, G., Nunes-do Prado, I. (2016). Effect of edible and active coating (with rosemary and oregano essential oils) on beef characteristics and consumer acceptability. *PLoS ONE, 11(VIII):* e0160535. Doi: 10.1371/journal.pone.0160535.

Pilau, M. R., Alves, S. H., Weiblen, R., Arenhart, S., Cueto, A. P., Lovato, L. T. (2011). Antiviral activity of the *Lippia graveolens* (Mexican oregano) essential oil and its main compound carvacrol against human and animal viruses. *Brazilian journal of microbiology, 42:* 1616-1624.

Rao, S., Timsina, B., Nadumane, V. K. (2014). Evaluation of the anticancer potentials of *Origanum marjorana* on fibrosarcoma (HT-1080) cell line. *Asian pacific journal of tropical disease, 4(I):* S389-S394.

Ribeiro, J. S., Santos, M. J. M. C., Silva, L. K. R., Pereira, L. C. L., Santos, I. A., da Silva Lannes, S. C., da Silva, M. V. (2019). Natural antioxidants used in meat products: A brief review. *Meat Science, 148:* 181-188.

Rodríguez-García, I., Silva-Espinoza, B. A., Ortega-Ramirez, L. A., Leyva, J. M., Siddiqui, Md. W., Cruz-Valenzuela, M. R., González-Aguilar, G. A., Ayala-Zavala, J. F. (2015). Oregano essential oil as an antimicrobial and antioxidant additive in food products. *Critical reviews in food science and nutrition, 56(X):* 1717-1727.

Shan, B., Cai, B., Sun, M., Corke, H. (2005). Antioxidant capacity of 26 spice extracts and characterization of their phenolic constituents. *Journal of Agriculture and Food Chemistry, 53:* 7749-7759.

Shange, N., Makasi, T., Gouws, P., Hoffman, L. C. (2019). Preeservation of previously frozen black wildebeest meat (*Connochaetes gnou)* using oregano *(Oreganum vulgare)* essential oil. *Meat science, 148:* 88-95.

Skendi, A., Irakli, M., Chatzopoulou, P. (2017). Analysis of phenolic compounds in greek plants of Lamiaceae family by HPLC. *Journal of applied research on medicinal and aromatic plants, 6:* 62-69.

Soubra, L., Sarkis, D., Hilan, C., & Verger, Ph. (2007). Dietary exposure of children and teenagers to benzoates, sulphites, butylhydroxyanisol (BHA) and butylhiddroxytoluen (BHT) in Beirut (Lebanon). *Regulatory Toxicology and Pharmacology, 47(I),* 68-77.

The International Agency for Research on Cancer (IARC). (2015). Q&A on the carcinogenicity of the consumption of red meat and processed meat. *Press Release Nº240. Monographs-Q&A, vol 114.*

Tsai, P., Tsai, T., Yu, C., Ho, S. (2007). Evaluation of No-supressing activity of several Mediterranean culinary spices. *Food chemistry & toxicology, 45:* 440-447.

Viuda-Martos, M., Ruiz-Navajas, Y., Fernández-López, J., Pérez-Álvarez, J. A. (2010). Effect of Orange dietary fibre, oregano essential oil and packaging conditions on shelf life of bologna sausages. *Food control, 21:* 436-443.

Xiong, Y. L. (2000). Chapter 4: Protein oxidation and implications for muscle food quality. In: "Decker, E. A., Faustman, C., Lopez-Bote, C. J. (2010). Antioxidants in muscle foods: nutritional strategies to improve quality. *John Wiley & Sons, Inc.* ISBN 0-471-31454-4," 85-112.

Xiong, Y. L., Blanchard, S. P., Ooizumi, T., Ma, Y. (2010). Hydroxyl radical and ferryl-generating systems promote gel network formation of myofibrillar protein. *Journal of Food Science, 75(II),* C215-C221.

Yan, F., Azizi, A., Janke, S., Schwarz, M., Zeller, S., Honermeier, B. (2016). Antioxidant capacity variation in the oregano (*Origanum vulgare* L.) collection of the German National Genebank. *Industrial crops and products, 92:* 19-25.

Zheng, W., Wang, S. (2001). Antioxidant activity and phenolic compounds in selected herbs. *Journal of agriculture and food chemistry, 49:* 5165-5170.

Zivanovic, S., Chi., S., Draughon, A. F. (2005). Antimicrobial activity of chitosan films enriched with essential oils. *Journal of food science, 70(I):* M45-M51.

Zou, Y., Hu, X. M., Zhang, T., Wei, H. K., Zhou, Y. F., Zhou, Z. X., Peng, J. (2017). Effects of dietary oregano essential oil and vitamin E supplementation on meat quality stress response and intestinal morphology in pigs following transport stress. *The journal of veterinary medical science, 79(II):* 328-335.

In: Oregano: Properties, Uses and Health Benefits
Editor: Gema Nieto Martínez
ISBN: 978-1-53616-284-4

Chapter 6

Chemical Compostion, Phytochemistry and Pharmacological Properties of Oregano

Farida Larit* and Sakal Akkal
Department of Chemistry, University of Mentouri Brothers Constantine 1, Constantine, Algeria

Abstract

Oregano (*Origanum vulgare* L.) is a popular aromatic herb that belongs to the mint family (Lamiaceae). This plant is originally from warm to temperate regions of Eurasia and the Mediterranean regions and has been naturalized in parts of America.

This popular medicinal plant is well known for its flavorful dried leaves and flowering tops. Oregano is a culinary herb and is widely used in kitchens all over the world, extensively through the Mediterranean cuisine. Furthermore, the oregano medicinal values were acknowledged by Greeks from ancient times.

The Oregano's essential oil has been largely studied and reported to have several biological properties, including, antioxidant, antimicrobial, and antimutagenic activities. It also has been found to have great potential in the food industry as a food additive. More specifically, oregano's essential oil contains carvacrol, thymol, ρ-cymene, thymoquinone, and γ-terpinene.

Currently, studying properties of this plant's extracts are attracting more interest due to the growing interest for the research of alternatives for potential treatment and prevention of certain diseases like cancer.

Therefore, there is much interest in investigating Oregano properties for medical purposes. In this chapter, the focus is laid on the chemical composition, pharmacological and biological properties of Oregano and its health benefits.

Keywords: oregano, essential oils, extracts, phytochemicals, biological activities

* Corresponding Author's E-mail: laritfarida@gmail.com.

ABBREVIATIONS

ABTS	2,20-azino-bis(3-ethylbenzothiazoline-6-sulphonic acid)
BHT	Butylated hydroxytoluene
CAA	Cellular *antioxidant* activity
COX-2	Cyclooxygenase-2
CUPRAC	Cupric ion reducing antioxidant capacity
DPPH	1,10-diphenyl-2-picrylhydrazyl radical
DW	Dried weight
DWE	Dried weight extract
ET	Electron transfer
FRAP	Ferric reducing-antioxidant power assay
HAT	Hydrogen atom transfer
iNOS	Nitric oxide synthase
IL-1β	Interleukin 1 beta
IL-6	Interleukin 6
IL-8	Interleukin 8
IL-10	Interleukin 10
LPS	Lipopolysaccharide
MCP-1	Monocyte chemoattractant protein 1
NF-κB	Nuclear factor kappa-light-chain-enhancer of activated B cells
NO	Nitric oxide
ORAC	Oxygen radical absorbance assay
ROS	Reactive oxygen species
SFE	supercritical fluid extraction
TAC	Total antioxidant capacity
TEAC	Trolox equivalent antioxidant capacity
TPC	Total phenolic content
TNF-	α Tumor necrosis factor alpha

INTRODUCTION

Origanum genus from the Lamiaceae family, is an important culinary herb. Based on morphological criteria, the genus *Origanum* has been classified into three groups, 10 sections, 38 species, 6 subspecies, and 17 hybrids, most of them are native to the Mediterranean region (Ietswaart and Ietswaart 1980, Vokou, Kokkini et al. 1993) . Oregano is morphologicaly characterized by the presence of glandular and nonglandular trichomes covering the aerial organs. The glandular trichoma responsible of the production of essential oil with its unique flavor, which is mainly due to certain major constituents such as carvacrol and thymol (Fleisher, Sneer et al. 1982).

Origanum vulgare L. (Oregano), is the most widespread and known species of Lamiaceae family and the most variable species of the genus *Oreganum*. Known as a flavoring herb, oregano is widely used in kitchens all over the world, extensively through the Mediterranean cuisine. Its flavoring properties have been attributed to its aromatic substances and compositions of essential oil. The chemical diversity of oregano can vary due to many factors, including geographical region of origin, climate, harvest time and genetic factors (Figuérédo, Cabassu et al. 2006, Béjaoui, Chaabane et al. 2013, Calvo-Irabién, Parra-Tabla et al. 2014, Martínez-Natarén, Parra-Tabla et al. 2014, Lukas, Schmiderer et al. 2015, Kosakowska and Czupa 2018), resultingin in different pharmacological properties.

Oregano has been used for centuries as a medicinal herb in ethnopharmacological preparations to treat various ailments such as coughs, respiratory and digestive disorders, menstrual problems, asthma, cramping, diarrhea, indigestion, and inflammation-related diseases (Sarikurkcu, Zengin et al. 2015, Pezzani, Vitalini et al. 2017). In many regions in the word, an oregano infusion is still used as a folk remedy against cold and upset stomach and to maintain general health.

In recent years, *Origanum vulgare* L. has been increasingly studied as valuable source of natural products. The aerial parts contain a wide array of bioactive components, including essential oil, phenolic glycosides, flavonoids, tannins, resins, sterols and high amounts of terpenoids (Milos, Mastelic et al. 2000, Chun, Vattem et al. 2005, Teixeira, Marques et al. 2013, Pezzani, Vitalini et al. 2017).

Phytochemicals are a heterogeneous class of compounds derived from the secondary metabolism of plants, thus most of them do not appear to participate in essential metabolic roles. Research indicates that the main physiological function of phytochemicals is to serve as a plant defense mechanism against plant pathogens, pests, herbivores, UV-light and oxidative stress (Briskin 2000, Shetty 2004, Liu 2007).

Numerous studies have shown that the pharmaceutical properties of oregano are due to its essential oil composition which consists mostly of phenolic monoterpenoides such as carvacrol and thymol (Lambert, Skandamis et al. 2001, Nostro, Blanco et al. 2004). Essential oil of oregano has shown to exhibit high antioxidant and antimicrobial activities (Chun, Vattem et al. 2005, Karakaya, El et al. 2011). Oregano essential oil has also been found to provid an interesting inhibitory effects on food-borne pathogens such as *Salmonella spp., E. coli and L. monocytogenes* (Şahin, Güllüce et al. 2004, Ozkalp, Sevgi et al. 2010, De Azeredo, Stamford et al. 2011).

Generally, the phytochemicals present in oregano are grouped depending on their hydrophilic and hydrophobic properties into two categories: essential oil and phenolic compounds. Previous research has often focused on the study of chemical composition of essential oil. On the other hand, the study of hydrophilic compounds such as phenolic compounds (flavonoids and phenolic acids) is frequently ignored.

Therefore, the present manuscript will review recent investigations regarding the composition of essential oil and phenolic compounds of different oregano subspecies and their biological activities, including the antimicrobial, antioxidant, anti-inflammatory, antiproliferative, and neuroprotective properties.

Classification, Description, Traditional Use and Benefits

Clasification

Kingdom Plantae – Plants
Subkingdom Tracheobionta – Vascular plants
Superdivision Spermatophyta – Seed plants
Division Magnoliophyta – Flowering plants
Class Magnoliopsida – Dicotyledons
Subclass Asteridae
Order Lamiales
Family Lamiaceae – Mint family
Genus Origanum L. – origanum P
Species Origanum vulgare L. – oregano P

Description and Geographical Distrubtion

Oregano, is a bushy, rhizomatous, woody-branched hairy perennial herb which typically grows to 30-80cm high on square stems clad with aromatic, glandular-spotted, rounded to ovate leaves (1.35-2.50 cm x 0.90-1.80cm), which are usually entire but sometimes have slightly toothed margins. Tiny, two-lipped, pinkish-purple or white flowers (typical mint family), each with 4 protruding stamens and leafy purple-toned bracts, bloom in axillary or terminal corymb-like spikelets which rise above the foliage in summer (Figure 1).

Without focusing on subspecies, oregano is indigenous to the Mediterranean regions, now it is widely distributed throughout Europe and the Mediterranean to West and Central Asia and Taiwan. It is also cultivated in many countries of the world, including South-East Asia and America.

Oregano is an extremely variable species. The taxonomic revision by Ietswaart (Ietswaart and Ietswaart 1980) divided Origanum vulgare L. into six subspecies: subsp.

hirtum (Link) Ietswaart, subsp. vulgare L., subsp. virens (Hoffmannsegg et Link) Ietswaart, subsp. viride (Boissier) Hayek, subsp. gracile (Kock) Ietswaart and subsp. glandulosum (Desfontaines) Ietswaart. Kokkini (Kokkini 1996) confirms this distribution, but identifies subsp. viride of Ietswaart as subsp. viridulum (Martin-Donos).

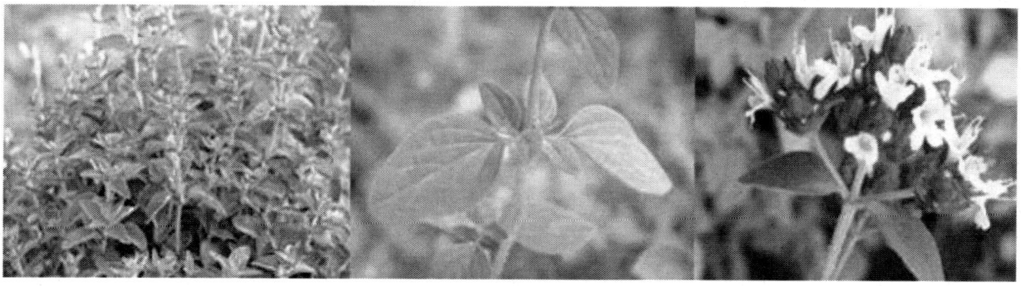

Figure 1. *Origanum vulgare* L. aerial parts, leaves and flowers.

Theses subspecies are distinguished from each other by some morphological characteristics such as the indumentums differences, number of sessile glands on leaves, and in size and colour of bracts and flowers.

Traditional Uses, Benefits and Side Effects

Oregano is one of the most economically and commercially important herbs. This is not only related to its use as a spice. Its essential oil is largely used because of its various pharmacological properties (Bakkali, Averbeck et al. 2008, Rubió, Motilva et al. 2013, Swamy, Akhtar et al. 2016). Recently, oregano has drawn more attention of researchers and consumers due to the many effects of this herb on human health (Singletary 2010).

Oregano has been used a long time for medicinal properties and food preparation purposes. It is mainly used as a culinary condiment and largely employed in popular medicine. Oregano mostly used in the Mediterranean cuisine as frequent addition to enhance the flavors of a variety of foods including legumes, fish, pizza, pasta sauce, chilis and several wordwild dishes. It has also been included in aromatic teas. It is also used as raw material in the pharmaceutical, cosmetic, and food industries.

As a medicinal plant, oregano has traditionally been used as a carminative, diaphoretic, expectorant, emmenagogue, stimulant, stomachic, and tonic. In addition, it has been used as a folk remedy to treat various diseases such as dysentery, colitis, bronco-pulmonary, gastric acidity, and gastro-intestinal diseases. Moreover, due to its antimutagenic and anticarcinogenic effects, oregano may represent a source for alternative potential treatment of certain chronic ailments, like cancer (Arcila-Lozano, Loarca-Pina et al. 2004).

The essential oil, aqueous infusion and decoction of oregano have been traditionally used for therapeutic applications. Essential oil of oregano is recognized to have many health benefits including treatment of parasitic and fungal infections, strengthening the immune system, and improving digestion. The benefits of oregano essential oil can be attribute to its constutents (carvacrol and thymol). Carvacrol may fight the growth of bacteria, including antibiotic-resistant bacteria (Magi, Marini et al. 2015). While thymol has antifungal effects, useful for treating oral thrush, or candidiasis (de Castro, de Souza et al. 2015).

There are a variety of methods used for the extraction of essential oils. Each method exhibits certain advantages and determining the biological and physicochemical properties of the extacted oils. Common extraction methods including Steam Distillation, Solvent Extraction, CO_2 Extraction, Maceration, Enfleurage, Cold Press Extraction, and Water Distillation are used to extract essential oils from plants. Advanced methods like supercritical fluid extraction (SFE) with CO_2, which is a high-pressure technology, subcritical extraction liquid, and solvent free microwave extraction, considered as attractive methods compared to conventional techniques such as steam distillation or Soxhlet extraction because due to less extraction time, low energy consumption, low solvent used and less carbon dioxide emission (Aziz, Ahmad et al. 2018). Thus, their use is in increasing demand to produce high-quality essential oils from plants material with therapeutical properties.

Despite their wide variety of applications, essential oils should be used with precaution. Essential oils tend to have potential toxic effects such as phototoxicity or photosensitivity. High doses of certain essential oils could have hepatotoxic, nephrotoxic and neurotoxic effects (Nath, Pandey et al. 2012). According to previous studies, oregano essential oil is never topically applied to mucous membranes in concentrations higher than 1%, due to the possible irritating effect to the skin and even a possible burning effect (Singletary 2010). Carvacrol and thymol, main compounds of oregano essential oil, can be toxic to liver, kidneys and nervous system if taken in excess. Carvacrol and thymol have been reported to show in *in vivo* mutagenicity and genotoxicity (Azirak and Rencuzogullari 2008, Llana-Ruiz-Cabello, Gutiérrez-Praena et al. 2015). On the other hand, It has been demonstrated that the use of infusion/decoction, by internal or external use, can avoid the toxic effects showed by other oregano fractions such as essential oil (Martins, Barros et al. 2014). Hence, the benefits of oregano and its components to human health will depend on the bioavailability of its bioactive phytochemicals and their possible potential toxicity and side effects on human cell.

CHEMICAL COMPOSTION AND ACTIVE CONSTITUENTS

The aroma, flavor, and pharmaceutical properties of oregano are resulted of its essential oil composition. According to the extensive phytochemical studies on the essential oil composition of oregano and other related species, a wide chemical diversity with a considerable intraspecific qualitative and quantitative variation in constituents is found (Mechergui, Jaouadi et al. 2016, Morshedloo, Salami et al. 2018)· (Béjaoui, Boulila et al. 2017).

Essential oil of Oregano is a very complex mixture of compounds which consist mostly of monoterpenes and sesquiterpenes. Previous studies reported that individuals rich in essential oil usually accumulate large amounts of phenolic monoterpenes such as carvacrol and thymol. Moreover, *γ*-terpinene and *p*-cymene have been detected in appreciable amounts, whereas the plants with poor essential oil content are often characterized by high amounts of sesquiterpenes (such as germacrene D, (E)-β-caryophyllene, γ-muurolene and caryophyllene oxide), acyclic monoterpenoids (such as linalool and/or linalyl acetate, β-ocimene or myrcene) and/or bicyclic sabinyl -type monoterpenoids (mainly sabinene and cis-/trans-sabinene hydrate) (Azizi, Yan et al. 2009, Lukas, Schmiderer et al. 2015).

The fragrance and chemical composition of essential oils of the different subspecies of oregano can vary depend on the geo-climatic location and growing conditions, including concentration of nutrients, temperature, humidity, soil type, climate, altitude, etc. (Azizi, Wagner et al. 2009, Gonceariuc, Balmuş et al. 2015, De Mastro, Tarraf et al. 2017, Morshedloo, Salami et al. 2018). The chemical composition of essential oil of oregano also depends on season or vegetative period of plant.

Essential oils extracted from the different subspecies of oregano are widely recognized for their antimicrobial and antifungal activities, as well as their antiviral, antioxidant, anti-inflammatory, antidiabetic and cancer suppressor agents properties (Singletary 2010, Leyva-López, Gutiérrez-Grijalva et al. 2017). These properties of oregano essential oil are of potential interest to the food, cosmetic and pharmaceutical industries. Several studies reported the relashionship between chemical composition and biological properties of essential oils and their application in various commercial and pharmacological preparations (Singletary 2010).

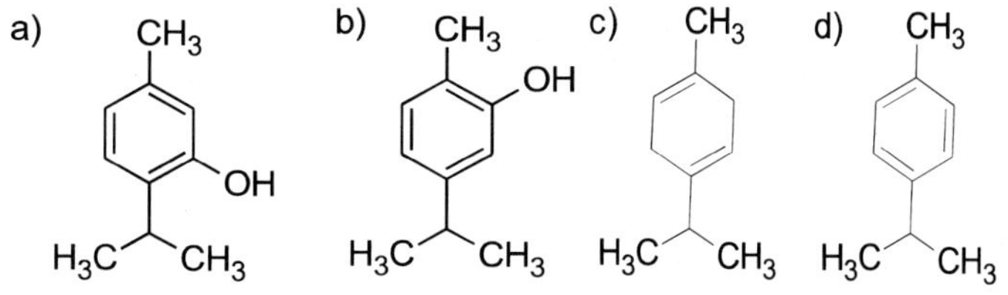

Figure 2. Chemical structures of the main compounds present in the essential oil of oregano (Origanum vulgare L. a) thymol, b) carvacrol, c) γ-Terpinene, d) p-Cymene.

In recent years, many researchers from all over the world have intensively investigated the essential oils of the diferrent subspecies of oregano for their chemical composition and pharmacological activities. These substances are responsible for the aroma and flavor of oregano, their pharmaceutical uses as antimicrobial and antiseptic agents, and its anti-oxidant activity, often touted as a health benefit.

Table 1. Chemical constituents of essential oils extracted from different subspecies of *Origanum vulgare* L.

***Oreganum vulgare* L. subspecies**	**Origin**	**Principal Constituents**	**Content %**	**Reference**
Origanum vilgare. L	Argentina	p-Cymene	26.00	(Werdin González, Gutiérrez et al. 2011)
		γ-Terpinene	21.89	
		Terpinen-4-ol	16.29	
		β-caryophyllene	8.25	
		Carvacrol	26.70	(Martucci, Gende et al. 2015)
		p-cymene	15.20	
		γ-Terpinene	15.10	
		Terpinene	7.50	
		γ-Terpinene	25.1	(Olmedo, Nepote et al. 2014)
		Terpinen-4-ol	16.7	
		Carvacrol	16.2	
		_α-Terpinene	8.54	
		γ-Terpinene	32.1	(Quiroga, Grosso et al. 2013)
		α-Terpinene	15.1	
		p-Cymene	8.0	
		Thymol	8.0	
		Carvacrol	81.92	(Wei, Chen et al. 2015)
		γ-Terpinene	4.49	
		Thymol	3.5	
		p-Cymene	3.07	
	Brazil	Carvacrol	73.9	(Waller, Madrid et al. 2016)
		γ-Terpinene	3.6	
		Thymol	3.0	
		β-Caryophyllene	2.8	
	Chile	cis-β-Terpineol	16.49	(Elizalde and Espinoza 2011)
		Thymol	13.26	
		Terpinen-4-ol	10.24	
		α-Terpineol	4.35	
	China	Carvacrol	30.73	(Han, Ma et al. 2017)
		Thymol	18.81	
		p-Cymene	10.88	
		β-caryophyllene	8.21	

***Oreganum vulgare* L. subspecies**	**Origin**	**Principal Constituents**	**Content %**	**Reference**
Origanum vilgare. L	China	β-Citronellol	85.3	(Gong, Liu et al. 2014)
		Citronellol acetate	5.2	
		β-Citronellal	1.2	
		Thymol	42.9	(Gong, Liu et al. 2014)
		Citronellol	12.2	
		β-caryophyllene	7.8	
		p-Cymen-2-ol	7.5	
		β-Citronellol	75.0	(Gong, Liu et al. 2014)
		Geraniol	7.7	
		Citronellol acetate	3.4	
		1,8-Cineole	20.8	(Gong, Liu et al. 2014)
		β-Caryophyllene	10.2	
		Eugenol methyl ether	9.8	
		Citronellol	8.8	
		Caryophyllene oxide _-	32.9	(Gong, Liu et al. 2014)
		caryophyllene	17.7	
		citronellol	10.2	
		germacrene D	9.8	
	Pakistan	β-Citronellol	72.7	(Gong, Liu et al. 2014)
		Thymol	7.2	
		Citronellol acetate	5.9	
	Colombia	Thymol	21.5	(Betancourt, Phandanauvong et al. 2012)
		p-Cymene	21.0	
		γ-Terpinene	20.3	
		α-Terpinene	5.9	
	Greece	Carvacrol	63.03	(Thomidis and Filotheou 2016)
		Thymol	15.09	
		p-Cymene	10.47	
		γ-terpinene	3.43	
	India	Carvacrol	35.02–62.81	(Verma, Rahman et al. 2010)
		p-Cymene	8.60–46.59	
		γ-Terpinene	2.49–19.11	
	Iran	Carvacrol	29.85	(Pirigharnaei, Zare et al. 2011)
		γ-Terpinene	20.94	
		α-Himachalene	12.17	
		β-Pinene	11.67	

Table 1. (Continued)

Oreganum vulgare L. subspecies	Origin	Principal Constituents	Content %	Reference
Origanum vilgare. L	Iran	Carvacrol γ-Terpinene Thymol Germacrene D-4-ol	23.54 20.50 15.41 9.26	(Pirigharnaei, Zare et al. 2011)
		Carvacrol γ-Terpinene Cedrene	59.37 18.36 6.65.	(Pirigharnaei, Zare et al. 2011)
		Carvacrol Humulene γ -Terpinene	58.51 11.46 9.56	(Pirigharnaei, Zare et al. 2011)
		Carvacrol γ-Terpinene Humulene	67.09 7.71 7.67	(Pirigharnaei, Zare et al. 2011)
	Italy	Cavacrol p-Cymene γ-terpinene β-Caryophyllene	65.94 9.33 5.25 3.72	(Fratini, Mancini et al. 2017)
		Carvacrol p-Cymene β-Caryophyllene Linalool	71.8 11.6 2.7 1.8	(Pesavento, Calonico et al. 2015)
	Morocco	Carvacrol γ-Terpinene p-Cymene Thymol	34.0 21.6 9.4 3.3	(Fouad, Bousta et al. 2015)
	Poland	Carvacrol Thymo γ-Terpinene p-Cymene	26.38–36.72 16.59–25.58 10.06–16.11 6.09–6.76	(Figiel, Szumny et al. 2010)
	Portugal	Carvacrol β-Fenchyl alcohol γ-Terpinene δ-Terpineol	14.5 12.8 11.6 7.5	(Teixeira, Marques et al. 2013)

***Oreganum vulgare* L. subspecies**	**Origin**	**Principal Constituents**	**Content %**	**Reference**
Origanum vilgare. L	Serbia	Sabinene Terpinen-4-ol 1,8-Cineole γ-Terpinene	10.2 9.3 5.8 5.6	(Ličina, Stefanović et al. 2013)
		Carvacrol p-Cymene γ-Terpinene Thymol	64.5 10.9 10.8 3.5	(Soković, Glamočlija et al. 2010)
		Carvacrol p-Cymene γ-Terpinene Thymol	64.5 10.9 10.8 3.5	(Stojković, Glamočlija et al. 2013)
		Carvacrol p-Cymene Trans-β-caryophyllene Linalool	77.6 5.14 2.45 2.44	(Boskovic, Zdravkovic et al. 2015)
	Spain	Terpinen-4-ol Carvacrol Thymol γ-Terpinene	24.57 16.09 9.03 6.20	(Bolechowski, Moral et al. 2011)
Origanum vulgare L.ssp. vulgare	Argentina	trans-Sabinene hydrate Thymol Terpinen-4-ol γ-terpinene	23.4–27.2 14.4–17.2 7.8–11.0 7.3–9.8	(Asensio, Grosso et al. 2015)
		trans-Sabinene hydrate Thymol γ-Terpinene Terpinen-4-ol	32.47 20.5 15.47 5.03	(Dambolena, Zunino et al. 2009)
	Iran	Thymol γ-Terpinene Carvacrol Carvacrol methyl ether	37.13 9.67 9.57 6.88	(Vazirian, Mohammadi et al. 2015)
	Italy	Spathulenol carvacrol β-Caryophyllene Terpinen-4-ol	18.6 11.7 8.8 5.6	(De Falco, Mancini et al. 2013)

Table 1. (Continued)

***Oreganum vulgare* L. subspecies**	**Origin**	**Principal Constituents**	**Content %**	**Reference**
Origanum vulgare L.ssp. vulgare	Italy	Carvacrol Spathulenol β-Caryophyllene Terpinen-4-ol	14.3 9.4 5.3 5.0	(De Falco, Mancini et al. 2013)
	Lithuania	Sabinene β-Caryophyllene E-β-ocimene allo-Ocimene	6.6–28.2 7.3–15.5 4.4–15.1 7.7–12.1	(Baranauskienė, Venskutonis et al. 2013)
	Turkey	Thymol Carvacrol p-Cymene γ-Terpinene	58.31 16.11 13.45 4.64	(Sarikurkcu, Zengin et al. 2015)
	Poland	Sabinene Z-(β)-Ocimene Germacrene D E-Caryophyllene	10.85–25.46 9.10–16.33 9.36–15.34 9.38–12.87	(Nurzyńska-Wierdak, Bogucka-Kocka et al. 2012)
Origanum vulgare L. ssp. hirtum	Germany	Carvacrol	77.4	(Azizi, Yan et al. 2009)
	Moldova	Carvacrol γ-Terpinene p-Cymene	77,61-85,88 3,64-9,33 8,22-5,30	(Gonceariuc, Balmuş et al. 2015)
	Argentina	trans-Sabinene hydrate Thymol γ-Terpinene Terpinen-4-ol	22.9 18.6 7.1 6.2	(Asensio, Grosso et al. 2015)
		trans-Sabinene hydrate thymol Terpinen-4-ol γ-Terpinene	17.9 17.1 9.5 8.0	(Asensio, Grosso et al. 2015)
		Terpinene Terpinen-4-ol α-terpinene trans-Sabinene hydrate	13.7 11.2 9.9 8.3	(Grondona, Gatti et al. 2014)

***Oreganum vulgare* L. subspecies**	**Origin**	**Principal Constituents**	**Content %**	**Reference**
Origanum vulgare L. ssp. hirtum	Colombia	Carvacrol Thymol p-Cymene γ-Terpinene	90.3 3.5 2.7 1.0	(Betancourt, Phandanauvong et al. 2012)
	Greece	Carvacrol p-Cymene γ-Terpinene β-Myrcene	70.38 8.17 7.78 2.37	(Rodríguez-Solana, Daferera et al. 2014)
		Carvacrol γ-Terpinene p-Cymene β-Caryophyllene	90.29 3.09 2.25 1.81	(Economou, Panagopoulos et al. 2011)
		Carvacrol p-Cymene γ-Terpinene β-Caryophyllene	81.28–91.21 1.52–6.40 0.49–4.01 0.94–2.03	(Paraskevakis, Tsiplakou et al. 2015)
		Carvacrol p-Cymene β-Disavolene	56.46–82.70 9.54–21.40 1.09–3.06	(Karamanos, Sotiropoulou et al. 2013)
	Hungary	Carvacrol p-Cymene γ-Terpinene	82.75 6.58 5.78	(Novák, Sipos et al. 2011)
	Italy	Thymol and Carvacrol	74.8	(Elshafie, Armentano et al. 2017)
		Terpinen-4-ol γ-Terpinene Carvacrol p-Cymene	13.27–17.51 14.58–14.95 12.31–14.58 8.43–10.07	(Tibaldi, Fontana et al. 2011)
		Thymol γ-Terpinene p-Cymene α-Terpinene	37.9 24.5 16.3 4.3	(Spagnoletti, Guerrinia et al. 2016)
		γ-Terpinene Thymol p-Cymene α-Terpinene	29.41 26.86 8.20 5.93	(Bonfanti, Iannì et al. 2012)

Table 1. (Continued)

Oreganum vulgare **L. subspecies**	**Origin**	**Principal Constituents**	**Content %**	**Reference**
Origanum vulgare L. ssp. hirtum	Italy	Thymol γ-Terpinene p-Cymene α-Terpinene	37.22 26.37 6.83 4.02	(Bonfanti, Iannì et al. 2012)
		Thymol -terpinene p-cymene carvacrol methyl ether	36.46 20.77 8.31 6.21	(Bonfanti, Iannì et al. 2012)
		Thymol γ-Terpinene p-Cymene Carvacrol methyl ether	30.25 25.89 7.62 5.63	(Bonfanti, Iannì et al. 2012)
		Thymol and carvacrol Linalool Carvacrol methyl ether	65.3–84.7 0.1–2.6 0.4–1.9	(Mancini, Camele et al. 2014)
		Thymol γ-Terpinene p-Cymene	18.16–56.37 12.70–32.70 8.22–10.30	(Baranauskienė, Venskutonis et al. 2013)
	Lithuania	Carvacrol γ-Terpinene p-Cymene β-caryophyllene	72.4–88.2 4.1–8.7 2.0–3.2 0.9–3.0	(Baranauskienė, Venskutonis et al. 2013)
	Serbia	Carvacrol p-Cymene γ-Terpinene trans-β-Caryophyllene	74.65 5.87 5.04 1.76	(Stamenic, Vulic et al. 2014)
	Turkey	Carvacrol p-Cymene Linalool	63.97 12.63 3.67	(Özkan, Güney et al. 2017)
		Linalool β-Caryophyllene	96.31 1.27.	(Sarikurkcu, Zengin et al. 2015)
		Carvacrol γ-Terpinene p-Cymene α-Terpinene	80.09 12.01 1.72 1.58	(Arslan, Uremis et al. 2012)

***Oreganum vulgare* L. subspecies**	**Origin**	**Principal Constituents**	**Content %**	**Reference**
Origanum vulgare ssp. gracile	Iran	Carvacrol, γ-Terpinene ρ-Cymene	46.5 -60.6 1.13- 6.88 13.91- 16.64	(Moradi, Hassani et al. 2014)
		Carvacrol γ-Terpinene p-Cymene Carvacrol methyl ether	46.86 14.16 11.63 5.97	(Morshedloo, Craker et al. 2017)
	Turkey	Thymol Carvacrol, γ-Terpinene p-Cymene	7.02–40.04 8.21–33.21 9.15–27.82 3.07–23.52	(Kilic and Özdemir 2016)
Origanum vulgare L.ssp. virens	Argentina	trans-Sabinene hydrate Thymol γ-Terpinene α-Terpinene	27.77 26.1 5.9 4.17	(Dambolena, Zunino et al. 2009)
	Iran	(Z)-α-Bisabolene Sabinene Carvacrol β-Bisabolene	39.17 11.52 5.23 4.24	(Morshedloo, Craker et al. 2017)
	Portugal	α-Terpineol γ-Terpinene Linalool Carvacrol E-Caryophyllene	0.1–65.1 0.3–34.25 2.0–27.4 0–34.2 2.4–11.0	(Vale-Silva, Silva et al. 2012)
Origanum vulgare var. creticum	Germany	Carvacrol	74.9	(Azizi, Yan et al. 2009)
Origanum vulgare var. samothrake		Carvacrol	70	(Azizi, Yan et al. 2009)

Two components of essential oils, the phenolic monoterpenes, thymol and carvacrol, which are especially known for their antimicrobial and antioxidant activities (Meeran, Fizur et al. 2017, Sharifi-Rad, Varoni et al. 2018), are generally the most abundant in essential oils of many species. However, the composition and quantity of essential oil varies strongly between populations and accessions of oregano (De Mastro, Tarraf et al. 2017, Morshedloo, Salami et al. 2018).

PHYTOCHEMICAL STUDY OF OREGANO

Previous studies on the oregano species from different regions of the world focused mainly on the study of the chemical composition and biological properties of oregano essential oil. In addition of these volatile constituents that significantly contribute to the aroma and flavour of oregano and in its pharmacological properties including antimicrobial and antioxidant activities, polyphenols like flavonoids and phenolic acids, are another kind of abundant constituents in oregano that possess diverse biological activities such as anti-ulcer, anti-inflammatory, antidiabetic, antiviral, cytotoxic and antitumour (Ghasemzadeh and Ghasemzadeh 2011), and they are suggested to be responsible in part for the health effects of oregano.

Bioactive compounds including phenolic acids such as caffeic acid, p-coumaric acid, rosmarinic acid and caffeoyl derivatives, ursolic acid, and carnosic acid, as well as a mixture of flavonoids have been identified in oregano (Hawas, El-Desoky et al. 2008, Radušienė, Ivanauskas et al. 2008, González, Luis et al. 2014, Zhang, Guo et al. 2014). Phenolics and flavonoids, constitute a major group of compounds, which act as primary antioxidants (Robards, Prenzler et al. 1999, Balasundram, Sundram et al. 2006), and are known to react with hydroxyl radicals (Husain, Cillard et al. 1987) and superoxide anion radicals (Yasuhisa, Hideki et al. 1993). They are also known to protect DNA from oxidative damage, inhibit growth of tumor cells and possess anti-inflammatory and antimicrobial properties. A significant positive correlation between the antioxidant activity and the contents of total flavonoid and total phenolic contents have been reported (Zheng and Wang 2001, Wojdyło, Oszmiański et al. 2007).

The content and distribution of flavonoids and phenolic acids in oregano can vary depending on the cultivar, geographical and environmental factors aforementioned. It has been indicated that the flavonoid and phenolic acids profile of oregano can be used to differentiate between oregano chemotypes within the same species (Gutiérrez-Grijalva, Picos-Salas et al. 2018). It can also be observed that oregano genotypes from the same species but from different places of origin can vary in their flavonoids and phenolic acids composition. Phytochemical investigations on oregano have shown that flavones including apigenin, luteolin and scutellarin and their derivatives are among the most abundant sub-group of flavonoids in oregano followed by flavonols, flavanones and flavanols (Gutiérrez-

Grijalva, Picos-Salas et al. 2018) (Figures 3-4). Among the most common phenolic acids in oregano are: hydroxycinnamic acid and hydrobenzoic acids derivatives (El-Seedi, El-Said et al. 2012) (Figures 5-6). A summary of the major flavonoids and phenolic acids recently found in oregano species are presented in Table 2.

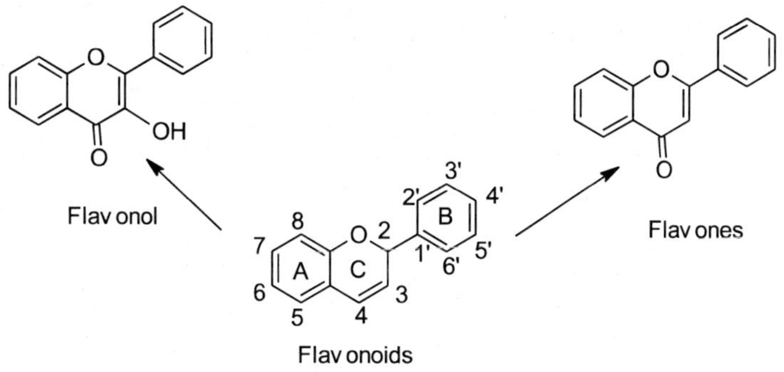

Figure 3. General structure of flavonoids, flavones and flavonols.

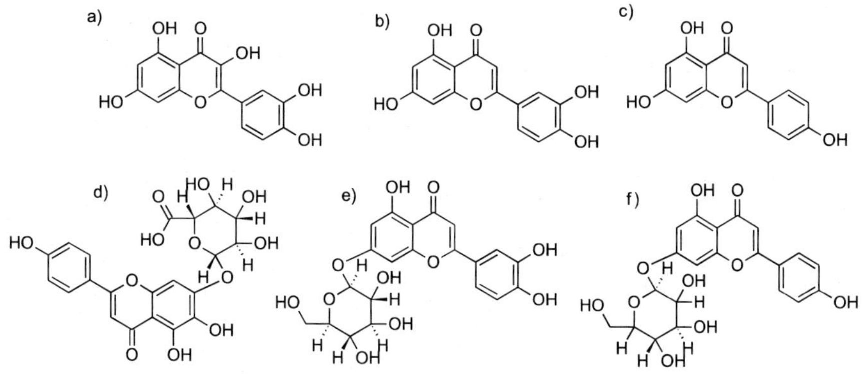

Figure 4. Chemical structure of certain flavonols and flavones commonly found in high abundance in oregano. a) Quercetin, b) luteolin, c) apigenin, d) scutellarin, e) luteolin-7-O-glucoside, f) apigenin-7-O-glucoside.

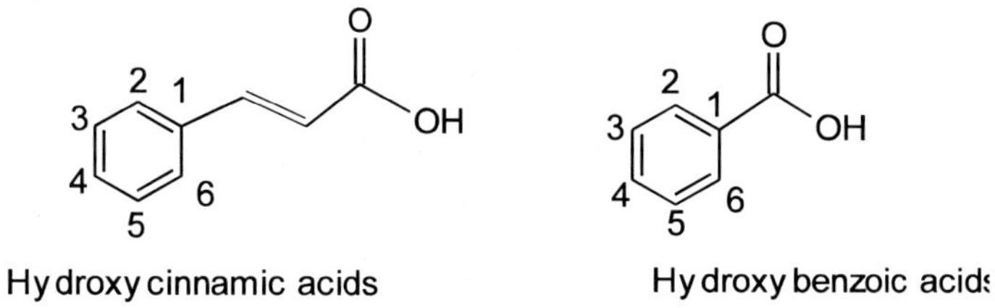

Figure 5. General structure of Hydroxycinnamic acids and hydroxybenzoic acids.

Table 2. Principal components of flavonoids and phenolic compounds of *Oreganum vulgare* L.

***Oreganum vulgare* L. subspecies**	**Origin**	**Extraction Solvent**	**Flavonoids and Phenolic Acids Constituents**	**Reference**
Origanum vulgare L. ssp. viride (Boiss.) Hayek	Turkey	Water Ethanol, ethanol, ethyl acetate and hexane	Gallic acid, caffeic acid, 4-hydroxybenzaldehyd, p-coumaric acid, apigenin-7-glucoside, rosmarinic acid, naringenin, quercetin, kaempferol and chicoric acid.	(Koldaş, Demirtas et al. 2015)
O. vulgare L. ssp. hirtum	Greece	Methanolic extract, aqueous extract	Salvianolic acid, Salvianolic acid B, Rosmarinic acid, Salvianolic acid C, Eriodictyol, Naringenin	(Vujicic, Nikolic et al. 2015)
Oreganum vulgare L.	China	Ethanolic extract	4-[[(2,5 -dihydroxybenzoyl)oxy]methyl] phenyl-O-β-D-glucopyranoside, 4-[[(3 ,4 -dihydroxybenzoyl)oxy]methyl]phenyl-O-β-D-[6-O-(3″,5″-dimethoxyl-4″-hydroxybenzoyl)] glucopyranoside, acacetin 7-O-[4‴-O-acetyl-β-D-apiofuransyl-(1→3)]- β-D-xylopyranoside, acacetin 7-O-[6-O-acetyl-β-D-galactopyranosyl-(1→3)]-β-D-xylopyranoside, apigenin 7-O-[6‴- O-acetyl-β-D-galactopyranosyl-(1→3)]-β-D-xylopyranoside, acacetin-7-O- [6‴-O-acetyl-β-D-galactopyranosyl-(1→2)]-β-D-glucopyranoside, 2,5-dihydroxybenzoic acid, rosmarinic acid, origanoside, maltol 6 -O-(5-O-pcoumaroyl)-β-D-apiofuranosyl-β-D-glucopyranoside	(Zhang, Guo et al. 2014)
	USA	Hydroalcholic extracts	Quercetin 3-O-glucoside, Quercetin 3 O-galactoside, Taxifolinc, Luteolin 7-O-glucoside, Rosmarinic acid	(Karimi, Min et al. 2014)
	Spain	Infusion, decoction, hydroalcoholic extract	3-O-Caffeolyquinic acid, Protocatechuic acid, 5-O-Caffeolyquinic acid, Rosmarinic acid, Lithospermic acid A, Apigenin 6,8-di-C-glucoside, Kaempferol O-hexosyl-O-hexoside, Myricetin 3-O-glucoside, Quercetin O-hexoside, 4-[[(2 ,5 Dihydroxybenzoyl)oxy]methyl]phenyl O-β-D-glucopyranoside, Taxifolin, Quercetin 3-O-rutinoside, Quercetin 7-O-hexoside, Luteolin O-glucuronide, Luteolin 7-O-glucoside, Apigenin 7-O-rutinoside, Apigenin 7-O-glucuronide, Kaempferol O-hexoside, Kaempferide O-glucuronide, Eridictyol, Methylapigenin O-glucuronide, Naringenin.	(Martins, Barros et al. 2014)
	Argentina	Hydroalcoholic extract	3-(3,4-dihydroxyphenyl)lactic acid, 3,4-dihydroxybenzoic acid, caffeic acid, 4-(3.4-dihydroxybenzoyloxymethyl)phenyl β-glucoside, rosmarinic acid	(González, Luis et al. 2014)
	Egypt	Methanolic extract	Apigenin, luteolin, salvagenin, cirsimartin, diosmetin, desmethoxycentauridin, 5-hydroxy-6,7,3,4 -tetramethoxy-abigenin, apigenin 7-O-glucoside, luteolin 7-O-glucoside, luteolin 7-O-glucoside-6″-methylester, luteolin 7-O-α-L-rhamnoside-4 -O-β-D-glucoside and quercetin 3-O-β-D-glucoside-4 -O-α-L-rhamnoside, 7-O-α-L-rhamnoside-4 -O-β-D-glucoside, 3-O-β-D-glucoside-4 -O-α-L-rhamnoside	(Hawas, El-Desoky et al. 2008)

***Oreganum vulgare* L. subspecies**	**Origin**	**Extraction Solvent**	**Flavonoids and Phenolic Acids Constituents**	**Reference**
Oreganum vulgare L.	Latvia	Methanol, Dietilether	Apigenin, Luteolin, Eriodictyol, Naringenin, Rosmarinic acid	(Kruma, Andjelkovic et al. 2008)
	Lithuania	ethanolic extracts	Rosemarinic acid, chlorogenic acid, caffeic acid, hyperozide, naringin, rutin, luteolin, astragalin, vitexin, isovitexin, eriodictol, quercetin, naringenin	(Radušienė, Ivanauskas et al. 2008)
	Taiwan	Aqueous ethanolic extract	Origalignanol, salvianolic acid A, salvianolic acid C, lithospermic acid, apigenin 7-O-β-D-glucuronide, apigenin 7-O-β-D-(6-methyl)glucuronide, luteolin, luteolin 7-O-β-D-glucopyranoside, luteolin 7-O-β-D-glucuronide, luteolin 7-O-β-D-xylopyranoside	(Lin, Wang et al. 2003)

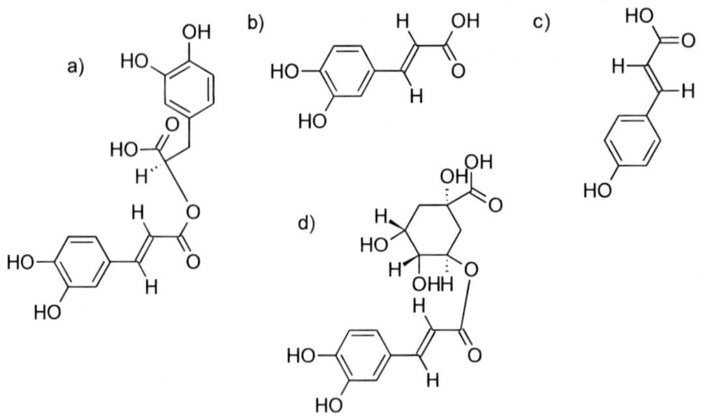

Figure 6. Chemical structures of phenolic acids commonly present in oregano. a) Rosmarinic acid, b) caffeic acid, c) p-coumaric acid d) Chlorogenic acid.

BIOLOGICAL/PHARMACOLOGICAL PROPERTIES

The biological activity of oregano depends on its composition. The polar phenols' thymol and carvacrol are responsible for many of the properties of the essential oil, as well as p-cymene and terpinene. The main known pharmacological activities of oregano were antibacterial, antifungal, antiparasitic, antioxidant, and anti-inflammatory (Leyva-López, Gutiérrez-Grijalva et al. 2017, Pezzani, Vitalini et al. 2017). Thymol is one of the most important dietary constituents in thyme and *Origanum* species. For centuries, it has been used in traditional medicine and has been shown to possess various pharmacological properties including antioxidant, free radical scavenging, anti-inflammatory, analgesic, antispasmodic, antibacterial, antifungal, antiseptic and antitumor activities (Meeran, Fizur et al. 2017). Carvacrol is widely used in food, pharmaceutical, nutraceutical, agricultural, and perfumery fields. It has been reported to exhibit antimutagenic activity, which seems to be mainly linked to the induction of mitochondrial dysfunction (Sharifi-Rad, Varoni et al. 2018).

Flavonoids isolated from oregano such as flavones, have been shown to posses many pharmacological properties such as anti-inflammatory, antioxidant, anti-asthmatic, anti-ulcer, decreased risk of cardiovascular diseases, anti-diabetic, anti-cancer, and neuroprotective (Zhang, Guo et al. 2014, Gutiérrez-Grijalva, Picos-Salas et al. 2018). Flavonols may have a rol in cardiovascular diseases prevention (Menezes, Rodriguez-Mateos et al. 2017). Phenolic acid derivatives have been linked with anti-diabetic, antioxidant and anti-cancer properties (Petersen and Simmonds 2003, Taofiq, González-Paramás et al. 2017).

In the following sub-sections, we will discuss studies regarding the pharmacological properties of oregano, including the antimicrobial, antioxidant, anti-inflammatory, anti-cancer and neuroprotective properties of oregano.

Antimicrobial Properties

Previous studies showed that oregano has important biological activities such as antibacterial, antifungal and anti-genotoxic effects (Leyva-López, Gutiérrez-Grijalva et al. 2017, Pezzani, Vitalini et al. 2017). Oregano possesses a broad spectrum of antimicrobial activity due, at least in part, to its high content of phenolic derivatives, such as carvacrol and thymol. Thymol and carvacrol are among the most active components against multiple foodborne pathogens. Their antibacterial activity and synergistic effect in combination with antibiotics against food-related bacteria have been reported (Meeran, Fizur et al. 2017, Sharifi-Rad, Varoni et al. 2018). There are a convincing number of studies that reveal that thymol alone or thymol in plants along with other metabolites possess potent antimicrobial, antifungal, antibacterial, and antiparasitic properties (Meeran, Fizur et al. 2017). Due to its potent antimicrobial properties, thymol is frequently used in dentistry for the treatment of oral cavity infections (Meeran, Fizur et al. 2017). Thymol was also shown to possess cytotoxic and antileishmanial activities (Robledo, Osorio et al. 2005). Previous studies reported that carvacrol showed strong antimicrobial activity against a wide range of Gram-positive and -negative bacteria (Magi, Marini et al. 2015).

In the assessment of antimicrobial activity of oregano preparations, it was shown that Gram-positive bacteria (*Micrococcus sp., Bacillus subtilis, Tetracoccus sp., Staphylococcus aureus, Enterococcus faecalis*) were more sensitive to the essential oil (Hac-Szymanczuk, Lipinska et al. 2014) and water extract of oregano than Gram-negative ones (*Proteus vulgaris, Proteus mirabilis, E. coli*, *Klebsiella* (K.) *pneumoniae, Salmonella Enteritidis*). The most resistant among the bacteria tested for the active components contained in the oregano oil were *E. coli* bacteria (Hac-Szymanczuk, Lipinska et al. 2014), and the lowest sensitivity to the activity of water extract from this plant was demonstrated by *K. pneumoniae* and *Salmonella Enteritidis* (Hac-Szymanczuk, Lipinska et al. 2014). The authors concluded that the antimicrobial activity of oregano oil was associated with the presence of compounds identified in it: carvacrol, camphor, linalol, R(+) limonene, 1,4-cineol and c-terpinene, and in the case of extract: chlorogenic and p-coumarin acid as well as mirycetin. Recently, some studies have demonstrated that the addition of oregano preparations may be an auxiliary factor in prolonging the storage stability of vacuum-packed BAADER meat from chickens stored frozen for 9 months (Hać-Szymańczuk, Cegiełka et al. 2018). The highest activity in inhibiting oxidative changes of lipids and limiting the growth of microflora in BAADER meat from chickens was demonstrated for oregano essential oil.

Oregano essential oil and certain of its constituents have been demonstrated to be antifungal *in vitro* and *in vivo* against yeasts of medical importance such as *Candida albicans*. The essential oil of oregano was found to be significantly active against the Gram-positive pathogens, among which *S. epidermidis* was the most affected (Sarikurkcu, Zengin et al. 2015). Cleff et al. (Cleff, Meinerz et al. 2010) demonstrated the antifungal effect of oregano essential oil against *Candida spp.* suggest its administration may represent an alternative treatment for candidiasis. Also, *O. vulgare* essential oil was exhibited antifungal activity against three Monilinia species(Mancini, Camele et al. 2014). Oregano essential oil and its components have been reported to show significant inhibition of some phytopathogenic fungi such as *Botrytis cinerea* Pers., *Penicillium italicum Wehmer*, *P. expansum* Link, *Phytophthora citrophthora* (R. E. Sm. & E. H. Sm.) *Leonian* and *Rhizopus stolonifer* (Ehrenb.: Fr.) Vuill. (Camele, Altieri et al. 2012) and *Aspergillus niger* Tiegh., *A. flavus* Link, *A. ochraceus* K. Wilh., *Fusarium oxysporum* W. C. Snyder & H. N. Hansen, *F. solani var. coeruleum* (Mart.) Sacc., *Penicillium sp.*, *Pseudomonas aeruginosa* J. Schrt. ATCC 2730, *Staphylococus aureus Rosenbach* ATCC 6538, *Clavibacter michiganensis* S., *P. infestans* Mont., *Sclerotinia sclerotiorum* Lib., and *Xanthomonas vesicatoria* Doidge (Adebayo, Dang et al. 2013).

A recent study has demonstrated the insect-repellent activity of oregano essential oils against *S. oryzae*, *T. confusum* adults and *Tribolium* adults (La Pergola, Restuccia et al. 2017). According to the report, these results were attributed to the activity of its main components, precisely, carvacrol.

Antioxidant Properties

The oxidative stress imposed by reactive oxygen species (ROS) plays an important role in many oxidative stress-related diseases, such as cardiovascular diseases, cancer, ageing, diabetes mellitus and neurodegenerative diseases. The high antioxidant activity of polyphenols is mainly due to their redox properties, which allows them to act as reducing agents, hydrogen donors, and singlet oxygen quenchers. In this context, oxidative stress plays an important role in the progression of neurodegenerative conditions, including rheumatic and cardiovascular disorders, metabolic syndrome and other diseases (Uttara, Singh et al. 2009). Phenolic compounds can be extracted using different polar solvents like water, methanol and ethanol to obtain antioxidant-rich extracts (Garcia-Salas, Morales-Soto et al. 2010). The antioxidant capacity of pure compounds, fractions and crud extracts can be tested using a wide variety of methods like hydrogen atom transfer (HAT) and electron transfer (ET). For instance, the oxygen radical absorbance assay (ORAC) is among the most common HAT assay used. On the other hand, the most commonly used ET methods are: the inhibition of the 1,10-diphenyl-2-picrylhydrazyl radical (DPPH), the Trolox equivalent antioxidant capacity (TEAC) method/ABTS radical cation decolorization assay (also known as ABTS assay), the ferric reducing-antioxidant power assay (FRAP), the cupric ion reducing antioxidant capacity method (CUPRAC) and total phenolic content assay. These assays have frequently been used by researchers to assess antioxidant capacity of different food products (Thaipong, Boonprakob et al. 2006, Ak and Gülçin 2008, Alam, Bristi et al. 2013). The cellular Antioxidant Activity Assay (CAA

Assay) is a more biologically relevant method than a chemical assay because it represents the complexity of biological system and accounts for cellular uptake, bioavailability, and metabolism of the antioxidant agent (Chandra, Khan et al. 2014).

Based on current litterature, oregano contains several potent antioxidants that may contribute to the findings in preliminary studies that oregano exhibits benefits toward the cardiovascular and nervous systems, relieves symptoms of inflammation, and modulates blood sugar and lipids (Singletary 2010). Numerous studies on oregano antioxidant properties revealed that either its essential oils and extracts have high antioxidative effect, which may be attributed to their high polyphenolic content. Essential oil of oregano has demonstrated to have efficacy as antioxidant. Non-polar phenolic compounds like thymol and carvacrol, which are major components of essential oil of Origanum taxa, possess remarkable antioxidant properties (Lagouri, Blekas et al. 1993). Antioxidant properties from essential oil of oregano offers the possibility of using this oil as preservatives and flavor for food or nutraceutical products (Tuttolomondo, La Bella et al. 2013).

Carvacrol and thymol, two monoterpenes commonly found in oregano, may induce oxidative stress in several Caco-2 cells when used in high concentrations (>230 μM), since these terpenes might increase the level of reactive oxygen species and decrease the content of glutathione (Llana-Ruiz-Cabello, Gutiérrez-Praena et al. 2015). These results suggest that essential oil of oregano can be useful for the management of lipid oxidation in food industry. Many authors reported that thymol-rich essential oils from oregano or other plant species exerted strong inhibitory activity on the oxidation of linoleic acid(Amiri and Medicine 2012). The antioxidant properties of thymol have been well documented in various preclinical studies including cell lines and animal models. One of the most studied effects of thymol includes the scavenging of free radicals by increasing the activities of several endogenous antioxidant enzymes levels viz. superoxide dismutase (SOD), catalase, glutathione peroxidase (GPx), glutathione-S-transferase (GST) along with non-enzymatic antioxidants such as vitamin C, vitamin E and reduced glutathione (GSH) (Nagoor Meeran, Stanely Mainzen Prince et al. 2012). A comparative study revealed that thymol has superior reducing power, DPPH, superoxide and hydroxyl radical scavenging activity and bestows protection against oxidative damage to lipids (Meeran, Fizur et al. 2017). Thymol was shown to exhibit potent superoxide anion, hydroxyl and DPPH radical scavenging and reducing capacity in a concentration dependent (Meeran, Fizur et al. 2017). Thymol attenuated the production of reactive oxygen species (ROS) and showed myeloperoxidase inhibitory activity in human neutrophils (Meeran, Fizur et al. 2017). Similarly, carvacrol has shown to have high antioxidant potential. Carvacrol has been reported to induce a significant hepatoprotective and antioxidant effect improving the activity of enzymatic antioxidants (superoxide dismutase, catalase, and glutathione peroxidase) and the levels of nonenzymatic antioxidants (vitamin C, vitamin E, and reduced glutathione), as demonstrated in the plasma of rats with D-galactosamine-induced hepatotoxicity (Aristatile, Al-Numair et al. 2009). A study in animal models has shown that carvacrol may improve acute pancreatitis through its antioxidative mechanisms (Bakır, Geyikoglu et al. 2016). An other study on rats revealed that carvacrol treatment ameliorated the oxidative stress damage in the brain, liver, and kidney (Samarghandian, Farkhondeh et al. 2016). In addition, an antioxidant synergism between thymol and carvacrol, both compounds present in oregano and most lamiaceae plants, have been investigated (Milos and Makota 2012). Thus, thymol and to a lesser extend carvacrol may be responsible for the strong inhibitory capacity of the essential oils. However, further pre-clinical and clinical studies are needed with special focus on their possible toxic effects in order to establish safe doses.

The phenolic compounds including flavonoids and phenolic acids, another kind of abundant constituent in oregano, are responsible for its antioxidant activity (Zhang, Guo et al. 2014). These phenolic antioxidants possess strong antioxidant acticity due to their potential function as reducing agents and free radical scavengers. Yan et al. (Yan, Azizi et al. 2016) conducted analysis of the hydro-methanolic extract of the leaves from oregano by total phenolic content (TPC) and Oxygen radical absorbance capacity (ORAC), with the fellowing results : 79–147 mg GAE/g DW and 1.59–3.39 mmol TE/g DW, respectively. Other studies partially attributed the high antioxidant capacity (DPPH, ABTS and FRAP) of the same kind of extract to the large quantity of rosmarinic acid (23.53 mg/g of dry extract) and the presence of other active compounds as well (Gonçalves, Moreira et al. 2017). Likewise, Kolda et al. (Koldaş, Demirtas et al. 2015) have reported that the presence rosmarinic, chicoric and caffeic acid in oregano extracts may be associated with the antioxidant capacity of samples. Furthermore, flavonoids such as eriodictyol, naringenin luteolin-7-O-glucoside and apigenin-7-O-glucoside that were also found in the extract of oregano leaves, have exhibited high TPC and a positive correlation with the ORAC and FRAP values (Hossain, Barry-Ryan et al. 2011). Moreover, Balkan et al. (Balkan, Balkan et al. 2017) found a correlation between the total phenolic content (TPC) and DPPH scavenging activity with the presence of eriodictyol, apigenin and caffeic acid in the aqueous extract of oregano.

Anti-Inflammatory Propertises

Inflammation is also trigger with the increase of oxidative stress, is considered as a risk factor for hypertension, diabetes and several types of cancer, and can be involved in Alzheimer's disease pathogenesis. NF-κB, iNOS, and ROS have long been considered as important targets for new anti-inflammatory drugs. NF-κB plays a central role in inflammation through its ability to induce transcription of proinflammatory genes. Excessive generation of nitric oxide (NO) and reactive oxygen species (ROS) contribute significantly to the progress of inflammation. Inhibition of inducible nitric oxide synthase (iNOS) can reduce the intracellular NO production (Zhao, Khan et al. 2014). Plant natural compounds, such as antioxidants have been associated with reduced risks of cancer, cardiovascular disease, diabetes, and other disorders associated with age.

Oregano is rich in antioxidants, which can help neutralize free radicals and reduce inflammation. Its essential oil contains compounds like carvacrol that have been shown to have anti-inflammatory properties. Oregano bioactive compounds and essential oil have been demonstrated to have the ability to supress inflammation and improve blood glucose and lipid regulation (Leyva-López, Gutiérrez-Grijalva et al. 2017). Previous research suggested that the significant inhibitory effect of oregano essential oils on proliferation as well as inflammatory and tissue remodeling biomarkers indicates that oregano essential oil may possess anti-inflammatory, immunomodulatory, tissue remodeling, and pro-wound healing properties (Han and Parker 2017). An other study conducted by A. Ocaña-Fuentes et al. (Ocana-Fuentes, Arranz-Gutierrez et al. 2010) reported that oregano essentials oils inhibit TNF-α-induced increases in the secretion of pro-inflammatory adipokines (IL-1β, IL-6 and leptin) and the TNF-α-induced decreases of IL-10 and adiponectin secretion. Recently, a study conducted by Han and Parker (Han and Parker 2017) showed that essential oil obtained from oregano significantly inhibited the levels of the inflammatory biomarkers monocyte chemoattractan protein-1 (MCP-1), the vascular cell adhesion molecule-1 (VCAM-1) and the intracellular cell adhesion molecule-1 (ICAM-1) on activated-primary human neonatal fibroblasts. These findings suggest that the essential oil of oregano has anti-inflammatory properties.

The oregano essential oil components such as thymol, carvacrol, p-cymene, β-caryophyllene and other components, have demonstrated anti-inflammatory properties. The individual components of essential oil of oregano have also been studied to better understand their effect on inflammation. For exemple, Thymol have been reported to attenuate bleomycin induced genotoxicity in human ovarian cells (SKOV-3) by virtue of its antioxidant and anti-inflammatory properties (Arab, Fathi et al. 2015). Ku and Lin (Ku and Lin 2013) reported the anti-inflammatory nature of thymol by its inhibiting of the T cell immune response and improved T-helper cells-1 (Th1) (interleukin-2 (IL-2) and IFN-g/T-helper cells-2 (Th2) (interleukin-4 (IL-4), interleukin-5 (IL-5) and interleukin-10 (IL-10) ratio in mouse primary splenocytes. Thymol (40 mg/ml) inhibited the LPS stimulated inflammatory response in mouse mammary epithelial cells mediating the down regulation of mitogen-activated protein kinases (MAPK) and nuclear factor-kB (NF-kB) signaling pathways (Liang, Li et al. 2014). Carvacrol also possesses analgesic and anti-inflammatory effects. Lima et al. (da Silva Lima, Quintans-Júnior et al. 2013) demonstrated that carvacrol exerts anti-inflammatory activity on a typical mice inflammation model. When carvacrol was administrated to mice (at 50 and 100 mg/kg), presenting paw edema, the levels of IL-1β and prostaglandin E2 (PGE2) prostaglandins were diminished. The reduction on the mRNA expression of IL-1β and cyclooxygenase-2 (COX-2) might be responsible for the effects mentioned. On the other hand, the levels of the cytokine IL-10 in the swollen paw were improved by carvacrol.

Oregano is a rich source of polyphenols such as flavonoids and phenolic acids. It is generally recognized that polyphenols have anti-inflammatory and antibiotic properties and may in addition activate the transcription factor Nrf2 which plays a key role in cellular protection against oxidative stress and inflammation (Cardozo, Pedruzzi et al. 2013). In a study conducted by Kogiannou et al. (Kogiannou, Kalogeropoulos et al. 2013), aqueous infusion of Oregano have been evaluated for their effect on IL-8 secretion, a pro-inflammatory and cancer promoting cytokine, in the cancerous cell lines HT-29 and PC3. The phenolic acid and flavonoid profile of the infusion from oregano was also determined. The anti-IL-8 activity was attributed to caffeic acid present in the infusion part of oregano.

Anticancer Properties

Cancer is the name given to a group of more than 100 diseases. In all types of cancer, some of the body's cells begin to divide without stopping and spread from the site of origin, or primary site into surrounding tissues to other sites in the body. Several factors are involved in the onset of cancer sauch as aging, tobacco, sun exposure, radiation exposure, cancer-causing substances, some viruses and bacteria, certain hormones, family history of cancer, alcohol, poor diet, lack of physical activity, obesity.etc. and they may play a direct or indirect role in the development and progressions of different types of cancers. Carcinogenesis includes five known steps: initiation, promotion, progression, invasion and metastasis.

Many studies have shown that the increased presence of antioxidants prevents free radical damage that has been associated with cancer development.

Essential oils constituents such as terpenoids could exert antiproliferative effect. Different mechanisms such antioxidant, antimutagenic, antiproliferative, among others are responsible for their chemopreventive properties (Bhalla, Gupta et al. 2013). Essential oils have been reported to show antiproliferative effects in diverse cancer cell models through several pathways (Sharifi-Rad, Sureda et al. 2017). Polyphenols are well known to display many anticarcinogenic properties including their inhibitory effects on cancer cell proliferation, tumor growth, angiogenesis, metastasis, and inflammation as well as inducing apoptosis.

Oregano main constituents have been reported to exert antimutagenic, antigenotoxic, and antiproliferative properties. Previous studies reported that, thymol and carvacrol, two main constituents found in oregano, explicated promising results against hepatocarcinoma cells (Elshafie, Armentano et al. 2017). Carvacrol may suppress proliferation and induce apoptosis in porcine enterocytes and lymphocytes in a significant manner (Bimczok, Rau et al. 2008). Thymol showed anticancer properties in different types of cell lines mimicking human cancer and it demonstrated its potential as a chemopreventive or anticancer agent in various types of cancers. The major mechanisms of anticancer actions of thymol include induction of apoptosis, anti-proliferation, inhibition of angiogenesis and migration as well as the diminution of umourigenesis by modulating the activity of carcinogen metabolizing enzymes(Meeran, Fizur et al. 2017).

The flavonoids and phenolic acids from oregano have been evaluated by Marrelli et al. (Marrelli, Conforti et al. 2016) for their antiproliferative activity against human breast cancer cells (MFC-7), hepatic cancer cells (HepG2) and colorectal cancer (LoVo) cells. According to authors, oregano extracts seemed to exhibit a selective antiproliferative activity against HepG2. (Savini, Arnone et al. 2009) evaluated the ethanolic extracts from *Origanum vulgare* on cell proliferation and cell death in colon adenocarcinoma (Caco-2) cells; finding that at a concentration of 300 μg/mL oregano extract cell viability of decreased approximately 30% after 24 h; however, at a concentration of 500 μg/mL death time-dependently occurred. They also suggested that the mix of phenolic compounds found in Oregano extracts is more effective than individual phenolics, indicating a synergistic effect between compounds. A study carried out by Nile et al. (Nile, Nile et al. 2017) has found that that the high cytotoxicity of oregano extracts against breast cancer cells (MFC-7) is related to its high phenolic content. Rosmarinic acid, a predominant compound in oregano, has shown potential against a variety of cancers including colon and skin cancer. This phenolic acid may helps modulate tumor necrosis factor, an immune system substance that plays a role in cancer treatment and prevention (Rui, Tong et al. 2017).

In an *in vivo* study, Mice treated orally with thymol and carvacrol (200 mg/kg body weight) evidenced significant increases in liver activities of glutathione-S-transferase, NAD(P)H-quinone reductase, and 7-ethoxycoumarin-O-deethylase (Sasaki, Wada et al. 2005). Rosmarinic acid blocked processes associated with cancer invasion and metastasis (Huang and Zheng 2006, Jankun, Selman et al. 2006). Also, rosmarinic acid administered topically (1.3 mg per mouse) inhibited epidermal inflammatory responses in a murine 2-stage model of skin cancer(Osakabe, Yasuda et al. 2004).

Begnini et al. (Begnini, Nedel et al. 2014) have conducted a study to evaluate the *in vitro* antiproliferative effect of essential oil of oregano against human breast adenocarcinoma [MCF-7], and human colon adenocarcinoma [HT-29]. The results show that the oregano essential oil is composed mostly of 4-terpineol and induces a high cytotoxicity effect in HT-29. In the MCF-7 cell line, the essential oil was less effective than its main component 4-terpineol in inducing cancer cell growth inhibition. Furthermore, in human breast (MCF-7) and prostate (LNCaP) cancer cell lines, essential oil of oregano showed an inhibitory effect on cancer cell viability in a range of 79–88% at 0.5 mg/Ml (24 h) (Hussain, Anwar et al. 2011). In a human study, anti- lung cancer effect of aqueous extract of oregano was investigated and it showed that the biosynthesized nanoparticles were found to be impressive in inhibiting human pathogens in a dose -dependent manner (Adams, Kanaya et al. 2011). The cytotoxic effect of the crude essential oil extracted from *Origanum vulgare* subsp hirtum and its main constituents (carvacrol, thymol, citral and limonene) on hepatocarcinoma HepG2 and healthy human renal cells HEK293 have been evaluated. Results showed that oregano essential oil and its main constituents could be potentially utilized as anticancer therapeutic agents (Elshafie, Armentano et al. 2017). In a recent study, it has been demonstrated that immunomodulatory biomarker, macrophage colony-stimulating factor (MCSF), was strongly inhibited by oregano essential oil treatment. In addition, oregano essential oil significantly modulated global gene expression and altered signaling pathways, many of which are critical in inflammation, tissue remodeling, and cancer signaling processes (Han and Parker 2017). The authors suggested that oregano essential oil, with carvacrol as the major active component, is a promising candidate for use in skin care products with anti-inflammatory and anticancer properties.

Neuroprotective Properties

Diseases of the nervous system can range from the nerve disorder that causes Tourette's to the serious CNS disease of Alzheimer's. The report, *Neurological disorders: Public health challenges,* reveals that of the one billion people affected worldwide. Neurological disorders affect people in all countries, irrespective of age, sex, education or income. An estimated 6.8 million people die every year as a result of neurological disorders. Alzheimer's disease (AD) is the most common neurodegenerative disorder. According to the World Health Organization (WHO), this disease is one of top 10 diseases causing the most deaths worldwide. Worldwide, nearly 44 million people have Alzheimer's or a related dementia (WHO 2018). Several herbs used in the folk medicine have been suggested as important source for treatment of depression, Alzheimer and Parkinson s diseases and other neuropsychiatric as well as neurological disorders (Schrader 2000, Adams, Gmünder et al. 2007, Song, Sze et al. 2012).

Because of the anti-inflammatory and anti-oxidative stress potentials of the oregano essential oil and its components, oregano essential oil has been used as a neuroprotective dietary supplement to promote mood, motivation and mental wellbeing. Oregano has been suggested to possess an antidepressant-like activity and reversed behavioral alterations observed in the CUS model (Amiresmaeili, Roohollahi et al. 2018). A previous study demonstrated that oregano extract inhibits the reuptake and degradation of the monoamine neuro-transmitters in a dose-dependent manner (Mechan, Fowler et al. 2011). Some constituents of oregano such as carvacrol, thymol, known by their anti-inflammatory and antioxidant potentials, can be used as a health promoting substances in the prevention of chronic diseases and neurodegenerative disorders which are linked to oxidative stress. These compounds have been reported in preliminary studies to influence nervous system chemistry and its diverse functions. Thymol (15 and 30 mg/kg) has been shown to up regulate the levels of central neurotransmitters and inhibit the expressions of proinflammatory cytokines in unpredictable mild stress (CUMS) mice model (Deng, Li et al. 2015). In an earlier study conducted by Azizi et al. (Azizi, Yan et al. 2009), thymol

(0.5–2 mg/kg) has been shown to inhibit cognitive impairments caused by increased Ab levels or cholinergic hypofunction in Ab (25–35) or scopolamine treated rats attributed to its antioxidant, anti-inflammatory and anticholine esterase properties. Lee et al. (Lee, Nam et al. 2015) demonstrated that thymol (0.39–25 mg/mL) may inhibit H_2O_2 induced oxidative stress in PC-12 cells whereas thymol (100 and 1000 mg/ml) also inhibited both AChE and butyrylcholinesterase (BChE) in a dose dependent manner. Moreover, It have been reported that thymol (10–100 ppm) in combination with gamma terpinene or para-cymene attenuated cholinergic dysfunction, which is manifested in a plethora of neurodegenerative and psychiatric disorders such as Alzheimers, Parkinsons, and Huntington s diseases, by enhancing synaptic levels of acetyl choline (Ach) and the responsiveness of nicotinic acetylcholine receptor (nAchR) in the Caenorhabditis elegans model (Sammi, Trivedi et al. 2017). The data that have been reported by M. Zotti et al. (Zotti, Colaianna et al. 2013) suggested that carvacrol is a brain-active molecule that clearly influences neuronal activity through modulation of neurotransmitters. Carvacrol was screened for pharmacological effects on the central nervous system and found to have anxiolytic activity when administered orally to mice. Antidepressant effects were observed in mice after carvacrol administration (12.5 to 50 mg/kg, oral). According to researchers, the observed result is most likely due to an increase in dopamine levels. In a study carried out by Maximilian Peters et al. (Peters, Trembovler et al. 2012), carvacrol was given to mice after TBI and its effect on their functional recovery was followed for several weeks. The results showed that neurological recovery after TBI was significantly enhanced by application of carvacrol. The authors found that neurological recovery after TBI was significantly enhanced by combining carvacrol with TRPC1 elimination.

As previously shown, oregano have high amounts of polyphenols, such as flavonoids and phenolic acids, which act as potent antioxidants. Thus, these compounds could potentially be beneficial for brain aging and neurodegenerative disorders. For example, rosmarinic acid and caffeic acid which are major phenolic acids identified in oregano, have been reported to exert neuroprotective effects. Rosmarinic acid have showed anti-epileptic Activity, by increasing the latency and decreasing the percentage of seizure incidents, reducing the levels of free radicals and DNA damage in the kindling CF-1 male mice model of epilepsy induced by PTZ (rosmarinic acid at 1, 2 or 4 mg/kg b.w., i.p.) (Coelho, Vieira et al. 2015). The Anti-epileptic activity of caffeic acid have been shown in the reduction of the levels of free radicals and DNA damage in the kindling CF-1 male mice model of epilepsy induced by PTZ (caffeic acid at 1, 4 or 8 mg/kg b.w., i.p.) (Coelho, Vieira et al. 2015). The administration of rosmarinic acid for 7 days at 5 and 10 mg/kg b.w./day, led to downregulation of mitogen-activated protein kinase phosphatase-1, upregulation of BDNF and modulation of dopamine and corticosterone synthesis in TST in a model of depression in mice with bupropion as a positive control (Kondo, El Omri et al. 2015). In addition, rosmarinic acid has shown to exhibit anti-tauopathy activity (Shan, Wang et al. 2016). Previous studies have suggested caffeic acid as a potent neuroprotective agent against the development of Parkinson s disease and other neurodegenerative disorders (Tsai, Chao et al. 2011, Kim, Wang et al. 2015). This phenolic acid has been reported to inhibit (in a dose-dependent manner) α-synuclein fibrillation in the presence of escitalopram (Fazili and Naeem 2015). Moreover, some flavonoids like quercetin, kaempferol, luteolin and apigenin, which were found in abundance in oregano, exhibited neuroprotection properties and are identified as potent MAOs inhibitors (Larit, Elokely et al. 2018).

Other Pharmacological Properties

Although oregano is reported as an effective treatment for several illenesses, there is limited evidence that oregano extracts or constituents have the potential to benefit the management of diabetes and cardiovascular diseases. Only few researches have been carried out to study the effects of oregano in diabetic, cardiovascular and hepatotoxicity liver diseases. As previously demonstrated, oregano is a rich source of several potent antioxidants that may contribute to the findings in preliminary studies that oregano exhibits benefits towards the cardiovascular and nervous systems and relieves inflammation and modulates blood sugar and lipids (Singletary 2010). For exemple, oral administration of the aqueous extract of oregano leaves (20 mg/kg) produced a significant decrease in blood-glucose levels, glycosylated haemoglobin, pancreatic amylase in STZ diabetic rats (Béjaoui, Chaabane et al. 2013). The results of this study showed that the treatment with the aqueous extracts of oregano leaves decreased liver weights/body weight ratios in diabetic rats, while kidney weight/body weight ratios, urea, uric acid, creatinine levels were partially improved. According to Milica Vujicic et al. (Vujicic, Nikolic et al. 2015) methanolic extract of oregano can protected mice from diabetes development due to its antioxidant, anti-apoptotic and immunomodulatory potentials. Rosmarinic acid, one of the predominant compounds in oregano, has been reported to inhibit porcine pancreatic amylase (PPA) activity (McCue and Shetty 2004). Other reports have been demonstrated that extracts of *Origanum* species and their individual constituents such as thymol, carvacrol and γ-terpinene, have been shown to inhibit blood platelet aggregation and adhesion, decrease cholesterol biosynthesis, and reduce serum total cholesterol and triglyceride levels (Singletary 2010). In normotensive rats, administration of carvacrol (100 2g/kg intraperitoneally) decreased systolic and diastolic blood pressures (Aydin, Kutlay et al. 2007). Carvacrol (100 microg/kg, I. P.) decreased heart rate, mean arterial pressure and systolic and diastolic blood pressures of the anesthetized rats and was observed to exhibit hypotension and to inhibit N((omega))-nitro- L-arginine methyl ester (L-NAME)-induced hypertension (Aydin, Kutlay et al. 2007). Some studies reported that oregano oil, rosmarinic acid, or carvacrol (73 mg/kg body weight) may protect liver cells in rodents from lead toxicity and to stimulate liver regeneration following partial hepatectomy (Singletary 2010). Carvacrol (73mg/kg body weight) also has shown to protecte rat liver from defects caused by ischemia and reperfusion and was not hepatotoxic (Singletary 2010). Rosmarinic acid (100-200 μM) can protect cardiomyocytes in culture from doxorubicin and adriamycin-induced toxicity and thus was suggested as a potential chemotherapeutic agent to inhibit cardiotoxicity in patients undergoing drug treatments (Singletary 2010).

Conclusion

In conclusion, it would seem that oregano represents a rich source of bioactive natural products. Oregano s phytochemicals have been of particular interest for their potential bioactive properties and promising role as alternative treatment in several illnesses, because of the anticancer, anti-inflammatory, antioxidant and antimicrobial activities. In this chapter we have summarized the most recent studies focusing on the characterization of oregano essential oil and its components as well as the phenolic compounds (flavonoids and phenolic acids) and their antimicrobial, antioxidant, anti-inflammatory, anti-cancer and neuroprotective properties.

Interestingly, the majority of reports regarding oregano pharmacological properties such as antimicrobial activity have used essential oil and its main components. Therefore, the identification and characterization of other bioactive molecules (e.g., phenolic compounds) is demanded. Most studies have been carried out with single, pure compounds. Combined effects are likely to be different fom those observed using single compounds. The combined effect of complex matrixes such as extracts and essential oils seem to be more relevent, possibly due to synergistic and/or additive interactions among the various constituents. In fact, most of the studies are based on *in vitro* approaches, the potential toxicity and the exact side effects of the studied substances were rarely taken into consideration, limiting its extrapolation to human health. Hence, the use of oregano and its bioactive compounds in therapeutical purposes need more research on oral bioavailability of oregano constituents as well as on their safety, pharmacokinetics and mechanism of action, side and adverse effects, toxicological risks and interactions with pharmaceuticals is necessary. Furthermore, the confirmation of certain therapeutic potentials of oregano towards some diseases like diabetic, cardiovascular and hepatotoxicity liver diseases, in particular the potential capacity of oregano to decrease hyperglycemia and enhance insulin sensitivity, need further investigations.

REFERENCES

Adams, L. S., N. Kanaya, S. Phung, Z. Liu and S. J. T. J. o. n. Chen. 2011. "Whole blueberry powder modulates the growth and metastasis of MDA-MB-231 triple negative breast tumors in nude mice." *The Journal of Nutrition* 141(10): 1805-1812.

Adams, M., F. Gmünder and M. Hamburger. 2007. "Plants traditionally used in age related brain disorders—A survey of ethnobotanical literature." *Journal of Ethnopharmacology* 113(3): 363-381.

Adebayo, O., T. Dang, A. Bélanger and S. J. J. o. F. R. Khanizadeh. 2013. "Antifungal studies of selected essential oils and a commercial formulation against Botrytis cinerea." *Journal of Food Research* 2(1): 217.

Ak, T. and İ. Gülçin. 2008. "Antioxidant and radical scavenging properties of curcumin." *Chemico-biological interactions* 174(1): 27-37.

Alam, M. N., N. J. Bristi and M. Rafiquzzaman. 2013. "Review on *in vivo* and *in vitro* methods evaluation of antioxidant activity." *Saudi Pharmaceutical Journal* 21(2): 143-152.

Amiresmaeili, A., S. Roohollahi, A. Mostafavi and N. J. R. i. p. s. Askari. 2018. "Effects of oregano essential oil on brain TLR4 and TLR2 gene expression and depressive-like behavior in a rat model." *Res Pharm Sci* 13(2): 130.

Amiri, H. J. E. B. C. and A. Medicine. 2012. "Essential oils composition and antioxidant properties of three thymus species." *Evidence-Based Complementary and Alternative Medicine* 2012. http://dx.doi.org/10.1155/2012/728065.

Arab, H. A., M. Fathi, E. Mortezai and S. J. Hosseinimehr. 2015. "Chemoprotective effect of thymol against genotoxicity induced by bleomycin in human lymphocytes." *Pharmaceutical and Biomedical Research.* DOI: 10.18869/acadpub.pbr.1.1.26.

Arcila-Lozano, C. C., G. Loarca-Pina, S. Lecona-Uribe and E. J. A. l. d. n. de Mejía González. 2004. "Oregano: properties, composition and biological activity." *Archivos Latinoamericanos de Nutricion* 54(1): 100-111.

Aristatile, B., K. S. Al-Numair, C. Veeramani, K. V. J. F. Pugalendi and c. pharmacology. 2009. "Effect of carvacrol on hepatic marker enzymes and antioxidant status in d-galactosamine-induced hepatotoxicity in rats." *Fundamental & Clinical Pharmacology* 23(6): 757-765.

Arslan, M., I. Uremis and N. J. E. a. Demirel. 2012. "Effects of sage leafhopper feeding damage on herbage colour, essential oil content and compositions of turkish and greek oregano." *Experimental agriculture* 48(3): 428-437.

Asensio, C. M., N. R. Grosso, H. R. J. I. C. Juliani and Products. 2015. "Quality characters, chemical composition and biological activities of oregano (Origanum spp.) Essential oils from Central and Southern Argentina." *Industrial Crops and Products* 63: 203-213.

Aydin, Y., Ö. Kutlay, S. Ari, S. Duman, K. Uzuner and S. J. P. m. Aydin. 2007. "Hypotensive effects of carvacrol on the blood pressure of normotensive rats." *Planta Medica* 73(13): 1365-1371.

Azirak, S. and E. J. E. T. A. I. J. Rencuzogullari. 2008. "The *in vivo* genotoxic effects of carvacrol and thymol in rat bone marrow cells." *Environmental Toxicology* 23(6): 728-735.

Aziz, Z. A., A. Ahmad, S. H. M. Setapar, A. Karakucuk, M. M. Azim, D. Lokhat, M. Rafatullah, M. Ganash, M. A. Kamal and G. M. J. C. d. m. Ashraf. 2018. "Essential Oils: Extraction Techniques, Pharmaceutical and Therapeutic Potential-A Review." *Current Drug Metabolism* 19(13): 1100-1110.

Azizi, A., C. Wagner, B. Honermeier, W. J. P. s. Friedt and evolution. 2009. "Intraspecific diversity and relationship between subspecies of Origanum vulgare revealed by comparative AFLP and SAMPL marker analysis." *Plant Systematics and Evolution* 281(1-4): 151-160.

Azizi, A., F. Yan, B. J. I. c. Honermeier and products. 2009. "Herbage yield, essential oil content and composition of three oregano (Origanum vulgare L.) populations as affected by soil moisture regimes and nitrogen supply." *Industrial crops and products* 29(2-3): 554-561.

Bakır, M., F. Geyikoglu, S. Colak, H. Turkez, T. O. Bakır and M. J. C. Hosseinigouzdagani. 2016. "The carvacrol ameliorates acute pancreatitis-induced liver injury via antioxidant response." *Cytotechnology* 68(4): 1131-1146.

Bakkali, F., S. Averbeck, D. Averbeck, M. J. F. Idaomar and c. toxicology. 2008. "Biological effects of essential oils–a review." *Food and Chemical Toxicology* 46(2): 446-475.

Balasundram, N., K. Sundram and S. Samman. 2006. "Phenolic compounds in plants and agri-industrial by-products: Antioxidant activity, occurrence, and potential uses." *Food chemistry* 99(1): 191-203.

Balkan, B., S. Balkan, H. Aydoğdu, N. Güler, H. Ersoy, B. J. A. J. f. S. Aşkın and Engineering. 2017. "Evaluation of antioxidant activities and antifungal activity of different plants species against pink mold rot-causing Trichothecium roseum." *Arabian Journal for Science and Engineering* 42(6): 2279-2289.

Baranauskienė, R., P. R. Venskutonis, E. Dambrauskienė, P. J. I. c. Viškelis and products. 2013. "Harvesting time influences the yield and oil composition of Origanum vulgare L. ssp. vulgare and ssp. hirtum." *Industrial Crops and Products* 49: 43-51.

Begnini, K. R., F. Nedel, R. G. Lund, P. H. Carvalho, M. R. Rodrigues, F. T. Beira and F. A. Del-Pino. 2014. "Composition and antiproliferative effect of essential oil of Origanum vulgare against tumor cell lines." *J Med Food* 17(10): 1129-1133.

Béjaoui, A., A. Boulila, A. Sanaa, M. Boussaid and X. J. J. o. f. b. Fernandez. 2017. "Antioxidant Activity and α-Amylase Inhibitory Effect of Polyphenolic-Rich Extract from Origanum Glandulosum Desf." *Journal of food Biochemistry* 41(1): e12271. https://doi.org/10.1111/jfbc.12271.

Béjaoui, A., H. Chaabane, M. Jemli, A. Boulila and M. J. J. o. m. f. Boussaid. 2013. "Essential oil composition and antibacterial activity of Origanum vulgare subsp. glandulosum Desf. at different phenological stages." *Journal of Medicinal Food* 16(12): 1115-1120. https://doi.org/10.1089/jmf.2013.0079.

Berrehal, D., T. Boudiar, L. Hichem, A. Khalfallah, A. Kabouche, A. Al-Freihat, A. Ghannadi, E. Sajjadi, M. Mehrabani and J. J. N. p. c. Safaei-Ghomi. 2010. "Comparative composition of four essential oils of Oregano used in Algerian and Jordanian folk medicine." *Natural Product Communications* 5(6): 957-960.

Betancourt, L., V. Phandanauvong, R. Patiño, C. Ariza-Nieto and G. J. R. d. l. F. d. M. V. y. d. Z. Afanador-Téllez. 2012. "Composition and bactericidal activity against beneficial and pathogenic bacteria of oregano essential oils from four chemotypes of Origanum and Lippia genus." *Rev. Med. Vet. Zoot* 59(1): 21-31.

Bhalla, Y., V. K. Gupta, V. J. J. o. t. S. o. F. Jaitak and Agriculture. 2013. "Anticancer activity of essential oils: a review." *Journal of the Science of Food and Agriculture* 93(15): 3643-3653. https://doi.org/10.1002/jsfa.6267.

Bimczok, D., H. Rau, E. Sewekow, P. Janczyk, W. B. Souffrant and H. J. J. T. i. v. Rothkötter. 2008. "Influence of carvacrol on proliferation and survival of porcine lymphocytes and intestinal epithelial cells *in vitro*." *Toxicology in Vitro* 22(3): 652-658.

Bolechowski, A., R. Moral, M. A. Bustamante, C. Paredes, E. Agulló, J. Bartual and Á. A. J. J. o. E. O. R. Carbonell-Barrachina. 2011. "Composition of oregano essential oil (Origanum vulgare) as affected by the use of winery-distillery composts." *Journal of Essential Oil Research* 23(3): 32-38.

Bonfanti, C., R. Iannì, A. Mazzaglia, C. M. Lanza, E. M. Napoli, G. J. I. c. Ruberto and products. 2012. "Emerging cultivation of oregano in Sicily: Sensory evaluation of plants and chemical composition of essential oils." *Industrial Crops and Products* 35(1): 160-165.

Boskovic, M., N. Zdravkovic, J. Ivanovic, J. Janjic, J. Djordjevic, M. Starcevic and M. Z. J. P. F. S. Baltic. 2015. "Antimicrobial activity of thyme (Tymus vulgaris) and oregano (Origanum vulgare) essential oils against some food-borne microorganisms." *Procedia Food Science* 5: 18-21.

Boughendjioua, H., R. J. J. o. P. Seridi and P. Research. 2017. "Antimicrobial Efficacy of the Essential Oil of Origanum Vulgare from Algeria." *Journal of Pharmacy and Pharmacology Research* 1(1): 19-27.

Briskin, D. P. J. P. p. 2000. "Medicinal plants and phytomedicines. Linking plant biochemistry and physiology to human health." *Plant physiology* 124(2): 507-514.

Calvo-Irabién, L. M., V. Parra-Tabla, V. Acosta-Arriola, F. Escalante-Erosa, L. Díaz-Vera, G. R. Dzib, L. M. J. C. Peña-Rodríguez and biodiversity. 2014. "Phytochemical

Diversity of the Essential Oils of Mexican Oregano (Lippia graveolens Kunth) Populations along an Edapho-Climatic Gradient." *Chemistry & Biodiversity* 11(7): 1010-1021.

Camele, I., L. Altieri, L. De Martino, V. De Feo, E. Mancini and G. L. J. I. j. o. m. s. Rana. 2012. "*In vitro* control of post-harvest fruit rot fungi by some plant essential oil components." *International Journal of Molecular Sciences* 13(2): 2290-2300.

Cardozo, L. F., L. M. Pedruzzi, P. Stenvinkel, M. B. Stockler-Pinto, J. B. Daleprane, M. Leite Jr and D. J. B. Mafra. 2013. "Nutritional strategies to modulate inflammation and oxidative stress pathways via activation of the master antioxidant switch Nrf2." *Biochimie* 95(8): 1525-1533.

Chandra, S., S. Khan, B. Avula, H. Lata, M. H. Yang, M. A. ElSohly and I. A. Khan. 2014. "Assessment of total phenolic and flavonoid content, antioxidant properties, and yield of aeroponically and conventionally grown leafy vegetables and fruit crops: A comparative study." *Evidence-Based Complementary and Alternative Medicine.* http://dx.doi.org/10.1155/2014/253875.

Chun, S. S., D. A. Vattem, Y. T. Lin and K. J. P. B. Shetty. 2005. "Phenolic antioxidants from clonal oregano (Origanum vulgare) with antimicrobial activity against Helicobacter pylori." *Process Biochemistry* 40(2): 809-816.

Cleff, M. B., A. R. Meinerz, M. Xavier, L. F. Schuch, M. C. A. Meireles, M. R. A. Rodrigues and J. R. B. d. J. B. J. o. M. Mello. 2010. "*In vitro* activity of Origanum vulgare essential oil against Candida species." *Brazilian Journal of Microbiology* 41(1): 116-123.

Coelho, V. R., C. G. Vieira, L. P. de Souza, F. Moysés, C. Basso, D. K. M. Papke, T. R. Pires, I. R. Siqueira, J. N. Picada and P. J. L. s. Pereira. 2015. "Antiepileptogenic, antioxidant and genotoxic evaluation of rosmarinic acid and its metabolite caffeic acid in mice." *Life Sciences* 122: 65-71.

da Silva Lima, M., L. J. Quintans-Júnior, W. A. de Santana, C. M. Kaneto, M. B. P. Soares and C. F. J. E. j. o. p. Villarreal. 2013. "Anti-inflammatory effects of carvacrol: evidence for a key role of interleukin-10." *European Journal of Pharmacology* 699(1-3): 112-117.

Dambolena, J. S., M. P. Zunino, E. I. Lucini, R. Olmedo, E. Banchio, P. J. Bima, J. A. J. J. o. a. Zygadlo and f. chemistry. 2009. "Total phenolic content, radical scavenging properties, and essential oil composition of Origanum species from different populations." *Journal of agricultural and Food Chemistry* 58(2): 1115-1120.

De Azeredo, G. A., T. L. M. Stamford, P. C. Nunes, N. J. G. Neto, M. E. G. De Oliveira and E. L. J. F. R. I. De Souza. 2011. "Combined application of essential oils from Origanum vulgare L. and Rosmarinus officinalis L. to inhibit bacteria and autochthonous microflora associated with minimally processed vegetables." *Food Research International* 44(5): 1541-1548.

de Castro, R. D., T. M. P. A. de Souza, L. M. D. Bezerra, G. L. S. Ferreira, E. M. M. de Brito Costa, A. L. J. B. c. Cavalcanti and a. medicine. 2015. "Antifungal activity and mode of action of thymol and its synergism with nystatin against Candida species involved with infections in the oral cavity: an *in vitro* study." *BMC Complementary and Alternative Medicine* 15(1): 417. https://doi.org/10.1186/s12906-015-0947-2.

De Falco, E., E. Mancini, G. Roscigno, E. Mignola, O. Taglialatela-Scafati and F. J. M. Senatore. 2013. "Chemical composition and biological activity of essential oils of Origanum vulgare L. subsp. vulgare L. under different growth conditions." *Molecules* 18(12): 14948-14960.

De Mastro, G., W. Tarraf, L. Verdini, G. Brunetti and C. J. F. c. Ruta. 2017. "Essential oil diversity of Origanum vulgare L. populations from Southern Italy." *Food Chemistry* 235: 1-6.

Deng, X. Y., H. Y. Li, J. J. Chen, R. P. Li, R. Qu, Q. Fu and S. P. J. B. b. r. Ma. 2015. "Thymol produces an antidepressant-like effect in a chronic unpredictable mild stress model of depression in mice." *Behavioural Brain Research* 291: 12-19.

Economou, G., G. Panagopoulos, P. Tarantilis, D. Kalivas, V. Kotoulas, I. Travlos, M. Polysiou, A. J. I. C. Karamanos and Products. 2011. "Variability in essential oil content and composition of Origanum hirtum L., Origanum onites L., Coridothymus capitatus (L.) and Satureja thymbra L. populations from the Greek island Ikaria." *Industrial Crops and Products* 33(1): 236-241.

El-Seedi, H. R., A. M. El-Said, S. A. Khalifa, U. Göransson, L. Bohlin, A.-K. Borg-Karlson, R. J. J. o. a. Verpoorte and f. chemistry. 2012. "Biosynthesis, natural sources, dietary intake, pharmacokinetic properties, and biological activities of hydroxycinnamic acids." *Journal of agricultural and Food Chemistry* 60(44): 10877-10895.

Elezi, F., F. Plaku, A. Ibraliu, G. Stefkov, M. Karapandzova, S. Kulevanova and S. J. A. S. Aliu. 2013. "Genetic variation of oregano (Origanum vulgare L.) for etheric oil in Albania." *Agricultural Sciences* 4(09): 449. DOI: 10.4236/as.2013.49060

Elizalde, J. J. and M. J. J. o. E. O. B. P. Espinoza. 2011. "Effect of ionizing irradiation on Origanum leaves (Origanum vulgare L.) essential oil composition." *Journal of Essential Oil Bearing Plants* 14(2): 164-171.

Elshafie, H., M. Armentano, M. Carmosino, S. Bufo, V. De Feo and I. J. M. Camele. 2017. "Cytotoxic activity of Origanum vulgare L. on hepatocellular carcinoma cell line HepG2 and evaluation of its biological activity." *Molecules* 22(9): 1435.

Fazili, N. A. and A. J. B. Naeem. 2015. "Anti-fibrillation potency of caffeic acid against an antidepressant induced fibrillogenesis of human α-synuclein: Implications for Parkinson s disease." *Biochimie* 108: 178-185.

Figiel, A., A. Szumny, A. Gutiérrez-Ortíz and Á. A. J. J. o. F. E. Carbonell-Barrachina. 2010. "Composition of oregano essential oil (Origanum vulgare) as affected by drying method." *Journal of Food Engineering* 98(2): 240-247.

Figuérédo, G., P. Cabassu, J. C. Chalchat, B. J. F. Pasquier and f. journal. 2006. "Studies of Mediterranean oregano populations. VIII—Chemical composition of essential oils of oreganos of various origins." *Flavour and Fragrance Journal* 21(1): 134-139.

Fleisher, A., N. J. J. o. t. S. o. F. Sneer and Agriculture. 1982. "Oregano spices and Origanum chemotypes." *Journal of the Science of Food and Agriculture* 33(5): 441-446.

Fouad, R., D. Bousta, A. E. O. Lalami, F. O. Chahdi, I. Amri, B. Jamoussi and H. J. J. o. E. O. B. P. Greche. 2015. "Chemical Composition and Herbicidal Effects of Essential Oils of Cymbopogon citratus (DC) Stapf, Eucalyptus cladocalyx, Origanum vulgare L and Artemisia absinthium L. cultivated in Morocco." *Journal of Essential Oil Bearing Plants* 18(1): 112-123.

Fratini, F., S. Mancini, B. Turchi, E. Friscia, L. Pistelli, G. Giusti and D. J. M. r. Cerri. 2017. "A novel interpretation of the Fractional Inhibitory Concentration Index: The case Origanum vulgare L. and Leptospermum scoparium JR et G. Forst essential oils against Staphylococcus aureus strains." *Microbiological Research* 195: 11-17.

Garcia-Salas, P., A. Morales-Soto, A. Segura-Carretero and A. J. M. Fernández-Gutiérrez. 2010. "Phenolic-compound-extraction systems for fruit and vegetable samples." *Molecules* 15(12): 8813-8826.

Ghasemzadeh, A. and N. J. J. o. m. p. r. Ghasemzadeh. 2011. "Flavonoids and phenolic acids: Role and biochemical activity in plants and human." *Journal of Medicinal Plants Research* 5(31): 6697-6703.

Gonçalves, S., E. Moreira, C. Grosso, P. B. Andrade, P. Valentão, A. J. J. o. f. s. Romano and technology. 2017. "Phenolic profile, antioxidant activity and enzyme inhibitory activities of extracts from aromatic plants used in Mediterranean diet." *Journal of Food Science and Technology* 54(1): 219-227.

Gonceariuc, M., Z. Balmuş, A. Benea, V. Barsan and T. J. B. A. Sandu, Ştiinţele vieţii. 2015. "Biochemical diversity of the Origanum vulgare ssp. vulgare L. and Origanum vulgare ssp. hirtum (link) ietswaart genotypes from Moldova." *Buletinul Academiei de Ştiinţe a Moldovei. Ştiinţele vieţii* (2): 326.

Gong, H., W. Liu, G. Lv and X. J. R. B. d. F. Zhou. 2014. "Analysis of essential oils of Origanum vulgare from six production areas of China and Pakistan." *Revista Brasileira de Farmacognosia* 24(1): 25-32.

González, M., C. Luis and P. J. P. Lanzelotti. 2014. "Profile of polyphenols of Origanum vulgare L. ssp. viridulum from Argentina." *Phyton (Buenos Aires)* 83(1): 179-184.

Grondona, E., G. Gatti, A. G. López, L. R. Sánchez, V. Rivero, O. Pessah, M. P. Zunino and A. A. J. P. f. f. h. n. Ponce. 2014. "Bio-efficacy of the essential oil of oregano (Origanum vulgare Lamiaceae. ssp. Hirtum)." *Plant Foods for Human Nutrition* 69(4): 351-357.

Gutiérrez-Grijalva, E., M. Picos-Salas, N. Leyva-López, M. Criollo-Mendoza, G. Vazquez-Olivo and J. J. P. Heredia. 2018. "Flavonoids and phenolic acids from oregano: occurrence, biological activity and health benefits." *Plants* **7**(1): 2. https://doi.org/10.3390/plants7010002.

Hać-Szymańczuk, E., A. Cegiełka, M. Karkos, M. Gniewosz, K. J. F. S. Piwowarek and Biotechnology. 2018. "Evaluation of antioxidant and antimicrobial activity of oregano (Origanum vulgare L.) preparations during storage of low-pressure mechanically separated meat (BAADER meat) from chickens." *Food Science and Biotechnology* 1-9.

Hac-Szymanczuk, E., E. Lipinska and A. J. Z. P. P. N. R. Chlebowska-Śmigiel. 2014. "Comparison of antimicrobial activity of essential oils from sage (Salvia officinalis L.) and oregano (Origanum vulgare L.)." *Zeszyty Problemowe Postępów Nauk Rolniczych* 577.

Han, F., G. Q. Ma, M. Yang, L. Yan, W. Xiong, J. C. Shu, Z. D. Zhao and H. L. J. J. o. Z. U. S. B. Xu. 2017. "Chemical composition and antioxidant activities of essential oils from different parts of the oregano." *Journal of Zhejiang University-SCIENCE B*18(1): 79-84.

Han, X. and T. L. J. B. o. Parker. 2017. "Anti-inflammatory, tissue remodeling, immunomodulatory, and anticancer activities of oregano (Origanum vulgare) essential oil in a human skin disease model." *Biochimie* 4: 73-77.

Hawas, U. W., S. El-Desoky, S. Kawashty and M. J. N. p. r. Sharaf. 2008. "Two new flavonoids from Origanum vulgare." *Natural Product Research* 22(17): 1540-1543.

Hossain, M., C. Barry-Ryan, A. B. Martin-Diana and N. J. F. C. Brunton. 2011. "Optimisation of accelerated solvent extraction of antioxidant compounds from rosemary (Rosmarinus officinalis L.), marjoram (Origanum majorana L.) and oregano (Origanum vulgare L.) using response surface methodology." *Food Chemistry* 126(1): 339-346.

Huang, S. S. and R. L. J. C. l. Zheng. 2006. "Rosmarinic acid inhibits angiogenesis and its mechanism of action *in vitro*." *Cancer letters* 239(2): 271-280.

Husain, S. R., J. Cillard and P. Cillard. 1987. "Hydroxyl radical scavenging activity of flavonoids." *Phytochemistry* 26(9): 2489-2491.

Hussain, A. I., F. Anwar, S. Rasheed, P. S. Nigam, O. Janneh and S. D. Sarker. 2011. "Composition, antioxidant and chemotherapeutic properties of the essential oils from two Origanum species growing in Pakistan" *Revista Brasileira de Farmacognosia* 21: 943-952.

Ietswaart, J. H. and J. Ietswaart. 1980. A taxonomic revision of the genus Origanum (Labiatae), Citeseer.

Jankun, J., S. H. Selman, J. Aniola and E. J. O. r. Skrzypczak-Jankun. 2006. "Nutraceutical inhibitors of urokinase: potential applications in prostate cancer prevention and treatment." *Oncology Reports* 16(2): 341-346.

Karakaya, S., S. N. El, N. Karagözlü and S. J. J. o. m. f. Şahin. 2011. "Antioxidant and antimicrobial activities of essential oils obtained from oregano (Origanum vulgare ssp.

hirtum) by using different extraction methods." *Journal of Medicinal Food* 14(6): 645-652.

Karamanos, A. J., D. E. J. I. c. Sotiropoulou and products. 2013. "Field studies of nitrogen application on Greek oregano (Origanum vulgare ssp. hirtum (Link) Ietswaart) essential oil during two cultivation seasons." *Industrial Crops and Products* 46: 246-252.

Karimi, A., B. Min, C. Brownmiller and S. O. J. J. o. F. R. Lee. 2014. "Effects of extraction techniques on total phenolic content and antioxidant capacities of two oregano leaves." *Journal of Food Research* 4(1): 112.

Khan, M., S. T. Khan, N. A. Khan, A. Mahmood, A. A. Al-Kedhairy and H. Z. J. A. j. o. c. Alkhathlan. 2018. "The composition of the essential oil and aqueous distillate of Origanum vulgare L. growing in Saudi Arabia and evaluation of their antibacterial activity." *Arabian Journal of Chemistry* 11(8): 1189-1200.

Kilic, Ö. and F. A. J. J. o. E. O. B. P. Özdemir. 2016. "Variability of essential oil composition of Origanum vulgare L. subsp. gracile populations from Turkey." *Journal of Essential Oil Bearing Plants* 19(8): 2083-2090.

Kim, J. H., Q. Wang, J. M. Choi, S. Lee, E. J. J. N. r. Cho and practice. 2015. "Protective role of caffeic acid in an Aβ25-35-induced Alzheimer s disease model." *Nutrition Research and Practice* 9(5): 480-488.

Kogiannou, D. A., N. Kalogeropoulos, P. Kefalas, M. G. Polissiou, A. C. J. F. Kaliora and c. toxicology. 2013. "Herbal infusions; their phenolic profile, antioxidant and anti-inflammatory effects in HT29 and PC3 cells." *Food and Chemical Toxicology* 61: 152-159.

Kokkini, S. 1996. Taxonomy, diversity and distribution of Origanum. Oregano: proceedings of the IPGRI international workshop on oregano.

Koldaş, S., I. Demirtas, T. Ozen, M. A. Demirci, L. J. J. o. t. s. o. f. Behçet and agriculture. 2015. "Phytochemical screening, anticancer and antioxidant activities of Origanum vulgare L. ssp. viride (Boiss.) Hayek, a plant of traditional usage." *Journal of the Science of Food and Agriculture* 95(4): 786-798.

Kondo, S., A. El Omri, J. Han and H. J. J. o. f. f. Isoda. 2015. "Antidepressant-like effects of rosmarinic acid through mitogen-activated protein kinase phosphatase-1 and brain-derived neurotrophic factor modulation." *Journal of Functional Foods* 14: 758-766.

Kosakowska, O. and W. J. H. P. Czupa. 2018. "Morphological and chemical variability of common oregano (Origanum vulgare L. subsp. vulgare) occurring in eastern Poland." *Herba Polonica* 64(1): 11-21.

Kruma, Z., M. Andjelkovic, R. Verhe, V. Kreicbergs, D. Karklina and P. J. F. Venskutonis. 2008. "Phenolic compounds in basil, oregano and thyme." *Foodbalt* 5(7): 99-103.

Ku, C. M. and J. Y. J. F. C. Lin. 2013. "Anti-inflammatory effects of 27 selected terpenoid compounds tested through modulating Th1/Th2 cytokine secretion profiles using murine primary splenocytes." *Food Chemistry* 141(2): 1104-1113.

Kula, J., T. Majda, A. Stoyanova and E. J. J. o. e. o. B. P. Georgiev. 2007. "Chemical composition of Origanum vulgare L. essential oil from Bulgaria." *Journal of Essential Oil Bearing Plants* 10(3): 215-220.

La Pergola, A., C. Restuccia, E. Napoli, S. Bella, S. Brighina, A. Russo and P. J. J. o. E. O. R. Suma. 2017. "Commercial and wild Sicilian Origanum vulgare essential oils: chemical composition, antimicrobial activity and repellent effects." *Journal of Essential Oil Bearing Plants* 29(6): 451-460.

Lagouri, V., G. Blekas, M. Tsimidou, S. Kokkini and D. J. Z. f. L. U. u. F. Boskou. 1993. "Composition and antioxidant activity of essential oils from oregano plants grown wild in Greece." *Zeitschrift für Lebensmittel-Untersuchung und Forschung* 197(1): 20-23.

Lambert, R., P. N. Skandamis, P. J. Coote and G. J. J. J. o. a. m. Nychas. 2001. "A study of the minimum inhibitory concentration and mode of action of oregano essential oil, thymol and carvacrol." *Journal of Applied Microbiology* 91(3): 453-462.

Larit, F., K. M. Elokely, N. D. Chaurasiya, S. Benyahia, M. A. Nael, F. León, M. S. Abu-Darwish, T. Efferth, Y. H. Wang and D. J. P. Belouahem-Abed. 2018. "Inhibition of human monoamine oxidase A and B by flavonoids isolated from two Algerian medicinal plants." *Phytomedicine* 40: 27-36.

Lee, B. H., T. G. Nam, W. J. Park, H. Kang, H. J. Heo, D. K. Chung, G. H. Kim, D.-O. J. F. S. Kim and Biotechnology. 2015. "Antioxidative and neuroprotective effects of volatile components in essential oils from Chrysanthemum indicum Linné flowers." *Food Science and Biotechnology* 24(2): 717-723.

Leyva-López, N., E. Gutiérrez-Grijalva, G. Vazquez-Olivo and J. J. M. Heredia. 2017. "Essential oils of oregano: Biological activity beyond their antimicrobial properties." *Molecules* 22(6): 989.

Liang, D., F. Li, Y. Fu, Y. Cao, X. Song, T. Wang, W. Wang, M. Guo, E. Zhou and D. J. I. Li. 2014. "Thymol inhibits LPS-stimulated inflammatory response via down-regulation of NF-κB and MAPK signaling pathways in mouse mammary epithelial cells." *Inflammation* 37(1): 214-222.

Ličina, B. Z., O. D. Stefanović, S. M. Vasić, I. D. Radojević, M. S. Dekić and L. R. J. F. c. Čomić. 2013. "Biological activities of the extracts from wild growing Origanum vulgare L." *Food control* 33(2): 498-504.

Lin, Y. L., C. N. Wang, Y. J. Shiao, T. Y. Liu and W. Y. J. J. o. t. C. C. S. Wang. 2003. "Benzolignanoid and polyphenols from Origanum vulgare." *Journal of the Chinese Chemical Society* 50(5): 1079-1083.

Liu, R. H. J. J. o. C. S. 2007. "Whole grain phytochemicals and health." *Journal of Cereal Science* 46(3): 207-219.

Llana-Ruiz-Cabello, M., D. Gutiérrez-Praena, M. Puerto, S. Pichardo, Á. Jos and A. M. J. T. i. v. Cameán. 2015. "*In vitro* pro-oxidant/antioxidant role of carvacrol, thymol and their mixture in the intestinal Caco-2 cell line." *Toxicology in Vitro* 29(4): 647-656.

Lukas, B., C. Schmiderer and J. J. P. Novak. 2015. "Essential oil diversity of European Origanum vulgare L. (Lamiaceae)." *Phytochemistry* 119: 32-40.

Magi, G., E. Marini and B. J. F. i. m. Facinelli. 2015. "Antimicrobial activity of essential oils and carvacrol, and synergy of carvacrol and erythromycin, against clinical, erythromycin-resistant Group A Streptococci." *Frontiers in Microbiology* 6: 165. https://doi.org/10.3389/fmicb.2015.00165.

Mancini, E., I. Camele, H. S. Elshafie, L. De Martino, C. Pellegrino, D. Grulova, V. J. C. De Feo and biodiversity. 2014. "Chemical composition and biological activity of the essential oil of Origanum vulgare ssp. hirtum from different areas in the Southern Apennines (Italy)." *Chemistry & Biodiversity* 11(4): 639-651.

Marrelli, M., F. Conforti, C. Formisano, D. Rigano, N. A. Arnold, F. Menichini and F. J. N. p. r. Senatore. 2016. "Composition, antibacterial, antioxidant and antiproliferative activities of essential oils from three Origanum species growing wild in Lebanon and Greece." *Natural Product Research* 30(6): 735-739.

Martínez-Natarén, D. A., V. Parra-Tabla, M. M. Ferrer-Ortega, L. M. J. P. s. Calvo-Irabién and evolution. 2014. "Genetic diversity and genetic structure in wild populations of Mexican oregano (Lippia graveolens HBK) and its relationship with the chemical composition of the essential oil." *Plant Systematics and Evolution* 300(3): 535-547.

Martins, N., L. Barros, C. Santos-Buelga, M. Henriques, S. Silva and I. C. J. F. c. Ferreira. 2014. "Decoction, infusion and hydroalcoholic extract of Origanum vulgare L.: different performances regarding bioactivity and phenolic compounds." *Food Chemistry* 158: 73-80.

Martucci, J. F., L. B. Gende, L. Neira, R. A. J. I. C. Ruseckaite and Products. 2015. "Oregano and lavender essential oils as antioxidant and antimicrobial additives of biogenic gelatin films." *Industrial Crops and Products* 71: 205-213.

McCue, P. P. and K. J. A. P. J. o. C. N. Shetty. 2004. "Inhibitory effects of rosmarinic acid extracts on porcine pancreatic amylase *in vitro*." *Asia Pacific Journal of Clinical Nutrition* 13(1).

Mechan, A. O., A. Fowler, N. Seifert, H. Rieger, T. Wöhrle, S. Etheve, A. Wyss, G. Schüler, B. Colletto and C. J. B. j. o. n. Kilpert. 2011. "Monoamine reuptake inhibition and mood-enhancing potential of a specified oregano extract." *British Journal of Nutrition* 105(8): 1150-1163.

Mechergui, K., J. A. Coelho, M. C. Serra, S. B. Lamine, S. Boukhchina, M. L. J. J. o. t. S. o. F. Khouja and Agriculture. 2010. "Essential oils of Origanum vulgare L. subsp. glandulosum (Desf.) Ietswaart from Tunisia: chemical composition and antioxidant activity." *Journal of the Science of Food and Agriculture* 90(10): 1745-1749.

Mechergui, K., W. Jaouadi, J. P. Coelho, M. L. J. I. C. Khouja and Products. 2016. "Effect of harvest year on production, chemical composition and antioxidant activities of essential oil of oregano (Origanum vulgare subsp glandulosum (Desf.) Ietswaart) growing in North Africa." *Industrial Crops and Products* 90: 32-37.

Mechergui, K., S. Khaldi, W. Jaouadi and M. J. S. f. P. R. Khouja. 2015. "Vegetative Multiplication of Oregano (Origanum vulgare subsp. glandulosum desf.) Letswaart from Cuttings of Tunisian Wild Populations." *Vegetos* 28 (3): 98-102.

Meeran, N., M. Fizur, H. Javed, H. Al Taee, S. Azimullah and S. K. J. F. i. p. Ojha. 2017. "Pharmacological properties and molecular mechanisms of thymol: prospects for its therapeutic potential and pharmaceutical development." *Frontiers in Pharmacology* 8: 380.

Menezes, R., A. Rodriguez-Mateos, A. Kaltsatou, A. González-Sarrías, A. Greyling, C. Giannaki, C. Andres-Lacueva, D. Milenkovic, E. Gibney and J. J. N. Dumont. 2017. "Impact of flavonols on cardiometabolic biomarkers: a meta-analysis of randomized controlled human trials to explore the role of inter-Individual variability." *Nutrients* 9(2): 117.

Milos, M. and D. J. F. c. Makota. 2012. "Investigation of antioxidant synergisms and antagonisms among thymol, carvacrol, thymoquinone and p-cymene in a model system using the Briggs–Rauscher oscillating reaction." *Food Chemistry* 131(1): 296-299.

Milos, M., J. Mastelic and I. J. F. C. Jerkovic. 2000. "Chemical composition and antioxidant effect of glycosidically bound volatile compounds from oregano (Origanum vulgare L. ssp. hirtum)." *Food Chemistry* 71(1): 79-83.

Moradi, M., A. Hassani, A. Ehsani, M. Hashemi, M. Raeisi, S. J. J. o. f. q. Naghibi and h. control. 2014. "Phytochemical and antibacterial properties of Origanum vulgare ssp. gracile growing wild in Kurdistan province of Iran." *Journal of Food Quality and Hazards Control* 1(4): 120-124.

Morshedloo, M. R., L. E. Craker, A. Salami, V. Nazeri, H. Sang, F. J. P. p. Maggi and biochemistry. 2017. "Effect of prolonged water stress on essential oil content, compositions and gene expression patterns of mono-and sesquiterpene synthesis in two oregano (Origanum vulgare L.) subspecies." *Plant Physiology and Biochemistry* 111: 119-128.

Morshedloo, M. R., S. A. Salami, V. Nazeri, F. Maggi, L. J. I. C. Craker and Products. 2018. "Essential oil profile of oregano (Origanum vulgare L.) populations grown under similar soil and climate conditions." *Industrial Crops and Products* 119: 183-190.

Nagoor Meeran, M. F., P. J. J. o. b. Stanely Mainzen Prince and m. toxicology. 2012. "Protective effects of thymol on altered plasma lipid peroxidation and nonenzymic antioxidants in isoproterenol-induced myocardial infarcted rats." *Journal of Biochemical and Molecular Toxicology* 26(9): 368-373.

Nath, S. S., C. Pandey and D. J. I. j. o. a. Roy. 2012. "A near fatal case of high dose peppermint oil ingestion-Lessons learnt." *Indian Journal of Anaesthesia* 56(6): 582.

Nile, S. H., A. S. Nile and Y.-S. J. B. Keum. 2017. "Total phenolics, antioxidant, antitumor, and enzyme inhibitory activity of Indian medicinal and aromatic plants extracted with different extraction methods." *3 Biotech* **7**(1): 76.

Nostro, A., A. R. Blanco, M. A. Cannatelli, V. Enea, G. Flamini, I. Morelli, A. Sudano Roccaro and V. J. F. M. L. Alonzo. 2004. "Susceptibility of methicillin-resistant staphylococci to oregano essential oil, carvacrol and thymol." *FEMS Microbiology Letters* 230(2): 191-195.

Novák, I., L. Sipos, Z. Kókai, K. Szabó, Z. Pluhár and S. J. A. A. Sárosi. 2011. "Effect of the drying method on the composition of Origanum vulgare L. subsp. hirtum essential oil analysed by GC-MS and sensory profile method." *Acta Alimentaria* 40(1): 130-138.

Nurzyńska-Wierdak, R., A. Bogucka-Kocka, I. Sowa and G. J. F. Szymczak. 2012. "The composition of essential oil from three ecotypes of Origanum vulgare L. ssp. vulgare cultivated in Poland." *Farmacia* 60(4): 571-577.

Ocana-Fuentes, A., E. Arranz-Gutierrez, F. Senorans, G. J. F. Reglero and C. Toxicology. 2010. "Supercritical fluid extraction of oregano (Origanum vulgare) essentials oils: anti-inflammatory properties based on cytokine response on THP-1 macrophages." *Food and Chemical Toxicology* 48(6): 1568-1575.

Olmedo, R., V. Nepote and N. R. J. F. c. Grosso. 2014. "Antioxidant activity of fractions from oregano essential oils obtained by molecular distillation." *Food Chemistry* 156: 212-219.

Osakabe, N., A. Yasuda, M. Natsume and T. J. C. Yoshikawa. 2004. "Rosmarinic acid inhibits epidermal inflammatory responses: anticarcinogenic effect of Perilla frutescens extract in the murine two-stage skin model." *Carcinogenesis: Integrative Cancer Research* 25(4): 549-557.

Ozkalp, B., F. Sevgi, M. Ozcan and M. M. J. J. F. A. E. Ozcan. 2010. "The antibacterial activity of essential oil of oregano (Origanum vulgare L.)." *Journal of Food, Agriculture and Environment* 8(2): 272-274.

Özkan, O. E., K. Güney, M. Gür, E. S. Pattabanoğlu, E. Babat, M. M. J. I. J. O. P. E. Khalifa and RESEARCH. 2017. "Essential Oil of Oregano and Savory; Chemical Composition and Antimicrobial Activity." *Indian Journal of Pharmaceutical Education and Research* 51(3): S205-S208.

Pande, C. and C. J. J. o. E. O. R. Mathela. 2000. "Essential oil composition of Origanum vulgare L. ssp. vulgare from the Kumaon Himalayas." *Journal of Essential Oil Research* 12(4): 441-442.

Paraskevakis, N., E. Tsiplakou, D. Daferera, K. Sotirakoglou, M. Polissiou and G. J. J. o. E. O. R. Zervas. 2015. "Changes in essential oil content and composition of Origanum vulgare spp. hirtum during storage as a whole plant or after grinding and mixing with a concentrate ruminant diet." *Journal of Essential Oil Research* 27(3): 264-270.

Pesavento, G., C. Calonico, A. Bilia, M. Barnabei, F. Calesini, R. Addona, L. Mencarelli, L. Carmagnini, M. Di Martino and A. L. J. F. C. Nostro. 2015. "Antibacterial activity of Oregano, Rosmarinus and Thymus essential oils against Staphylococcus aureus and Listeria monocytogenes in beef meatballs." *Food Control* 54: 188-199.

Peters, M., V. Trembovler, A. Alexandrovich, M. Parnas, L. Birnbaumer, B. Minke and E. J. J. o. n. Shohami. 2012. "Carvacrol together with TRPC1 elimination improve functional recovery after traumatic brain injury in mice." *Journal of Neurotrauma* 29(18): 2831-2834.

Petersen, M. and M. S. J. P. Simmonds. 2003. "Rosmarinic acid." *Phytochemistry* 62(2): 121-125.

Pezzani, R., S. Vitalini and M. J. P. R. Iriti. 2017. "Bioactivities of Origanum vulgare L.: an update." *Phytochemistry Reviews* 16(6): 1253-1268.

Pirigharnaei, M., S. Zare, R. Heidari, J. Khara, R. E. Sabzi and F. J. I. J. F. A. E. Kheiry. 2011. "The essential oil composition of Iranian oregano (Origanum vulgare L.) populations in field and provenance from Piranshahr district, West Azarbaijan province, Iran." *Journal of Food, Agriculture and Environment* 9: 89-93.

Quiroga, P. R., N. R. Grosso, A. Lante, G. Lomolino, J. A. Zygadlo, V. J. I. J. o. F. S. Nepote and Technology. 2013. "Chemical composition, antioxidant activity and anti-lipase activity of O riganum vulgare and L ippia turbinata essential oils." *International Journal of Food Science +Technology* 48(3): 642-649.

Radušienė, J., L. Ivanauskas, V. Janulis and V. J. B. Jakštas. 2008. "Composition and variability of phenolic compounds in Origanum vulgare from Lithuania." *Biologija* 54(1): 45-49.

Robards, K., P. D. Prenzler, G. Tucker, P. Swatsitang and W. Glover. 1999. "Phenolic compounds and their role in oxidative processes in fruits." *Food Chemistry* 66(4): 401-436.

Robledo, S., E. Osorio, D. Munoz, L. M. Jaramillo, A. Restrepo, G. Arango, I. J. A. a. Vélez and chemotherapy. 2005. "*In vitro* and *in vivo* cytotoxicities and antileishmanial activities of thymol and hemisynthetic derivatives." *Antimicrobial Agents and Chemotherapy* 49(4): 1652-1655.

Rodríguez-Solana, R., D. J. Daferera, C. Mitsi, P. Trigas, M. Polissiou, P. A. J. I. C. Tarantilis and Products. 2014. "Comparative chemotype determination of Lamiaceae plants by means of GC–MS, FT-IR, and dispersive-Raman spectroscopic techniques and GC-FID quantification." *Industrial Crops and Products* 62: 22-33.

Rubió, L., M. J. Motilva, M. P. J. C. r. i. f. s. Romero and nutrition. 2013. "Recent advances in biologically active compounds in herbs and spices: a review of the most effective antioxidant and anti-inflammatory active principles." *Critical Reviews in Food Science and Nutrition* 53(9): 943-953.

Rui, Y., L. Tong, J. Cheng, G. Wang, L. Qin, Z. J. F. Wan and n. research. 2017. "Rosmarinic acid suppresses adipogenesis, lipolysis in 3T3-L1 adipocytes, lipopolysaccharide-stimulated tumor necrosis factor-α secretion in macrophages, and inflammatory mediators in 3T3-L1 adipocytes." *Food & Nutrition Research* 61(1): 1330096. https://doi.org/10.1080/16546628.2017.1330096.

Şahin, F., M. Güllüce, D. Daferera, A. Sökmen, M. Sökmen, M. Polissiou, G. Agar and H. J. F. c. Özer. 2004. "Biological activities of the essential oils and methanol extract of Origanum vulgare ssp. vulgare in the Eastern Anatolia region of Turkey." *Food Control* 15(7): 549-557.

Samarghandian, S., T. Farkhondeh, F. Samini and A. J. B. r. i. Borji. 2016. "Protective effects of carvacrol against oxidative stress induced by chronic stress in rat s brain, liver, and kidney." *Biochemistry Research International* 2016. http://dx.doi.org/10. 1155/2016/2645237.

Sammi, S. R., S. Trivedi, S. K. Rath, A. Nagar, S. Tandon, A. Kalra and R. J. M. n. Pandey. 2017. "1-Methyl-4-propan-2-ylbenzene from Thymus vulgaris attenuates cholinergic dysfunction." *Molecular Neurobiology* 54(7): 5468-5481.

Sarikurkcu, C., G. Zengin, M. Oskay, S. Uysal, R. Ceylan, A. J. I. C. Aktumsek and Products. 2015. "Composition, antioxidant, antimicrobial and enzyme inhibition activities of two Origanum vulgare subspecies (subsp. vulgare and subsp. hirtum) essential oils." *Industrial Crops and Products* 70: 178-184.

Sasaki, K., K. Wada, Y. Tanaka, T. Yoshimura, K. Matuoka and T. J. J. o. m. f. Anno. 2005. "Thyme (Thymus vulgaris L.) leaves and its constituents increase the activities of xenobiotic-metabolizing enzymes in mouse liver." *Journal of Medicinal Food* 8(2): 184-189.

Savini, I., R. Arnone, M. V. Catani and L. Avigliano. 2009. "Origanum vulgare induces apoptosis in human colon cancer caco2 cells." *Nutr Cancer* 61(3): 381-389.

Schrader, E. 2000. "Equivalence of St John s wort extract (Ze 117) and fluoxetine: a randomized, controlled study in mildmoderate depression." *International Clinical Psychopharmacology* 15(2): 61-68.

Shan, Y., D. D. Wang, Y. X. Xu, C. Wang, L. Cao, Y. S. Liu and C. Q. J. J. o. A. s. D. Zhu. 2016. "Aging as a precipitating factor in chronic restraint stress-induced tau aggregation pathology, and the protective effects of rosmarinic acid." *Journal of Alzheimer's Disease* 49(3): 829-844.

Sharifi-Rad, J., A. Sureda, G. Tenore, M. Daglia, M. Sharifi-Rad, M. Valussi, R. Tundis, M. Sharifi-Rad, M. Loizzo and A. J. M. Ademiluyi. 2017. "Biological activities of essential oils: From plant chemoecology to traditional healing systems." *Molecules* 22(1): 70.

Sharifi-Rad, M., E. M. Varoni, M. Iriti, M. Martorell, W. N. Setzer, M. del Mar Contreras, B. Salehi, A. Soltani-Nejad, S. Rajabi and M. J. P. R. Tajbakhsh. 2018. "Carvacrol and human health: A comprehensive review." *Phytotherapy Research* 32(9): 1675-1687.

Shetty, K. J. P. B. 2004. "Role of proline-linked pentose phosphate pathway in biosynthesis of plant phenolics for functional food and environmental applications: a review." *Process Biochemistry* 39(7): 789-804.

Singletary, K. J. N. T. 2010. "Oregano: overview of the literature on health benefits." Nutrition Today 45(3): 129-138.

Soković, M., J. Glamočlija, P. D. Marin, D. Brkić and L. J. J. M. van Griensven. 2010. "Antibacterial effects of the essential oils of commonly consumed medicinal herbs using an *in vitro* model." *Molecules* 15(11): 7532-7546.

Song, J. X., S. C. W. Sze, T. B. Ng, C. K. F. Lee, G. P. Leung, P. C. Shaw, Y. Tong and Y.-B. Zhang. 2012. "Anti-Parkinsonian drug discovery from herbal medicines: what have we got from neurotoxic models?" *Journal of ethnopharmacology* 139(3): 698-711.

Spagnoletti, A., A. Guerrinia, M. Tacchini, V. Vinciguerra, C. Leone, I. Maresca, G. Simonetti, G. Sacchetti and L. J. N. p. c. Angiolella. 2016. "Chemical Composition and Bio-efficacy of Essential Oils from Italian Aromatic Plants: Mentha suaveolens, Coridothymus capitatus, Origanum hirtum and Rosmarinus officinalis." *Natural Product Communications* 11(10): 1517-1520.

Stamenic, M., J. Vulic, S. Djilas, D. Misic, V. Tadic, S. Petrovic and I. J. F. c. Zizovic. 2014. "Free-radical scavenging activity and antibacterial impact of Greek oregano isolates obtained by SFE." *Food Chemistry* 165: 307-315.

Stojković, D., J. Glamočlija, A. Ćirić, M. Nikolić, M. Ristić, J. Šiljegović and M. J. A. B. S. Soković. 2013. "Investigation on antibacterial synergism of Origanum vulgare and Thymus vulgaris essential oils." Arch. *Biol. Sci., Belgrade* 65(2): 639-643.

Swamy, M. K., M. S. Akhtar, U. R. J. E.-B. C. Sinniah and A. Medicine. 2016. "Antimicrobial properties of plant essential oils against human pathogens and their mode of action: an updated review." *Evidence-Based Complementary and Alternative Medicine* 2016. http://dx.doi.org/10.1155/2016/3012462.

Taofiq, O., A. González-Paramás, M. Barreiro and I. J. M. Ferreira. 2017. "Hydroxycinnamic acids and their derivatives: cosmeceutical significance, challenges and future perspectives, a review." *Molecules* 22(2): 281.

Teixeira, B., A. Marques, C. Ramos, C. Serrano, O. Matos, N. R. Neng, J. M. Nogueira, J. A. Saraiva, M. L. J. J. o. t. S. o. F. Nunes and Agriculture. 2013. "Chemical composition and bioactivity of different oregano (Origanum vulgare) extracts and essential oil." *Journal of the Science of Food and Agriculture* 93(11): 2707-2714.

Thaipong, K., U. Boonprakob, K. Crosby, L. Cisneros-Zevallos and D. H. Byrne. 2006. "Comparison of ABTS, DPPH, FRAP, and ORAC assays for estimating antioxidant activity from guava fruit extracts." *Journal of food composition and analysis* 19(6): 669-675.

Thomidis, T. and A. J. C. P. Filotheou. 2016. "Evaluation of five essential oils as bio-fungicides on the control of Pilidiella granati rot in pomegranate." *Crop Protection* 89: 66-71.

Tibaldi, G., E. Fontana, S. J. I. C. Nicola and Products. 2011. "Growing conditions and postharvest management can affect the essential oil of Origanum vulgare L. ssp. hirtum (Link) Ietswaart." *Industrial Crops and Products* 34(3): 1516-1522.

Tsai, S.-j., C.-y. Chao and M.-c. J. E. j. o. p. Yin. 2011. "Preventive and therapeutic effects of caffeic acid against inflammatory injury in striatum of MPTP-treated mice." *European Journal of Pharmacology* 670(2-3): 441-447.

Tuttolomondo, T., S. La Bella, M. Licata, G. Virga, C. Leto, A. Saija, D. Trombetta, A. Tomaino, A. Speciale, E. M. J. C. Napoli and biodiversity. 2013. "Biomolecular characterization of wild sicilian oregano: phytochemical screening of essential oils and extracts, and evaluation of their antioxidant activities." *Chemistry & Biodiversity* 10(3): 411-433.

Uttara, B., A. V. Singh, P. Zamboni and R. J. C. n. Mahajan. 2009. "Oxidative stress and neurodegenerative diseases: a review of upstream and downstream antioxidant therapeutic options." *Current Neuropharmacology* 7(1): 65-74.

Vale-Silva, L., M. J. Silva, D. Oliveira, M. J. Gonçalves, C. Cavaleiro, L. Salgueiro and E. J. J. o. m. m. Pinto. 2012. "Correlation of the chemical composition of essential oils from Origanum vulgare subsp. virens with their *in vitro* activity against pathogenic yeasts and filamentous fungi." *Journal of Medical Microbiology* 61(2): 252-260.

Vazirian, M., M. Mohammadi, M. Farzaei, G. Amin and Y. J. R. J. o. P. Amanzadeh. 2015. "Chemical composition and antioxidant activity of Origanum vulgare subsp. vulgare essential oil from Iran." *Research Journal of Pharmacognosy* 2(1): 41-46.

Verma, R., L. Rahman, R. Verma, C. Chanotiya, A. Chauhan, A. Yadav, A. Yadav and A. J. C. s. Singh. 2010. "Changes in the essential oil content and composition of Origanum vulgare L. during annual growth from Kumaon Himalaya." *Current science* 98(8): 1010-1012.

Vokou, D., S. Kokkini, J. M. J. B. S. Bessiere and Ecology. 1993. "Geographic variation of Greek oregano (Origanum vulgare ssp. hirtum) essential oils." *Biochemical Systematics and Ecology* 21(2): 287-295.

Vujicic, M., I. Nikolic, V. G. Kontogianni, T. Saksida, P. Charisiadis, Z. Orescanin-Dusic, D. Blagojevic, S. Stosic-Grujicic, A. G. Tzakos and I. J. B. J. o. N. Stojanovic. 2015. "Methanolic extract of Origanum vulgare ameliorates type 1 diabetes through antioxidant, anti-inflammatory and anti-apoptotic activity." *British Journal of Nutrition* 113(5): 770-782.

Waller, S. B., I. M. Madrid, A. L. Silva, L. L. D. De Castro, M. B. Cleff, V. Ferraz, M. C. A. Meireles, R. Zanette and J. R. B. J. M. de Mello. 2016. "*In vitro* susceptibility of Sporothrix brasiliensis to essential oils of Lamiaceae family." *Mycopathologia* 181(11-12): 857-863.

Wei, H. K., G. Chen, R. J. Wang and J. J. J. o. F. F. Peng. 2015. "Oregano essential oil decreased susceptibility to oxidative stress-induced dysfunction of intestinal epithelial barrier in rats." *Journal of Functional Foods* 18: 1191-1199.

Werdin González, J. O., M. M. Gutiérrez, A. P. Murray and A. A. J. P. m. s. Ferrero. 2011. "Composition and biological activity of essential oils from Labiatae against Nezara viridula (Hemiptera: Pentatomidae) soybean pest." *Pest Management Science* 67(8): 948-955.

WHO. 2018. from http://www.who.int/.

Wojdyło, A., J. Oszmiański and R. Czemerys. 2007. "Antioxidant activity and phenolic compounds in 32 selected herbs." *Food Chemistry* 105(3): 940-949.

Yan, F., A. Azizi, S. Janke, M. Schwarz, S. Zeller, B. J. I. C. Honermeier and Products. 2016. "Antioxidant capacity variation in the oregano (Origanum vulgare L.) collection of the German National Genebank." *Industrial Crops and Products* 92: 19-25.

Yasuhisa, T., H. Hideki and Y. Muneyoshi. 1993. "Superoxide radical scavenging activity of phenolic compounds." *International Journal of Biochemistry* 25(4): 491-494.

Zhang, X. L., Y. S. Guo, C. H. Wang, G. Q. Li, J. J. Xu, H. Y. Chung, W. C. Ye, Y -L. Li and G.-C. J. F. c. Wang. 2014. "Phenolic compounds from Origanum vulgare and their antioxidant and antiviral activities." *Food Chemistry* 152: 300-306.

Zhao, J., S. I. Khan, M. Wang, Y. Vasquez, M. H. Yang, B. Avula, Y.-H. Wang, C. Avonto, T. J. Smillie and I. A. J. J. o. n. p. Khan. 2014. "Octulosonic acid derivatives from Roman chamomile (Chamaemelum nobile) with activities against inflammation and metabolic disorder." *Journal of Natural Products* 77(3): 509-515.

Zheljazkov, V. D., T. Astatkie and V. J. H. Schlegel. 2012. "Distillation time changes oregano essential oil yields and composition but not the antioxidant or antimicrobial activities." *HortScience* 47(6): 777-784.

Zheng, W. and S. Y. Wang. 2001. "Antioxidant activity and phenolic compounds in selected herbs." *Journal of Agricultural and Food Chemistry* 49(11): 5165-5170.

Zotti, M., M. Colaianna, M. G. Morgese, P. Tucci, S. Schiavone, P. Avato and L. Trabace. 2013. "Carvacrol: From Ancient Flavoring to Neuromodulatory Agent." *Molecules* 18(6): 6161.

In: Oregano: Properties, Uses and Health Benefits
Editor: Gema Nieto Martínez
ISBN: 978-1-53616-284-4

Chapter 7

OREGANO USES AND BENEFITS IN FOOD SCIENCE

Narimane Segueni[1,*] and Salah Akkal[2,*]
[1]Laboratory of Natural Products and Organic Synthesis,
Department of Chemistry, Faculty of Science,
University of Mentouri Constantine 1, Constantine, Algeria
[2]Valorization of Natural Resources,
Bioactive Molecules and Biological Analysis Unit,
Department of Chemistry, University of Mentouri Constantine 1,
Constantine, Algeria

ABSTRACT

Oregano is one of the most famous culinary herbs used all over the world. The genus *Origanum* L. is represented by several species. The most important is *Origanum vulgare* which predominate in occurrence. Oregano has been used in traditional medicine since ancient times. Greek and Roman used oregano for diarrhea, asthma and to maintain general health. Oregano contains many bioactive compounds such as essential oil.

Oregano essential oils present a characteristic odor due to the main compounds carvacrol and thymol. Oregano essential oils have been largely investigated for their potential as antimicrobial and antioxidant agents. In addition, they are used in food products and cosmetic. However oregano use and benefit is not limited to human but is also related to animal.

Natural products are gaining interest. They are considered as an alternative to synthetic ones. Moreover, the use of natural additives is considered more safety and will assure a better quality to food products. In the last recent years, products containing essential oil have been used as growth promoters and feed additives in animal nutrition. This chapter discusses actual and potential uses of oregano as an alternative food and feed additive.

Keywords: oregano, essential oil, food additive, feed additive

* Corresponding Author's E-mail: segueninarimane@yahoo.fr and salah4dz@yahoo.fr.

INTRODUCTION

Oregano is one of the most famous culinary herbs used all over the world. The word Oregano is derived from the Greek *"Oros"* and *"Ganos"* which means the *"beauty of the mountains"* [1]. The name Oregano designates a wide variety of plant with a typical aroma and flavor [2] including 60 species and 17 genera belonging to six botanical families. Lamiaceae and Verbenaceae families are the most interesting families due to their economic importance. Apiaceae, Asteraceae and Rubiaceae are the other families.

The genus *Origanum* is belonging to the Lamiaceae. In contrast, the genus *Lippia* is belonging to the Verbenaceae family [1,3]. *Origanum sp.* and *Lippia sp.* share the same name but differ widely in term of use and taste. *Origanum sp.* designed as European oregano is used as flavoring in meat, soups, sauce and salads. While, *Lippia sp.* designed as Mexican oregano is used in Mexican foods and pizza [1].

The genus *Origanum* is represented by 10 sections, 39 species, 6 subspecies and 17 hybrids and it is widely distributed in the Mediterranean region. Regarding commercial value, four groups with a characteristic odor and flavor can be distinguished. They are commonly used. Groups are named Greek oregano (*Origanum vulgare* subsp *hirtus* (Link) letswaart), Spanish oregano (*Coridohymus capitatu* (L) Hoffmanns and Links), Turkish oregano (*Origanum onites* L), and Mexican oregano (*Lippia graveolens* Kunth or *Lippia berlandieri*) [4]. But regarding occurrence, the most important is *Origanum vulgare* [5]. While, the genus *Lippia* is distributed in territories of tropical Africa and the South and Central America Countries with 200 species [6, 7].

Chemistry of oregano is well documented. Many publications referring to the chemical composition of *Origanum vulgare* are available. Four classes of active principle were identified namely: essential oil, polyphenols (flavonoids and phenolic acids), triterpenes and sterols [8, 9, 10, 11]. Chemical composition of oregano essential oils has been extensively studied. The major constituents are terpenes (mono and sesquiterpenes). Carvacrol, thymol, *p*-cymene and γ-terpinene are the principal terpenes identified. In addition, linalool, terpinen-4-ol, trans-sabinene hydrate, β-myrcene and β-caryophyllene are also identified. The proportion of these and other components in the essential oil within the same species defines the chemotype [12].

Many *Lippia* species have been investigated in order to determine their chemical composition. Research indicated the presence of several classes of chemical components such as: phenolic compounds (phenolic acids, flavonoids and caffeic acid derivatives) [12-20] naphtoquinoids [14, 21], terpenes (monoterpenes and sequiterpenes) [12]; iridoids [22-24], alkaloids, tannins and saponins [25, 26]. The essential oils from *Lippia* species have also been extensively investigated. β-caryophyllene, limonene, *p*-cymene, camphor, linalool, thymol and α-pinene were the most frequent components found. The variability in chemical composition of *Lippia* essential oil led to the identification of several chemotypes [6, 7].

Oregano has been used in traditional medicine since ancient times. Greek and Roman used oregano as antiseptic and to treat diarrhea, asthma, indigestion, and to maintain general health. Oregano was also used as antiseptic and for the treatment of skin sores [27, 28]. European Oregano was used as tonic, stimulant, expectorant, diaphonic and carminative. In addition, European oregano was also used as a natural remedy for nervousness, toothaches, headaches, colic and coughs [1, 11, 29]. Recent investigation on *Origanum vulgare* demonstrated a wide range of biological activities such as: antioxidant [30], antispasmodic [29], anti-inflammatory [11], antimicrobial [30, 31], neuroprotective [32], antiproliferative [8, 11] etc.

The most traditionally utilization of *Lippia* species is a remedy for respiratory disorders such as: asthma, bronchitis, colds and grippe and gastrointestinal remedy as a treatment of indigestion and stomach [6]. In addition, several species are used for the treatment of hepatic diseases, vesicule ache, cutaneous diseases, gonorrhea, syphilis [33], arterial hypertension [17], diarrhea and for abdominal pains [34]. Several studies demonstrated that some *Lippia* species are also used as carminatives [22]. Moreover, some *Lippia* species have shown antimalarial [22], anti-inflammatory, analgesic, antipyretic [34], diuretic, sedative and myorelaxing activities [6].

However oregano uses and benefits are not limited to human but are also related to animal. Natural products are gaining interest. They are considered as an alternative to synthetic ones. Moreover, the use of natural additives is considered more safety and will assure a better quality to food products. In the last recent years, products containing essential oil have been used as growth promoters and feed additives in animal nutrition. This chapter discusses potential uses of oregano as an alternative food and feed additive.

OREGANO AS FOOD ADDITIVE

The growing interest of some consumers in the use of minimally processed foods and their tendency to choose those containing natural additives or with fewer additives enhance the interest and the effort of food manufacturers to develop an alternative additives. As a consequence the use of natural products as food additives is gaining interest [35, 36]. Natural products are considered as an alternative to synthetic ones. Moreover, the use of natural additives is considered more safe and will assure a better quality to food products [37].

Herbs and spices have been used since ancient times for their healthy and nutritional properties. They are also used in food for their sensory characteristics. Most of their properties are attributed to their phytochemical constituents such as phenolic compounds and essential oil in particular antioxidant and antimicrobial activities. Many studies reported a high correlation between phenolic components and antioxidant [38-40] and antimicrobial activities of herbs and spices [35, 41]. Essential oils can act on bacteria, molds and yeasts causing their inhibition or reducing their growth [42, 43]. Several mechanisms of action are reported in the literature. They are varying according to the chemical composition of the tested oils and can be attributed to individual compound present in the mixture or a synergetic activity of several compounds. In general, membrane and cytoplasm targets are involved [44].

Spices and herbs are considered as an excellent source of antioxidants. Herbs and spices such as rosemary, sage and oregano are rich on phenolic compounds. Their high content on those components is responsible of their strong antioxidant effect [45]. Phenolics derived from herbs and spices can inhibit oxidative rancidity. Oxidative rancidity is causing rejection by consumers due to the formation of off-flavours and off-odours. In addition to the deterioration of foods, harmful compounds can be formed [46]. The chemical structure of phenolic compounds and their redox abilities are the main cause of their antioxidant properties. In general, the cited compounds can cause the neutralization of free radicals, chelating transitional metals or quenching oxygen [45]. As a consequence, spices and herbs are a great source of antioxidants for food preservation. The used forms might be ground spice/herb, encapsulated or emulsions [45].

In food technology microbial degradation and lipid peroxidation appearing in food products are the major concerns. They are responsible of the decrease in safety and nutritional quality. The dual functionality of herb and spices and their derivatives such as essential oil in preventing microbial spoilage and lipid oxidation is making theme a new source of natural and safe additive [47].

Antimicrobial Activity

Antimicrobial components play an important role in the safety of food, they prevent and control the growth of micro-organisms. In addition, they are used as a food preservative to control natural spoilage processes [48, 49].

The occurrence of microbial spoilage is possible in any stage of the chain production, starting from the raw material to the packaging of the final product. Bacteria and molds are the main organisms of spoilage. However, yeasts spoilage is often predictable in high acid foods, sugar or salt high content products or frozen products [50].

The analysis of the recent bibliography indicates that researchers in the field of the food industry pay particular attention to the use of natural antimicrobial agents, in particular essential oils (EOs) in fresh food such as fruit and vegetables. Recently, an increasing interest for the incorporation of natural antimicrobials in packaging materials has been observed [51-54].

Antimicrobial activity of Oregano essential oil (OEO) is well described in the literature. Numerous *in vitro* and *in vivo* investigations of the potential antifungal and antibacterial activities of OEO alone or in combination with other plants essential oils have been conducted [55]. In comparison with others essential oil such as thyme, rosemary, sage, mint, coriander, mustard, cinnamon and cilantro OEO was found to possess the strongest antimicrobial activity [56]. Carvacrol and thymol (Figure-1) are thought to be responsible of the high antimicrobial activity of OEO [57]. The majority of terpenoid antimicrobial activity in particular phenolic terpenoid antimicrobial activity is related to their hydroxyl group and the functional groups. In addition, an important element for such activity is the presence of delocalized electrons [58-61].

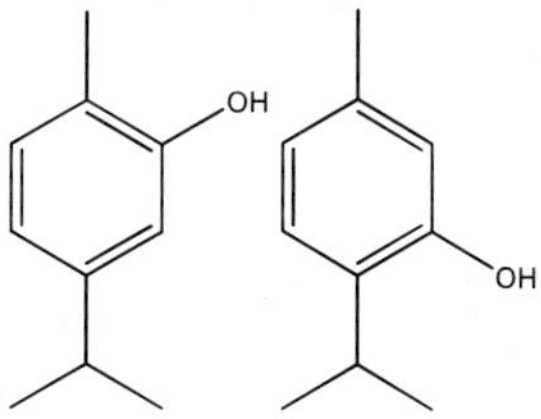

Carvacrol Thymol

Figure 1. Chemical structure of carvacrol and thymol.

Carvacrol is considered as a fast acting component. Cytoplasmic membrane is the site of action of carvacrol which increases the permeability of adenosine triphosphate. As a consequence, the passive permeability of the cell changes leading to inhibition and eventual cell death of Gram negative bacteria [62-64]. In general, essential oils are more active on Gram positive bacteria than Gram negative bacteria [44, 61, 65-67]. Mechanism of action of carvacrol on Gram negative bacteria is represented in Figure-2. The higher resistance of Gram negative bacteria can be attributed to differential membrane structure. Gram negative bacteria have an outer phospholipid membrane which is more complex than Gram positive bacteria. This rigid outer membrane rich on lipopolysaccharide (LPS) is impermeable to lipophilic constituents [44, 68-70]. Carvacrol is one of the few essential oil components that can act on Gram negative bacteria causing a disintegration of the outer membrane [71].

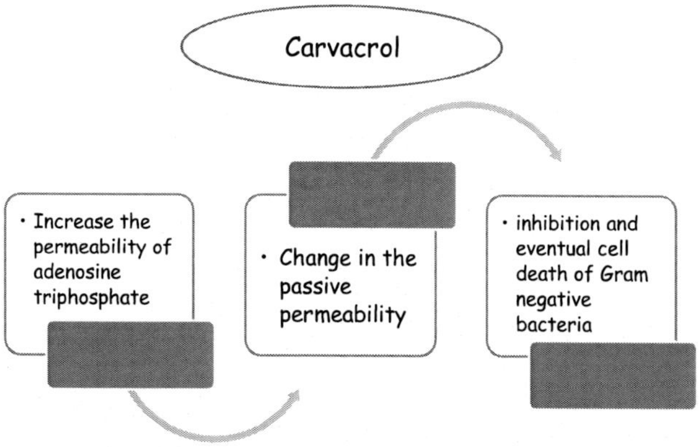

Figure 2. Mechanism of action of carvacrol on Gram Negative bacteria.

Thymol has a similar structure to carvacrol with a hydroxyl group in a different position on the phenolic ring (Figure 1). Antimicrobial activity of thymol represented in Figure 3 results also on alterations in the cytoplasmic membrane leading to disruption of outer and inner membranes [72, 73]. In addition, thymol can interact with membrane proteins and intracellular targets [69, 72, 74, 75].

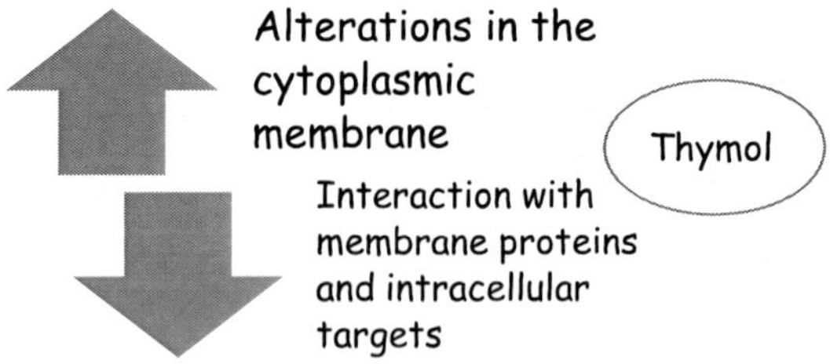

Figure 3. Mechanism of action of thymol.

The purpose of this chapter is not to provide a literature review of recent studies of the antimicrobial activity of oregano. However, it is important to highlight some work to better understand the potential use of oregano as a food additive.

The antimicrobial effects of OEO have been screened against a wide range of microorganisms and foodborn pathogens over the years. Cetin et al. 2011 screened the antibacterial activity of *Origanum rotundifolium, Origanum acutidens* and *Thymus sipyleus* subsp. *sipyleus* var. *rosulans* on 43 microorganisms, including 26 bacteria, 3 yeasts and 14 fungi. MIC and inhibition zones varied from 7.8-500 µg/ml and 8-72 mm respectively. *O rotundifolium* was most active on *S. aureus, S. pyogenes, E. coli, P. aeruginosa* and *P. pseudoalkaligenes*. While, *O acutidens* exhibited the strongest activity on *B. subtilis, S. pyogenes* and *P. aeruginosa*. *T sipyleus* subsp. *sipyleus* var. *rosulans* showed the highest inhibitory activity on *P. pseudoalkaligenes*, *S. aureus, B. subtilis, P. aeruginosa, S. pyogenes* and *P. vulgaris* [57]. Cattelan et al. 2013 evaluated the antibacterial activity of OEO on *S. aureus* (ATCC 25923), *B. cereus* (ATCC 11778), *B. subtilis* (ATCC 6633), *P. aeruginosa* (ATCC 9027), *S. typhimurium* (ATCC 14028) and *E. coli* (ATCC 8739). OEO were most actives on *S. aureus.* While, *P. aeruginosa* was resistant to all tested concentrations [76]. Boskovic et al. 2015 investigated the antibacterial activity of oregano and thyme essential oils on some foodborne pathogens. The tested oils exhibited antibacterial activity against *Salmonella Thyphimurium, Salmonella Enteritidis, Escherichia coli, Staphylococcus aureus*, methicillin resistant *Staphylococcus aureus* and *Bacillus cereus* [77]. Teixeira et al. 2013 evaluated the antimicrobial activity of ethanolic extract, hot and cold water extracts of the aerial part of *O vulgare* on foodborne spoilage and pathogenic bacteria. The tested strains were: *Escherichia coli* (ATCC 25922), *Pseudomonas putida* (CECT 7005), *Shewanella putrefaciens* (CECT 5346), *Salmonella typhimurium* (ATCC 14028), *Listeria monocytogenes* (CECT 5873), *Listeria innocua* (CECT 910) and *Brochothrix thermosphacta* (CECT 847). All tested bacteria were resistant to both hot and cold water except *B. thermosphacta* and *S. putrefaciens.* While, ethanolic extract was able to inhibit all studied bacteria, except *S. putrefaciens* and *B. thermosphacta.* Essential oil was the most effective extract inhibiting the growth of all tested bacteria [78].

Food commodities and stored food are frequently contaminated by moulds, fungal infestations, toxins and mycotoxins generated by some species during post-harvest processing, storage and transportation. Therefore, the control of molds, fungi and toxins is required to enhance the shelf life of food commodities [79, 80]. The antifungal activity and anti-aflatoxigenic potency of essential oil was found to be related to the chemical structure of the most abundant components of the tested oil [80, 81]. The presence of nucleus, the presence and position of hydroxyl group, special orientation and solubility in fats also affect essential oil antifungal activity. Aromatic nucleus compounds with phenolic OH group are characterized by high antimicrobial activity [82]. Several study concerning essential oil components and their mechanisms of action suggest an action on the structure and the functionality of cell membrane [83]. The observed activity depend on the used concentration. High concentrations might cause severe membrane damage and loss of homeostasis leading to cell death. On the contrast, low concentrations act on the permeability of the membrane causing changes in the cell structure and inhibiting respiration [82]. In addition to their action on cell membrane, essential oil components interact with some enzymes in particular those involved in synthesis of structural compounds and energy production [82].

Terpenes antifungal activity is due to their ability to act on membrane permeability and their interaction with intracellular structures. Phenolic components form hydrogen bonds between their hydroxyl groups and active sites of cellular enzymes [84, 85]. Monoterpenes cause the inhibition of mycelia growth of fungi and increase the concentration of lipid peroxydation such as hydroxyl, alkoxyl and alkoperoxy radicals [85]. Concerning the effects on mycotoxin biosynthesis, it is considered that active components of essential oils inhibit one or more steps in the mycotoxin biosynthesis pathway [82]. Carvacrol and thymol, the most abundant components of oregano essential oil exhibit a strong antifungal activity. They interract whit ergosterol causing damage in the cell membrane [44, 87-89]. In addition, thymol affects mycelium morphology, with changes in the localization of chitin within the hyphae [44]. Phenol compounds exhibit the strongest antifungal and antimycotoxigenic activity, followed by alcohols, aldehydes, ketones, ethers and hydrocarbons [82].

In comparaison with others oregano chemotypes, carvacrol/thymol chemotypes exhibited the highest inhibitory activity against fungal growth, conidial germination and production of *Penicillium* species such as *P. digitatum* [90]. They also have a synergetic effect in the inhibition of *P. digitatum* as reported by Daferera *et al.* 2000 which compared the antifungal activities of *O. dictamus* (78% thymol), *O. vulgare* (71% carvacrol-thymol) and *Thymus vulgaris* (66% carvacrol-thymol) and observed a more pronounced activity for *O. vulgare* and *T. vulgaris* [85].

OEO were found to inhibit the growth of several spoilage fungi such as: *A. niger, A. ochraceus, A. flavus* [91-93], *A. parasiticus, A. terreus, A. fumigates* [93], *Aspergillus sp, Penicillium sp, Rhizopus* sp. Rh18 [94], *Fusarium sp, Penicillium. Citrinum, Mucor sp* [91]. Moreover, *in vitro* tests on Mexican oregano essential oil fractions with different concentrations of thymol and carvacrol in a medium representative of bakery product contamined by *Aspergillus sp, Penicillium sp* and *Rhizopus* sp. demonstrated that the tested fractions have antifungal effects. The observed effect is dependent on the concentration of essential oil in the culture medium suggesting the use of Mexican oregano essential oil (*L. berlandieri* Schauer) as a natural antimicrobial agent to prevent fungal growth. Further study on the effect on mycelium structure and spore production might help to better understand the mechanism of action of the tested oil fractions [94].

In general evaluation of antimicrobial activity of essential oil is performed in aqueous system by direct contact. In the last recent years several studies regarding gaseous contact of essential oil in particular OEO are available. The use of vapor phase seems to be more effective against fungi. Lopez et al. 2007 demonstrated that *Origanum vulgare* essential oil possesses antifungal activity on *A. flavus* by gaseous contact [95]. Gomez-Sanchez et al. 2011 reported important antifungal activity of Mexican oregano (*Lippia berlandieri* Schauer) on the growth of *A. flavus after* using gas phase application [96].

Some authors showed that antifungal activity of essential oil is more effective in the vapor state on comparison with the liquid state [97,98]. Therefore, they can be used to develop an alternative desinfection strategie in the food industry. Puškárová et al. 2017 studied the antifungal and antibacterial properties of six essential oil : oregano, lavender, clary sage, clove, thyme and arborvitae against *Penicillium chrysogenum, Chaetomium globosum, Aspergillus fumigates, Alternaria alternate* and *Cladosporium cladosporoides* (fungi), *Escherichia coli, Yersinia enterocolitica, Salmonella typhimurium, Staphylococcus aureus, Enterococcus faecalis and Listeria Monocytogenes* (pathogenic bacteria), *Bacillus cereus, Pseudomonas fragi, Arthrobacter protophormiae* (environmental bacteria). Oregano, clove, thyme and arborvitae exhibited a strong antibacterial activity against all tested bacteria. The antifungal activity of the mentioned oils varied when tested by direct application and in vapor phase. The combined antibacterial and antifungal properties of these oils suggest their use as agent in decontamination on indoor environment [99].

Antifungal activity of OEO is not limited to the inhibition of the growth of spoilage fungi but also affected their production of aflatoxin and ochratoxin. Bluma et al. 2008 reported a reduction effect on the biosynthesis of aflatoxins B1 by *A. flavus, A. parasiticus* and *A. nomius* cultured on SMKY broth, PKB or on wheat grains [100]. Basilico and Basilico 1999 reported also a good inhibition of the synthesis of ochratoxin A in what grains and YES broth [101]. In addition, Marín et al. 2004, Velluti et al. 2003 and 2004, reported an inhibitory effect of oregano essential oil on the production of *Fusarium* toxins (fumonisin B1, deoxynivalenol, and zearalenone) by *F. graminearum, F. verticillioides, F. proliferatum* on the grains of corn and wheat [102-104].

In addition to bacteria and molds, yeasts are also able to cause the spoilage of many foods such as cheese, meat and beverages [105]. In general, yeasts are very important in the food industry in particular in the elaboration of fermented products. In contrast, yeasts are also considered nowadays as classic contaminants of food. Their abilities to grow in low PH levels and low water activity environment, in addition to the presence of some chemical preservatives is causing a huge losses to the food industry [50].

Corner and Beuchat 1984 screened the inhibitory activity of thirty-two plants essential oils on 13 food spoilage yeasts. The most active oils: allspice, clove, cinnamon, onion, oregano, garlic, savory and thyme were then tested for their effects on biomass production and pseudomycelium formation of *Cancida lipolytica, Debaryomyces hansenii, Hansenula anomala, Kloeckera apiculata, Lodderomyces elongisporus, Rhodotorula rubra, Saccharomyces cerevisiae* and *Torulopsis glabrata*. Garlic oil was the most active oil followed by oregano and thyme oils. All tested oils delayed pseudomycelium formation. Among the eight active oils, garlic and onion oils were the most inhibitory to yeast biomass production [106].

Souza et al. 2007 investigated the anti-yeast activity of *O. vulgare*. L essential oil on the survival and the growth inhibition of may yeasts causing food spoilage namely: *Candida albicans* ATCC 7645, *C. tropicalis* MD 37, *C. krusei* ATCC 6258, *P. ohmeri* ATCC 46053, *Pichia minuscula* NI 7638, *Saccharomyces cerevisae* ATCC 2601 and *Rhodotorula rubra* LBFHC 1096. MIC were determined using solid diffusion method and microplate bioassay. MIC values varied from 0,6 μL/mL to 20 μL/ML. *P. minuscule* was the most sensitive yeast. While, *S. cerevisae* and *C. krusei* were the least sensitive yeasts [107].

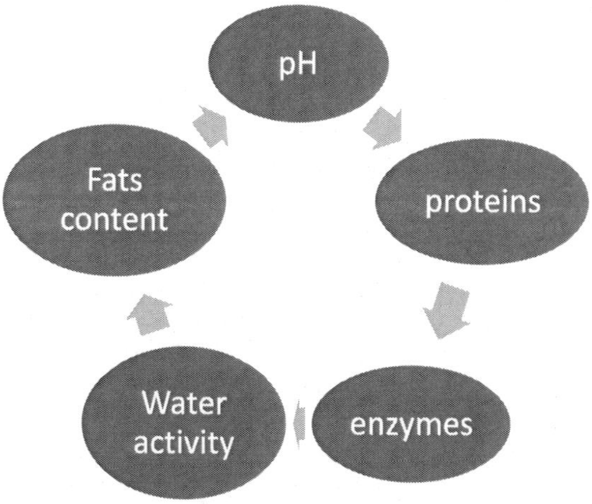

Figure 4. Factors affecting the efficacy of essential oil in food matrices.

Many studies have conclusively established the effectiveness of OEO or its compounds as a potent antimicrobial with a broad spectrum of action including a large number of microorganisms incriminated in food contamination. However, most of these studies are related to *in vitro* tests. In addition, the amounts required to the use of such substances in food system were 1 to 3% higher. In some cases they are much higher with a great disadvantage. The taste and aroma of oregano will be noticeable. Which will undoubtedly modify the final and usual aspect of the food product [49, 108]. In addition, factors present in food matrices represented in Figure 4 such as pH, proteins, enzyme, water activity and fats content can potentially diminish the efficacy of essential oils [49,109, 110].

Antioxidant Activity

Oxidation degradation is a major problem in the storage of fatty foods. Lipid oxidation causes the development of rancidity, decreases the nutritional quality and generates toxic compounds. Fats, oils and related compounds are highly vulnerable to oxidation. Oxidation can involve both enzymatic and non-enzymatic mechanisms [111]. Rancidity of fats and oils caused by oxidation is in most cases due to the penetration of air oxygen in food [112]. Antioxidants are added to food to delay lipid oxidation. The antioxidants used in food industries can be natural or synthetic compounds. It is well accepted and documented that natural antioxidants are safer than synthetic antioxidants [111]. BHA and BHT, two of the most common synthetic antioxidants used showed carcinogenic effects on animals. Hockman et al. 1981 reported lesion formation in rat stomach [111] and Botteweck et al. 2000 reported a carcinogenic effect in rats and mice livers [113]. However, both natural and synthetic antioxidants have some limitations. Natural antioxidants can be affected by processing conditions like boiling, evaporation or sterilization, etc [112]. While, synthetic antioxidants like gallates can't be used in food requiring severe thermal treatment because of their decomposition [111].

In conjunction with the antimicrobial activity of oregano, there are abundant literatures on the antioxidant activity of OEO or oregano components. The available literature on this subject is quite considerable, so that only some representative cases can be mentioned within the scope of the present chapter.

Similar to antimicrobial components identified in OEO and thought to be responsible of the antimicrobial activity of the cited oil, carvacrol and thymol are the main antioxidant compounds pointed to be responsible of the antioxidant activity of OEO. Those compounds act as antioxidant agents by scavenging free radicals, chelating metal or quenching oxygen. As a result lipid oxidation will be retarded [56]. In this context, Quiroga et al. 2011 investigated the antioxidant activity of four Argentinean OEO (*O. vulgare ssp. vulgare, vulgare ssp. virens, O. appli, O. majoricum*) using DPPH method. The highest activity was obtained by the oils that containing the highest amounts of thymol (*O. vulgare ssp. virens* and *ssp. Vulgare*). The authors concluded that the investigated OEO might be used as antioxidants in high content lipids food products [114]. In addition, the occurrence of thymol and carvacrol and others monoterpenes was related to the good radical scavenging activity of 51 Sicilian OEO. IC50 in UV-IP test (UV radiation-induced peroxidation in liposomal membranes) varied from 3.8 to 11.0 μg/mL [115].

Martinez-Tome et al. 2001 evaluated and compared the antioxidant effects of some Mediterranean food spices (annatto, cumin, oregano, sweet and hot paprika, rosemary, and saffron) at 5% with three common food additives: butylated hydroxyanisole (BHA), butylated hydroxytoluene (BHT), and propyl gallate at 100 μg/g. The highest inhibition of lipid peroxidation was observed with rosemary and oregano. All tested spices inhibit lipid peroxidation better than BHT and protect deoxyribose better than BHT and BHA. In addition, the tested spices are able to scavenge HOCl. Oxidative stability of refined olive oil was also evaluated using the Rancimat method during (72 h, 2, 4, and 6 months) at room temperature and compared with BHT, BHA and propyl gallate. The spices extracts demonstrated a significant stabilizing effect [116]. Alinkina et al. 2013 also compared the antioxidant activity of *O. vulgare* and ionol using DPPH assay. The main constituents were carvacrol and thymol. The antiradical effect was slightly smaller than ionol [117]. In another report, Gavaric et al. 2015 compared the antioxidant activity of *O. vulgare L.* to BHT using DPPH and OH radical scavenging assays. IC50 values were 0,2 and 1,12 g/mL respectively. Thymol and carvarcrol were also tested. The antiradical activity seems to be the result of synergetic effects of the main compounds of the essential oil [118].

Differences in antioxidant activity of OEO have been reported with relation to the phonological stages [119], mode of extraction, chemical composition, harvesting time and geographical origin [56, 120]. Asensio et al. 2016 investigated the antioxidant activity of four Argentinean oregano (*O. x majoricum, O. vulgare ssp. vulgare* and *ssp. Hirtum*) using FRAP (ferric reducing power), ABTS (2,2 azinobis (3-ethylbenzothiazoline-6-sulfonic acid)) and ORAC (oxygen radical absorbance capacity) assays. The obtained values were 0.184-0.072, 0.234-0.163 and 1.708-1.024mM Trolox/mg respectively. β-carotene assay was also used [121].

Mechergui et al. 2010 determined the IC50 and total phenolic content of essential oil of *O. vulgare L.* sp. *glandulosum* collected from three different localities (Bargou, Krib and Nefza) situated in the north of Tunisia using DPPH. IC50 varied from 59 to 80 mg/L. While, phenolic content varied from 9.37 to 17.70 mg of gallic acid equivalents/g [122]. In another hand, Mechergui et al. 2016 evaluated the influence of the harvest year, the used part of the plant (leaves and flowers) and the location on the antioxidant activity of essential oil of *O. glandulosum*. All the cited parameters influenced the tested activity. Differences in composition and concentration of carvacrol, thymol, *p*-cymene and γ-tepinene might be responsible of the observed variation in antioxidant activity [120].

Bouyahya et al. 2017 evaluated the chemical composition, antioxidant, antibacterial and antileishmanial activities of *O. compactum* at three phenological stages (vegetative, flowering and post-flowering). The main components of the essential oil were carvacrol, thymol, p-cymene and γ-terpinene in the three phenoligical stages. However, the best antioxidant activity was found at the post-flowering stage. The findings highlighted in this study show that flowering stage is the best optimal harvesting times of *Origanum compactum* for food and pharmaceutical applications [119].

Oregano and its essential oil have been studied as an antioxidant in different kinds of food products. *O. vulgare ssp. Hirtum* (dry leaves) showed a high antioxidant effect in olive oil. In addition, the adjunction of oregano improved the organoleptic quality of olive oil [123]. Ruben et al. 2014 investigated the inhibition of lipid oxidation in sunflower oil by OEO and its fractions separated using short-path molecular distillation. Fractions showed higher antioxidant activity. Chemical analysis of the most active fractions indicated the presence of high content of terpenes with low boiling point and without a functional group. These fractions can be used as natural antioxidants. The used method can be an alternative in the separation of OEO and obtaining fractions with the strongest antioxidant effectiveness [124].

Oregano leaves were used for enrichment of virgin olive oil as natural antioxidant. The enrichment of olive oil was monitored using capillary electrophoresis method. Different mechanical methods were compared including sonication and stirring. Vertical stirring at 1000 r.p.m for 3 hours was the best extraction procedure. Stability and evolution of antioxidants (rosmarinic, *o*-coumaric and vanillic acids) in Virgin olive oil and the enriched oil were tested after 45 days under stress and storage at room temperature. Virgin oil enriched by exogenous antioxidant originated from oregano was found to be more stable [125].

Olmedo et al. 2009 demonstrated that the oxidative stability of fried salted peanuts during storage is enhanced using olive oil and 20 g/kg OEO [126]. The effectiveness of ground oregano and its petroleum ether extracts on the oxidative stability of fried chips was evaluated. Analysis of the rate of peroxide formation during storage at 63°C indicated a significant increase in the oxidative stability [127]. In addition, a combination of oregano extract and olive oil in fresh potatoes with 4412 and 1126 ppm respectively reduced the acrylamide content after heating [128]. Boroski et al. 2011 reported that the addition of oregano in 5-10% combined to carrot leaf in the same proportion to pasta formulations improved the nutritional parameters and increased the antioxidant activity. Omega-3 fatty acid content also increased [129].

Fasseas et al. 2007 assessed the antioxidant activity of 3% (w/w) oregano and 3% (w/w) sage essential oils in raw and cooked bovine and porcine meat samples. The antioxidant activity was determined after 1, 4, 8 and 12 days of storage at 4°C using DDPH, TBA (thiobarbituric acid) and a crocin assays. The used essential oils were much more effective in cooked meat. The oxidation was significantly reduced [130]. Hulankova et al. 2013 reported that the addition of OEO to stored minced beef improved the flavor, odor and color and was almost undetectable after cooking [131].

Jayasena et al. 2014 reported that essential oils from rosemary, oregano, sage, thyme, turmeric and many other essential oils used alone on in combination together or with other method used for preservation might extend the shelf-life of meat and meats products. Sensory quality was also improved. Chouliara et al. 2007 investigated the effect of packaging method and the adjunction of OEO on shelf life and sensory attributes of fresh chicken breast meat stored at 4°C. The addition of OEO at 1% affected the taste of the product. While, the color was not affected [108]. Unattractive odor and unacceptable damage to the appearance of carrot discs, lettuce, cabbage and dry coleslaw were also reported after application of undiluted thyme, oregano, and rosemary essential oils. However, undesirable organoleptic effects can be avoided by diluting essential oils or using a combination of essential oils. A combination of essential oils and plant material such as carrot or cabbage shreds can also be envisaged [132]. Al-Hijazeen et al. 2016 showed that OEO reduced significantly lipid and protein oxidation, and improved color stability of raw and cooked chicken breast meat [133].

Gutierrez et al. 2008 treated lettuce with oregano at 250 ppm. There was no differences between the treated lettuce with oregano and the washed ones with chlorinated water. Moreover, the sensory panel was acceptable [48]. Oregano and rosemary essential oils demonstrated a protective effect against lipid oxidation and fermentation in flavored cheese prepared with a cream cheese base. Fermentation parameters and peroxide and anisidine were used to evaluate the stability of samples during storage. Flavored cheese showed higher stability during storage, lower acidity and higher pH [126].

In more recent investigation, Dutra et al. 2019 reported an efficient control of *Alicyclobacillus spp* using OEO (*Origanum vulgare*). *Alicyclobacillus spp.* is the main cause of deterioration of citrus foods such as fruit juices, teas and tomato extract. Carvacrol acetate was determined in the chemical characterization of the essential oil of oregano as major compound. The good antioxidant activity of the compounds present in the oil is responsible of the control of this bacteria. However, future studies should be performed *in vivo* to verify such actions in food matrices [134].

In previous study, Boroski et al. 2012 reported that oregano (*Origanum minutiflorum*) extracts exhibited a better antioxidant activity than OEO on dairy beverages enriched with 2 g/100 g linseed oil. Both extracts reduced light and heat-induced oxidation of omega-3 fatty acids. The authors suggested the use of the tested extracts as natural antioxidants in dairy beverages enriched with omega-3 fatty acid to inhibit oxidation during storage. However, the impact on sensory properties and consumer acceptance before the use of these ingredients are in need [135].

Numerous studies concerning the antioxidant activity of OEO and oregano components certainly helped to better understand the mechanism involved. It is important to note that the majority of studies conducted to date are related to the antiradical effect. However, oxidation reactions in food systems are more complicated. On one hand, foods are also rich in endogenous antioxidants that also play a role in food protection. On the other hand, the antioxidant effect of OEO and its compounds considered as exogenous antioxidants is also related to the protection of proteins, food membranes, carbohydrates and nucleic acids [56].

Oregano as Feed Additive

Antibiotic-based growth promoters have been used as feed supplements during a long period. In-feed antibiotics have been used in subtherapeutic dosages for growth promotion and prophylaxis against enteric pathogens in large scale livestock production for the last almost 50 years [3]. The actual trends in food and feed additives are the use of natural products [136]. The main reason is the public awareness of the potential risks dealing with the use of such promoters which are suspected to contribute in the increasing resistance of human pathogens [3].

Herbs and spices and aromatic plants are a promising source of natural feed additives. Many herbal products are used as a sensory additives, flavoring and appetizing substances [3]. Moreover, products containing essential oils have been used in animal nutrition. Essential oils and aromatic compounds modulate the bacterial flora [137], increase gastric and intestinal motility, stimulate the secretion of digestive enzymes, increase the absorbance of nutrients and improve intake feed and flavor. They possess also antioxidant, antimicrobial anthelmintic, immunomodulator and coccidiostat activities [136, 137]. Herbs and spices main functions as feed additives are represented in Figure 5.

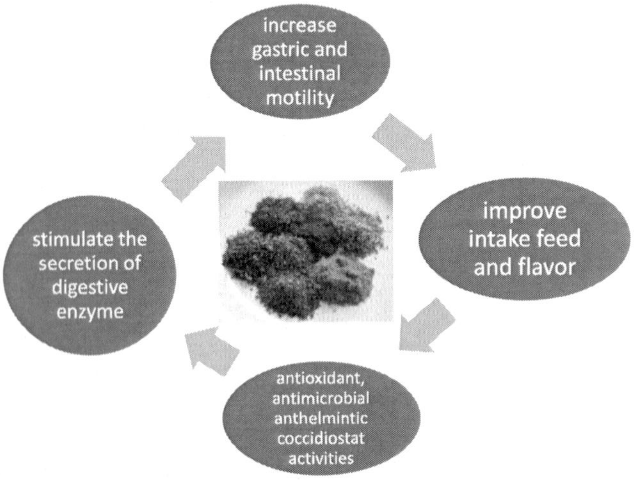

Figure 5. Herbs and spices main functions as feed additives.

Current trends, particularly in relation to food industry, have really pushed the field of research. Naturalness has been the key element. Animal production does not escape this new path. Nowadays, there is an increasing interest in the use of natural growth promoters such as symbiotics, oligosaccharides and phytogentic additives [136].

Many researches were performed on the use of phytogenic additives. However they are reduced to growth-promoting parameters: weight gain, feed intake and feed conversion rate [3].

Oregano can be used as dried plants, essential oil or as source of carvacrol and thymol. In general, the examined parameters were body-weight gain, feed consumption and mortality. In case of layer hens or ruminants eggs and milk production were also examined [136].

Effects in Poultry

In poultry, experiments conducted on the beneficial effects of essential oils showed that the feed conversion rate was improved. In most cases growth was enhanced but no significant change was observed in feed intake [3]. A mixture of essential oils of oregano, anise, sage, laurel and citrus showed a higher feed-to-gain ratio value compared to control group chicken without supplements [138]. Diet supplemented with a mixture of oregano, pepper, cinnamon, cayenne, thyme, and citrus resulted also in higher body-weight gain and higher feed intake [139].

OEO were reported to increase performance [136, 140], daily and final body weight in broilers [141], egg weight and production [142] and nutrient utilization [5].

Oregano at 50–100 mg/kg doses showed an antioxidant effect in chicken tissues [143]. Carvacrol resulted in lowered plasma triglyceride [144]. Feed supplementation with oregano decreased lipid peroxidation as expressed by malondialdehyde values in meat [145]. In contrast, some researches demonstrated that OEO had no effect on animal performance [142, 144, 146].

Plant essential oils are pointed to have a significant impact on intestinal architecture [147]. The suggested mechanism of action is to enhance the intestinal activities of major digestion enzymes [144]. Theron et al. 2007 reported that the supplementation of broiler chickens feed with 125 mg/kg of a mixture of oregano, citrus and anise essential oils improved ileal apparent fat digestibility [148]. Furthermore, Fonseca-García et al. 2017 reported a significant increase in the height of intestinal villi, especially in the duodenum, by using oregano oil in poultry feed [149].

Effects in Pigs

Many investigations on the effect of plant extracts and essential oils on the growth performance and meat quality indicated that they improved both of them. However the used plant seems to be of great importance. In comparison with ginger and oregano, pigs preferably consumed feed supplemented with rosemary and garlic [150].

Jugl-Chizzola et al. 2006 reported a preferably consumption of feed without supplement. Research on the beneficial effects of the inclusion of oregano extracts or OEO in pig diets are contradictory [151]. Bilkei et al. 2001 reported that a combinison of oregano and high levels of vitamin E showed a positive effect on daily weight gain [152]. Kyriakis et al. 1998 reported an improvement of up to 20% on zootechnical parameters in large-scale piggeries feed with 240-500 mg/kg oregano [153]. In contrast, feeding oregano diets to nursery pigs resulted in no improvement in performance [154, 155].

Henn et al. 2010 investigated the effect of dietary supplementation of OEO on the performance and the occurrence of diarrhea in weanling pigs. Antimicrobial and antioxidant ativities were also evaluated *in vitro*. OEO had no effect on the zootechnical performance and didn't prevent diarrhea. Results indicated that OEO exhibited a strong antimicrobial and antioxidant activities [156].

Oregano leave and flowers and OEO were reported to have a positive effect on mortality rate [157], a positive immune stimulation effect [158]. In sows, oregano was reported to increases reproductive performance [158, 159], decrease the mortality rate, increase the farrowing rate, decrease the weaning-to-oestrus interval [70] and reduce the oxidative stress [160].

Effects in Ruminants

In ruminants, researches are focused on the potential use of plant essential oils to improve the rumen microbial activity. Essential oils or their active components were found to potentially improve nitrogen and/or energy utilization. OEO can be used as feed additives in ruminant nutrition to improve performance of dairy or meat animals, increase feed efficiency, and support health [136]. Busquet et al. 2006 tested the effect of oragono, clove bud and cinnamon essential oils in rumen ammonia concentration. Some active components such as carvacrol, carvone, cinnamaldehyde and eugenol were also tested. At 3 g/l the tested oils and active components showed an up to 50% reduction in ammonia concentration [161]. Hristov et al. 2013 reported that oregano leaf induced a decrease in rumen ammonia concentration and methane production. The milk composition was not affected [162]. In contrast, Lejonklev et al. 2016 demonstrated that oregano improved milk flavor but didn't affect methane production [163].

REFERENCES

[1] Spiridon E, Kintzios. (2002). *Oregano: The genera Origanum and Lippia*. CRC Press.

[2] Calpouzos, L. (1954). Botanical aspects of oregano. *Economic Botany*, 8 (3): 222–233. https://link.springer.com/article/10.1007/BF02984891.

[3] Franz, C., Baser, K.H.C., Windisch, W. (2010). Essential oils and aromatic plants in animal feeding-a European perspective. A review. *Flavour and Fragrance Journal,* 25: 327–340. https://doi. org/10.1002/ffj.1967.

[4] Arcila-Lozano, C., Loarca-Piña, G., Lecona-Uribe, S., Gonzáles de Mejía, E. (2004). El orégano: propiedades, composición y actividad biológica de sus componentes. [Oregano:properties, composition and biological activity of its components]. *Archivos latinoamericanos de nutrición,* 54: 100–111. https://www. scienceopen. com /document?vid= af0772eb-2b4f-42e2-bfd3-e6920 35fbe4a.

[5] Vokou, D., Kokkini, S., Bessiere, J.M. (1993). Geographic variation of Greek oregano (*Origanum vulgare* ssp. *hirtum*) essential oils. *Biochemical Systematics and Ecology,* 21 (2): 287–295. doi:10.1016/0305-1978(93)90047-U.

[6] Pascual, M.E., Slowing, K., Carretero, E., Sanchez Mata, D., Villar, A. (2001). Lippia: Traditional uses, chemistry and pharmacology: A review. *Journal of Ethnopharmacology,* 76(3): 201-14. doi:10.1016/S0378-8741(01)00234-3.

[7] Terblanché, F.C., Kornelius, G. (1996). Essential oil constituents of the genus *Lippia* (Verbenaceae)-A literature review. *Journal of Essential Oil Research,* 8 (5): 471–485. doi:10.1080/10412905.1996.9700673.

[8] Elshafie, H.S., Armentano, M.F., Carmosino, M., Bufo, S.A., De Feo, V., Camele, I. (2017). Cytotoxic activity of *Origanum vulgare* L. on hepatocellular carcinoma cell line HepG2 and evaluation of its biological activity. *Molecules,* 22 (9): 1435. doi:10.3390/molecules22091435.

[9] Gutiérrez-Grijalva, E.P., Picos-Salas, M.A., Leyva-López, N., Criollo-Mendoza, M.S., Vazquez-Olivo, G., Heredia, J.B. (2018). Flavonoids and phenolic acids from oregano: occurrence, biological activity and health benefits. *Plants,* 7, 2. https://doi.org/10.3390/plants7010002

[10] Hawas, U.W., El-Desoky, S.K., Kawashty, S.A., Sharaf, M. (2008). Two new flavonoids from *Origanum vulgare*. *Natural Product Research*, 22 (17):1540-1543. doi:10.1080/14786410600898987.

[11] Pezzani, R., Vitalini, S., Iriti, M. (2017). Bioactivities of *Origanum vulgare* L.: An update. *Phytochemistry Reviews,* 16, 1253–1268. doi: 10.1007/s11101-017-9535-z.

[12] Leyva-Lopez, N., Nair, V., Bang, W.Y ., Cisneros-Zevallos. L., Heredia, J.B. (2016). Protective role of terpenes and polyphenols from three species of Oregano (*Lippia graveolens*, *Lippia palmeri* and *Hedeoma patens*) on the suppression of

lipopolysaccharide-induced inflammation in RAW 264.7 macrophage cells. *Journal of Ethnopharmacology,* 187: 302–312. doi:10.1016/j.jep. 2016.04.051.

[13] Cheng, L.C., Murugaiyah, V., Chan, K.L. (2015). Flavonoids and phenylethanoid glycosides from *Lippia nodiflora* as promising antihyperuricemic agents and elucidation of their mechanism of action. *Journal of Ethnopharmacology,* 176: 485–493. doi.org/10.1016/j.jep.2015.11.025.

[14] Dominguez, X.A., Sanchez, H., Suarez, M., Baldas, J.H., Gonzalez, M.R. (1989). Chemical constituents of *Lippia graveolens. Planta Medica,* 55: 208–209.

[15] Long-Ze. L., Mukhopadhyay, S., Robins, J. R., Harnly, M. J. (2007). Identification and quantification of flavonoids of Mexican oregano (*Lippia graveolens*) by LC-DAD-ESI/MS analysis. *Journal of Food. Composition and Analysis,* 20 (5): 361–369. https://doi.org/10. 1016/j.jfca.2006.09.005.

[16] Nakamura, T., Okuyama, E., Tsukada, A., Yamazaki, M., Satake, M., Nishibe, S., Deyama, T., Moriya, A., Maruno, M., Nishimura, H. (1997). Acteoside as the analgesic principle of Cedron (*Lippia triphylla*), a Peruvian medicinal plant. *Chemical and Pharmaceutical Bulletin,* 45(3):499-504. doi:10.1248/cpb.45.499.

[17] Pham, H. C, Koffi, Y., Pham, H.C.A. 1988. Comparative hypotensive effects of compounds extacted from *Lippia multiflora* leaves. *Planta. Medica,* 54 (4): 294–296. doi:10.1055/s-2006-962436.

[18] Skaltsa, H., Shammas, G. (1988). Flavonoids from *Lippia citriodora. Planta Medica,* 54, 465. doi:10.1055/s-2006-962505.

[19] Stashenko, E. E., Martınez, J.R., Cala, M.P., Duran, D.C., Caballero, D. (2013). Chromatographic and mass spectrometric characterization of essential oils and extracts from Lippia (Verbenaceae) aromatic plants. *Journal of Separation Science* 36: 36(1):192-202. doi: 10. 1002 / jssc. 201200877.

[20] Taoubi, K., Fauvel, M.T., Gleye, J., Moulis, C., Fourasté, I. (1997). Phenylpropanoid glycosides from *Lantana camara* and *Lippia multiflora*. Planta Medica, 63 (2): 192–193. doi:10.1055/s-2006-957647.

[21] Macambira, L.M.A, Andrade, C.H.S., Matos, F.J.A., Craveiro, A.A. (1986). Naphthoquinoids from *Lippia sidoides. Journal of Natural Products,* 49 (2): 310–312. doi:10.1021/np50044a019.

[22] Heinrich, M., Rimpler, H., Barrera, N.A. (1992). Indigenous phytotherapy of gastrointestinal disorders in a lowland mixe community (Oaxaca, Mexico): Ethnopharmacologic evaluation. *Journal of Ethnopharmacology,* 36 (1): 63–80. https://doi.org/10.1016/0378-8741(92)90062-V.

[23] Hennebelle, T., Sahpaz, S., Gressier, B., Joseph, H., Bailleul, F. (2008). Antioxidant and neurosedative properties of polyphenols and iridoids from *Lippia alba. Phytotherapy Research,* 22 (2): 256-8. doi: 10.1002/ptr.2266.

[24] Rastelli, L., Caceres, A., Morales, C., De Simone, F., Aquinos, R. (1998). Iridoids from *Lippia Graveolens. Phytochemistry,* 49 (6): 1829-1832. https://doi.org/10.1016/S0031-9422(98)00196-4.

[25] Arika, W.M., Abdirahman, Y.A., Mawia, M.M., Wambua, K.F., Nyamai, D.M., Ogola, P.E., Kiboi, N.G., Nyandoro, H.O., Njagi, S.M., Agyirifo, D.S., Ngugi, M.P., Njagi, E.N.M. (2015). Hypoglycemic Effect of *Lippia javanica* in Alloxan Induced Diabetic Mice. *Journal of Diabetes and Metabolism*, 6: 624. doi:10.4172/2155-6156.1000624.

[26] Forestieri, A.M., Monforte, M.T., Ragusa, S., Trovato, A., Iauk, L. (1996). Antiinflammatory, analgesic and antipyretic activity in rodents of plant extracts used in African medicine. *Phytotherapy Research,* 10 (2): 100–106. https://doi.org/10.1002/(SICI)1099-1573(199603)10:2<100::AID-PTR724>3.0.CO;2-I.

[27] Clark, M. (1997). Wild herbs in the marketplace. In Kardulias P and Shutes M, (eds). *Aegean Strategies: Studies of Culture and Environment on the European Fringe.* Lanham, MD: Rowman and Littlefield Publishers.

[28] Shan, B., Cai, Y.Z., Sun, M., Corke. H. (2005). Antioxidant capacity of 26 spice extracts and characterization of their phenolic constituents. *Journal of Agricultural and Food Chemistry,* 53 (20):7749-7759.doi: 10.1021/jf051513y

[29] Gonceariuc, M., Balmus, Z., Benea, A., Barsan, V., Sandu, T. (2015). Biochemical diversity of the *Origanum vulgare ssp. vulgare* L. and *Origanum vulgare ssp. hirtum* (link) ietswaart genotypes from Moldova. *Buletinul Academiei de Ştiinţe a Moldovei. Ştiinţele vieţii,* 2: 92–100. https://ibn.idsi.md/ro/vizualizare_articol/37588.

[30] Zhang, X.L., Guo, Y.S., Wang, C.H., Li, G.Q., Xu, J.J., Chung, H. Y., Ye, W.C., Li, Y.L., Wang, G.C. (2014). Phenolic compounds from *Origanum vulgare* and their antioxidant and antiviral activities. *Food Chemistry,* 152:300–306. https://doi.org /10 .1016/ j.foodchem.2013.11.153.

[31] Hêro, F.S.A., Rebwar, M.H. S., Pishtiwan, A.H. (2015). *In vitro* screening of antibacterial properties of Rhus coriaria and Origanum vulgare against some pathogenic bacteria. ARO: *The Scientific Journal of Koya University III,* (2): 35-41. doi: 10.14500/aro.10085.

[32] Gîrd, C.E., Dutu, L.E., Costea, T., Nencu, I., Popescu, M.L., Tudorel, O. O. (2016). Preliminary research concerning the obtaining of herbal extracts with potential neuroprotective activity note I. Obtaining and characterization of a selective *Origanum vulgare* L. dry extract. *Farmacia,* 64 (5): 680–687. http://www.revistafarmacia.ro/201605/art-06-Gird_Costea_680- 687.pdf.

[33] Zamora-Martinez, M.C, and Nieto de Pascual. C. (1992). Medicinal plants used in some rural populations of Oaxaca, Puebla and Veracruz, Mexico. *Journal of Ethnopharmacology,* 35 (3): 229–257. doi:10.1016/0378-8741(92)90021-I..

[34] Hutchings, A., Van Staden, J. (1994). Plants used for stress-related ailments in traditional Zulu, Xhosa and Sotho medicine. Part 1: Plants used for headaches. *Journal of Ethnopharmacology*,43 (2):89-124. doi: 10.1016/0378-8741(94)90008-6.

[35] Martinez-Gracia, C., Gonzalez-Bermudez, C.A., Cabellero-Valcarcel, A.M., Santaella Pascual, M., Frontela-Saseta, C. (2015). Use of herbs and spices for food preservation: advantages and limitations. *Current Opinion in Food Science,* 6: 38-43. doi:10.1016/j.cofs.2015.11.011.

[36] Mendonca, A., Jackson-Davis, A., Moutiq, R.., Thomas-Popo, E. Use of Natural Antimicrobials of Plant Origin to Improve the Microbiological Safety of Foods in *Food and Feed Safety Systems and Analysis*. 2018, Pages 249-272. Academc Press. https://doi.org/10.1016/B978-0-12-811835-1.00014-2.

[37] Ayala-Zavala, J.F., González-Aguilar, G.A., Del-Toro-Sánchez, L. (2009). Enhancing safety and aroma appealing of fresh-cut fruits and vegetables using the antimicrobial and aromatic power of essential oils. *Journal of Food Science,* 74: R84-R91. doi:org/10.1111/j.1750-3841. 2009. 01294.x.

[38] Wojdyło, A., Oszmianski, J., Czemerys, R. (2007). Antioxidant activity and phenolic compounds in 32 selected herbs. *Food Chemistry* 105 (3): 940–949. https://doi.org/ 10.1016 /j. foodchem .2007 . 04.038.

[39] Yashin, A., Yashin, Y., Xia, X., Nemzer, B. (2017). Antioxidant Activity of Spices and Their Impact on Human Health: A Review. *Antioxidants,* 6 (3), 70. doi:10.3390/antiox6030070.

[40] Zheng, W., Wang Shiow Y. (2001). Antioxidant activity and phenolic compounds in selected herbs. *Journal of Agricultural and Food. Chemistry* 94 (11): 5165-5170. doi:10.1021/jf010697n.

[41] Albayrak, S., Aksoy, A., Sagdic, O., Albayrak, S. (2012). Antioxidant and antimicrobial activities of different extracts of some medicinal herbs consumed as tea and spices in Turkey. *Journal of Food Chemistry*, 36 (5): 547- 554. doi: 10.1111/j.1745-4514.2011.00568.x.

[42] Burt, S.A., Reinders, R.D. (2003). Antibacterial activity of selected plant essential oils against *Escherichia coli* O157:H7. *Letters in Applied Microbiology,* 36 (3):162–167. https://www.ncbi.nlm.nih.gov/pubmed/12581376.

[43] De Martino, L., de Feo, V., Nazzaro, F. (2009). Chemical composition and *in vitro* antimicrobial and mutagenic activities of seven lamiaceae essential oils. *Molecules, 14 (10)*: 4213–4230. doi:10.3390/molecules14104213.

[44] Nazzaro, F., Fratianni, F., De Martino, L ., Coppola, R. ., De Feo, V. (2013). Effect of Essential Oils on Pathogenic Bacteria. *Pharmaceuticals,* 6(12): 1451–1474. doi:10.3390/ph6121451.

[45] Embuscado Milda, E. (2015). Spices and herbs: Natural sources of antioxidants – a mini review. *Journal of Functional food,* 18: 811–819. https://doi.org/10.1016/j.jff.2015.03.005.

[46] Decker, E., Elias, R., McClements Julian, D. (2010). *Oxidation in foods and beverages and antioxidant applications.* Oxford: Woodhead Publishing.

[47] Riuz-Navajas, Y., Viuda-Martos, M., Sendra, E., Perez-Alvarez, J.A., Fernandez-Lopez, J. (2013). *In Vitro* Antioxidant and Antifungal Properties of Essential Oils Obtained from Aromatic Herbs Endemic to the Southeast of Spain. *Journal of Food Protection,* 76 (7): 1218–1225. doi:10.4315/0362-028X.JFP-12-554.

[48] Gutierrez, J., Rodriguez, G., Barry-Ryan, C., Bourke, P. (2008). Efficacy of plant essential oils against food-borne pathogens and spoilage bacteria associated with ready to eat vegetables: antimicrobial and sensory screening. *Journal of Food. Protection,* 71 (9): 1846–1854. https://jfoodprotection.org/doi/pdfplus/10.4315/0362-028X-71.9.1846.

[49] Tajkarimi, M.M., Ibrahim, S.A., Cliver, D.O. (2010). Antimicrobial herb and spice compounds in food. *Food Control*, 21 (9): 1199–1218. doi:10.1016/j.foodcont.2010.02.003.

[50] Graham Fleet, H. (2011). Chapter 5. Yeast Spoilage of Foods and Beverages. In: *The Yeasts*, 53-63. Elsevier. doi: 10.1016/B978-0-444-52149-1.00005-7.

[51] Raybaudi-Massilia, R.M., Mosqueda-Melgar, J., Martin-Belloso, O. (2008). Edible alginate-based coating as carrier of antimicrobials to improve shelf-life and safety of fresh-cut melon. *International Journal of Food Microbiology,* 121(3): 313–327. doi:10.1016/j. ijfoodmicro . 2007.11.010.

[52] Suet-Yen, S., Tin Sin, L., Tiam-Ting, T., Soo-Tueen, B., Rahmat, A.R., Rahman, W.A.W.A, Ann-Chen, T., Vikhraman, M. (2013). Antimicrobial agents for food packaging applications. *Trends in Food Science and Technology*,33 (2): 110–123. https://doi.org/10.101 6/j. tifs. 2013.08.001.

[53] Teixeira, B., Marques, A., Pires, C., Ramos, Cr., Batista, I., Saraiva Jorge, A., Nunes Maria, L., (2014). Characterization of fish protein films incorporated with essential oils of clove, garlic and origanum: physical, antioxidant and antibacterial properties. *LWT—Food Science and Technology,* 59: 533–539. doi:10.1016/j.lwt.2014.04.024

[54] Zivanovic, S., Chi, S., Druaughon Ann. F. (2005). Antimicrobial activity of chitosan films enriched with essential oils. *Journal of Food Science*, 70 (1): M45–M51. doi:10.1111/j.1365-2621.2005.tb09045.x.

[55] Leyva-López, N., Gutiérrez-Grijalva, E.P., Vazquez-Olivo, G., Basilio Heredia, J. (2017). Essential Oils of Oregano: Biological Activity beyond Their Antimicrobial Properties. *Molecules,* 22: 989. doi:10.3390/molecules22060989.

[56] Rodriguez-Garcia, I., Silva-Espinoza, B.A., Ortega-Ramirez, L.A., Leyva, J.M., Siddiqui, M.W., Cruz-Valenzuela, M.R., Gonzalez-Aguilar, G.A., Ayala-Zavala, J.F. (2015). Oregano essential oil as an antimicrobial and antioxidant additive in

food products. *Critical Reviews in Food Science and Nutrition,* 56: 1717–1727. doi: 10.1080/10408398.2013.800832.

[57] Cetin, B., Cakmakci, S., Cakmakci, R. (2011). The investigation of antimicrobial activity of thyme and oregano essential oils. *Turkish Journal of Agriculture and Foresty,* 35:145–154. doi:10.3906/tar-0906-162

[58] Ben Arfa, A., Combes, S., Preziosi-Belloy, L., Gontard, N., Chalier, P. (2006). Antimicrobial activity of carvacrol related to its chemical structure. *Letters in Applied Microbiology,* 43:149–154. doi: 10.1111/j.1472-765X.2006.01938.x.

[59] Dorman HJD, and Deans SG. (2000). Antimicrobial agents from plants: Antibacterial activity of plant volatile oils. *Journal of Applied Microbiology 88*: 308–316. https://doi.org/10.1046/j.1365-2672.2000.00969.x.

[60] Ultee, A., Bennik,M.H., Moezelaar, R. (2002). The phenolic hydroxyl group of carvacrol is essential for action against the food-borne pathogen *Bacillus cereus. Applied and Environmental Microbiology*, 68 (4):1561–1568. doi: 10.1128/AEM. 68.4.1561-1568.2002.

[61] Zengin H, and Baysal AH. (2014). Antibacterial and Antioxidant Activity of Essential Oil Terpenes against Pathogenic and Spoilage-Forming Bacteria and Cell Structure-Activity Relationships Evaluated by SEM Microscopy. *Molecules, 19*: 17773-17798, doi:10.3390/molecules191117773.

[62] Di Pasqua, R., Betts, G., Hoskins, N., Edwards, M., Ercolini, D., Mauriello, G. (2007). Membrane toxicity of antimicrobial compounds from essential oils. *Journal of Agricultural and Food Chemistry,* 55: 4863–4870. doi:10.1021/ jf 0636465.

[63] Di Pasqua, R., Hoskins, N., Betts, G., Mauriello, G. (2006). Changes in membrane fatty acids composition of microbial cells induced by addiction of thymol, carvacrol, limonene, cinnamaldehyde, and eugenol in the growing media. *Journal of Agricultural and Food Chemistry,* 54: 2745–2749. doi:10.1021/jf052722l.

[64] Guarda, A., Rubilar, J.F., Miltz, J., Galotto, M.J. (2011). The antimicrobial activity of microencapsulated thymol and carvacrol. *International Journal of Food Microbiolog,.* 146(2):144-50. doi:10.1016/j.ijfoodmicro.2011.02.011.

[65] Anamaria Semeniuc, C., Rodica Pop, C., Mihaela Rotar, A. (2017). Antibacterial activity and interactions of plant essential oil combinations against Gram-positive and Gram-negative bacteria. *Journal of Food and Drug Analysis* 25 (2): 403-408. doi: Org/10.1016/j.jfda.2016.06.002Guarda

[66] Azhdarzadeh, F, and Hojjati, M. (2016). Chemical composition and antimicrobial activity of leaf, ripe and unripe peel of bitter orange (*Citrus aurantium*) essential oils. *Nutrition and Food Science Research,* 3: 43–50. http://nfsr.sbmu.ac.ir/article-1-118-en.html.

[67] Trombetta, D., Castelli, F., Sarpietro, M.G., Venuti, V., Cristani, M., Daniele, C., Saija A., Mazzanti, G., Bisignano, G. (2005). Mechanisms of antibacterial action of

three monoterpenes. *Antimicrobial Agents Chemotherapy,* 49 (6): 2474–2478. doi:10.1128/AAC.49.6.2474-2478.2005.

[68] Delamare, A.P.L., Moschen-Pistorello, I.T., Artico, L., Atti-Serafini, L., Echeverrigaray, S. (2007). Antibacterial activity of the essential oils of *Salvia officinalis* L. and *Salvia triloba* L. cultivated in South Brazil. *Food Chemistry* 100 (2): 603–8. https://doi.org/10.1016/j.f oodchem.2005.09.078.

[69] Chouhan, S., Sharma, K., Sanjay Guleria, S. (2017). Antimicrobial Activity of Some Essential Oils—Present Status and Future Perspectives. *Medicines,* 4, 58, doi: 10.3390/ medicines 4030058.

[70] Kovac, B, and Bilkei, G. (2003). Oregano (*Origanum vulgare*) dietary supplementation increases the reproductive performance of sows. *Folia Veterinaria,* 47: 207–209. https://eurekamag.com/research/004/258/004258119.php.

[71] La Storia, A., Ercolini, D., Marinello, F., Di Pasqua, R., Villani, F., Mauriello, G. (2011). Atomic force microscopy analysis shows surface structure changes in carvacrol-treated bacterial cells. *Research in Microbiology,* 162 (2): 164–172. doi:10.1016/j.resmic.2010.11.006.

[72] Juven, B.J., Kanner, J., Schved, F., Weisslowicz, H. (1994). Factors that interact with the antibacterial action of thyme essential oil and its active constituents. *Journal of Applied Bacteriology,*76: 626–631. https://doi.org/10.1111/j.1365-2672.1994.Tb 01661.x.

[73] Sikkema, J., de Bont, J.A.M., Poolman, B. (1995). Mechanisms of membrane toxicity of Hydrocarbons. *Microbiology Reviews,* 59: 201–222. https://www.ncbi. nlm.nih.gov/pmc/articles/ PMC239360/pdf/590201.pdf.

[74] Lambert, R.J.W., Skandamis, P.N., Coote, P.J., Nychas, G.J.E. 2001. A study of the minimum inhibitory concentration and mode of action of oregano essential oil, thymol and carvacrol. *Journal of Applied Microbiology,* 91: 453–462. https://doi.org/10.1046/j.1365-2672. 2001. 01428.x.

[75] Xu, J., Zhou, F., Ji, B.P., Pei, R.S., Xu, N. (2008). The antibacterial mechanism of carvacrol and thymol against *Escherichia coli. Letters in Applied Microbiology,* 47(3):174-9. doi: 10.1111/j.1472-765X.2008.02407.x.

[76] Cattelan, M.C., Machado de Castilhos, M.B., Pinsetta Sales, P.J., Hoffmann, F.L. (2013). Antibacterial activity of oregano essential oil against foodborne pathogens. *Nutrition & Food Science,* 43 (2): 169-174. doi.org/10.1108/00346651311313544.

[77] Boskovic, M., Zdravkovic, N., Ivanovic, J., Janjic, J., Djordjevic, J., Starcevic, M., Baltic, M.Z. (2015). Antimicrobial activity of Thyme (*Tymus vulgaris*) and Oregano (*Origanum vulgare*) essential oils against some food-borne microorganisms. *Procedia Food Science,* 5: 18 – 21. doi.org/10.1016/j.profoo.2015.09.005.

[78] Teixeira, B., Marques, A., Ramos, C., Serrano, C., Matos, O., Neng, N.R., Nogueira, J.M.F., Alexandre Saraiva, J., Nunes, M.L. (2013). Chemical composition and bioactivity of different oregano (*Origanum vulgare*) extracts and essential oil.

Journal of the Science of Food and Agriculture, 93(11): 2707-2714. doi: 10.1002/jsfa.6089.

[79] Prakash, B., Kedia, A., Mishra Prashunt, K., Dubey, N.K. (2015). Plant essential oils as food preservatives to control moulds, mycotoxin contamination and oxidative deterioration of agri-food commodities-Potentials and challenges. *Food. Control,* 47: 381-391. https://doi.org/ 10. 1016/ j.foodcont.2014.07.023

[80] Prakash, B., Mishra Prashant, K., Kedia, A., Dwivedy Abhishek, K., Dubey, N.K. (2015). Efficacy of some essential oil components as food preservatives against food contamination molds, aflotoxin B1 production and free radical generation. *Journal of Food Quality,* 38: 231–239. https://doi.org/10.1111/jfq.12145.

[81] Biondi, D, Cianci, P., Geraci, C., Ruberto, G., Piattelli, M. (1993). Antimicrobial activity and chemical composition of essential oils from Sicilian aromatic plants. *Flavour and Fragrance Journal,* 8 (6): 331–337. doi. org/10.1002/ffj.2730080608.

[82] Kocić-Tanackov, S.D, and Dimić, G.R. (2013). Antifungal activity of essential oils in the control of food-borne fungi growth and mycotoxin biosynthesis in food. *Microbial pathogens and strategies for combating them: science, technology and education* (A. MéndezVilas, Ed.) 838-849. http://formatex.info/microbiology4/ vol2/ 838-849.pdf.

[83] Viuda-Martos, M., Ruiz-Navajas, Y., Fernández-López, J., Pérez-Álvarez, J. (2008). Antifungal activity of lemon (*Citrus lemon* L.), mandarin (*Citrus reticulata* L.), grapefruit (*Citrus paradisi* L.) and orange (*Citrus sinensis* L.) essential oils. *Food Control,* 19 (12): 1130-1138. doi:10.1016/j.foodcont.2007.12.003.

[84] Cristani, M., d'Arrigo, M., Mandalari, G., Castelli, F., Sarpietro, M.G., Micieli, D., Venuti, V., Bisignano, G., Saija, A., Trombetta, D. (2007). Interaction of four monoterpenes contained in essential oils with model membranes: Implications for their antibacterial activity. *Journal of Agricultural and Food Chemistry,* 55 (15): 6300-6308. doi:10.1021/jf070094x.

[85] Daferera, D., Ziogas, B., Polissiou, G. (2000). GC-MS analysis of essential oils from some Greek aromatic plants and their fungitoxicity on *Penicillium digitatum. Journal of Agricultural and Food Chemistry,*48:2576–2581. https://www.ncbi.nlm. nih.gov / pubmed/10888587.

[86] Lucini Enric, I., Zunino Maria, P., Lopez, M.L., Zygadlo Julio, A. (2006). Effect of monoterpenes on lipid composition and sclerotial development of *Sclerotium cepivorum* Berk. *Journal of Phytopathology,* 154 (7-8): 441–446. doi: 10.1111/ j.1439-0434.2006.01126.x.

[87] Chavan Pradnya, S, and Tupe Santosh, G. (2014). Antifungal activity and mechanism of action of carvacrol and thymol against vineyard and wine spoilage yeasts. *Food Control,* 46: 115–120. doi.org/10.1016/j.foodcont.2014.05.007

[88] Lima Igra, O., De Oliveira Pereira, F., De Oliveira Wylly, A., De Oliveira Lima, E., Menezes Everardo, A., Cunha Francisco, A., de Fátima Margareth, F.M.D. (2013).

Antifungal activity and mode of action of carvacrol against Candida albicans strains. *Journal of Essential Oil Research*, 25 (2): 138–142. https://doi.org/10.1080/10412905.2012.754728.

[89] Nobrega Raffael,. D.O., Teixeira Anna Paola, D.C, De Oliveira Wylly, A., Lima Edeltrudes, O., Lima Igara, O. (2016). Investigation of the antifungal activity of carvacrol against strains of Cryptococcus neoformans. *Pharmaceutical Biology,* 54 (11): 2591 -2596. https://doi.org/ 10.3109/ 1388 0209.2016.1172319.

[90] Schmitz, S., Weidenbörner, M., Kunz, B. (1993). Herbs and spices as selective inhibitors of mould growth. *Chemie Mikrobiologie Technologie der Lebensmtell,* 15 (5/6): 175–7.

[91] Boudine, L., Louaste, B., Eloutassi, N., Chami, N., Chami, F., Remmal, A. (2016). Antifungal activity of oregano essential oil and thymol against some fungi isolated from corn grains. *International Journal of Innovation and Applied Studies,* 17 (4): 1120-1124. http://www.ijias.issr-journals.org/abstract.php?article=IJIAS-16-121-02.

[92] Mitchell, T.C., Stamford, T.L.M., Souza, E.L., Lima, E.O., Carmo, E.S. (2010). "Origanum vulgare L. essential oil as inhibitor of potentially toxigenic Aspergilli," *Ciência e Tecnologia de Alimentons,* 30 (3): 755-760. http://dx.doi.org/10.1590/S0101 - 20612010000300029.

[93] Santos Carmo, E., de Oliveira Lima, E., Leite de Souz,. E. (2008). The potential of *Origanum vlgare* L. (Lamiaceae) essential oil in inhibiting the growth of some food-related *Aspergillus* species. *Brazilian Journal of Microbiology,* 39 (2):362-367. doi:10.1590/S1517-83822008000200030.

[94] Portillo-Ruiz, M.C., Avila-Sosa Sanchez, R., Viramontes Ramos, S., Vinicio Torres Munoz, J., Nevarez-Moorillon Guadolipe, V. (2012). Antifungal Effect of Mexican Oregano (*Lippia berlandieri* Schauer) Essential Oil on a Wheat Flour-Based Medium. *Journal of Food Science,* 77 (8): M441- M445. doi: 10.1111/j.1750-3841.2012.02821.x.

[95] Lopez, P., Sanchez, C., Batlle, R, Nerın. C. (2007). Vapor-phase activities of cinnamon, thyme and oregano essential oils and key constituents against foodborne microorganisms. *Journal of Agricultural and Food Chemistry*,55: 4348–4356. doi:10.1021/jf063295u.

[96] Gomez-Sanchez, A., Enrique Palou, A., Lopez-Malo, A. (2011). Antifungal Activity Evaluation of Mexican Oregano (*Lippia berlandieri* Schauer) Essential Oil on the Growth of *Aspergillus flavus* by Gaseous Contact. *Journal of Food Protection,* 74 (12): 2192-8. doi:10.4315/0362-028X.JFP-11-308.

[97] Tyagi A. K, and Malik, A. (2011). Antimicrobial potential and chemical composition of Eucalyptus globulus oil in liquid and vapour phase against food spoilage microorganisms. *Food Chemistry*, 126: 228–235. https://doi.org/10.1016/j.food chem.2010.11.002.

[98] Tyagi, A. K, and Malik, A. (2010). Liquid and vapour-phase antifungal activities of selected essential oils against *Candida albicans*: microscopic observations and chemical characterization of *Cymbopogon citratus*. *BMC Complementary and Alternative Medecine,* 10: 1–11. doi:10.1186/1472-6882-10-65.

[99] Puškárová, A., Bučková, M., Kraková, L., Pangallo, D., Kozics, K.. (2017). The antibacterial and antifungal activity of six essential oils and their cyto/genotoxicity to human HEL 12469 cells. Scientific Report,7: 8211. doi:10.1038/s41598-017-08673-9.

[100] Bluma, R., Amaiden, M.R.: Daghero, J., Etcheverry, M. (2008). Control of *Aspergillus* section Flavi growth and aflatoxin accumulation by plant essential oils. *Journal of Applied Microbiology,* 105:203-214. doi: 10.1111/j.1365-2672.2008.03741.x.

[101] Basilico, M.Z, and Basilico, J.C. (1999). Inhibitory effects of some spice essential oils on *Aspergillus ochraceus* NRRL 3174 growth and ochratoxin A production. *Letter of Applied Microbiology,* 23: 238-241. https://www.ncbi.nlm.nih.gov/pubmed/10583751.

[102] Marín, S., Velluti, A., Ramos, A., Sanchis, V. (2004). Effect of essential oils on zearalenone and deoxynivalenol production by *Fusarium graminearum* in non-sterilized maize grain. *Food Microbioogy*,21 (3): 313-318. doi:10.1016/j.fm.2003.08.002.

[103] Velluti, A., Sanchis, V., Ramos, A.J., Egido, J., Marín, S. (2003). Inhibitory effect of cinnamon, lemongrass, oregano and palmarose essential oils on growth and fumonisin B1 production by *Fusarium proliferatum* in maize grain. *International Journal of Food Microbiology*, 89 (2-3):145-154. doi:10.1016/S0168-1605(03)00116-8.

[104] Velluti, A., Sanchis, V., Ramos, A.J., Turon, C., Marín, S.(2004). Impact of essential oils on growth rate, zearalenone and deoxynivalenol production by *Fusarium graminearum* under different temperature and water activity conditions in maize grain. *Journal of Applied Microbiology,* 96 (4):716-724. doi:10.1111/j.1365-2672.2004.02212.x.

[105] Ray, B, and Bhunia, A. (1996). *Fundamental food microbiology*. Boca Raton: CRC Press.

[106] Conner, D.E, and Beuchat, L.R. (1984). Effect of essential oils from plants on growth of food spoilage yeasts. *Journal of Food Science,* 49:429-434. https://doi.org/10.1111 /j. 1365-2621. 1984. tb12437.x.

[107] Souza, E.L., Stamford, T.L.M., Lim, E.O., Trajano, V.N. (2007). Effectiveness of *Origanum vulgare* L. essential oil to inhibit the growth of food spoiling yeasts. *Food Control,* 18 (5):409-413. https://doi.org/10.1016/j.foodcont. 2005. 11.008.

[108] Chouliara, E., Karatapanis, A., Savvaidis, I.N., Kontominas, M.G. (2007). Combined effect of oregano essential oil and modified atmosphere packaging on

shelf-life extension of fresh chicken breast meat, stored at 4 °C. *Food Microbiology,* 24 (6): 607–617. doi:10.1016/j.fm.2006.12.005.

[109] Firouzi, R., Shekarforoush, S.S., Nazer, A.H., Borumand, Z., Jooyandeh, A.R. (2007). Effects of essential oils of oregano and nutmeg on growth and survival of Yersinia enterocolitica and Listeria monocytogenes in barbecued chicken. *Journal of Food Protection,* 70 (11): 2626-30. doi:10.4315/ 0362-028X-70.11.2626.

[110] Friedly, E.C., Crandall, P.G., Ricke, S.C., Roman, M., O'Bryan, C., Chalova, V.I. (2009). *In vitro* antilisterial effects of citrus oil fractions in combination with organic acids. *Journal of Food. Science,* 74 (2): M 67–72. doi:10.1111/j.1750-3841.2009.01056.x.

[111] Thorat, Indrajt, D., Jagtap Dipali.,D., Mohapatra, D., Joshi, D.C., Sutar, R.F., Kapdi, S.S. (2013). Antioxidants, their properties, uses in food products and their legal implications. *International Journal of Food Studies,* 2: 81-104. https://www.iseki-food-ejournal.com/ojs/index.php/e-journal/article/view/134/84.

[112] Pokorny, J. (2008). Antioxidants in food preservation. In Rahman (eds.). *Handbook of Food Preservation* (2nd ed). p 259-286.U.S.A. CRC Press.

[113] Botterweck, A., Verhagen, H., Goldbohm, R., Kleinjans, J, Van den Brandt, P. (2000). Intake of butylated hydroxyanisole and butylated hydroxytoluene and stomach cancer risk: Results from analyses in the Netherlands cohort study. *Food and Chemical Toxicology,* 38 (7): 599-605. https://www.ncbi.nlm.nih.gov/pubmed/10942321.

[114] Quiroga, P.R., Riveros, C., Zygadlo, J. A., Grosso, N. R., Nepote, V. (2011). Antioxidant activity of essential oil of oregano species from Argentina in relation to their chemical composition. *International Journal of Food Science and Technology*, 46 (12): 2648–2655. doi:10.1111/j.1365-2621.2011.02796.x.

[115] Tuttolomondo, T., La Bella, S., Licata, M., Virga, G., Leto, C., Saija, A., Trombetta, D., Tomaino, A., Speciale, A., Napoli, E.M., Siracusu, L., Pasquate, A., Ruberto, G., Curcutito, G., Robero, G. (2013). Biomolecular characterization of wild sicilian oregano: Phytochemical screening of essential oils and extracts, and evaluation of their antioxidant activities. *Chemistry and Biodiversity,* 10(3): 411–433. doi:10.1002/cbdv.201200219.

[116] Martinez-Tome, M., Jimenez, A.M., Ruggieri, S., Frega, N., Strabbioli, R., Murcia, M.A. (2001). Antioxidant Properties of Mediterranean Spices Compared with Common Food Additives. *Journal of Food Protection,* 64 (9): 1412–1419. https://jfood protection.org/doi/ pdf/10. 4315/0362 -028X-64.9.1412.

[117] Alinkina, E.S., Misharina, T.A., Fatkullina, L.D. (2013). Antiradical properties of oregano, thyme, and savory essential oils. *Applied Biochemistry and Microbiology,* 49: 73–78. https://link.springer. com/article/10.1134/S000368381301002X.

[118] Gavaric, N., Mozina Sonja, S., Kladar Nebojsa, V., Bozin, B. (2015). Chemical profile, antioxidant and antibacterial activity of thyme and oregano essential oils,

thymol and carvacrol and their possible synergism. *Journal of Essential Oil-Bearing Plants,* 18 (4): 1013–1021. doi:10.1080/0972060X.2014.971069.

[119] Bouyahya, A., Dakka, N., Talbaoui, A, Et-Touys, A., El-Boury, H., Abrini, J., Bakri, Y. (2017). Correlation between phenological changes, chemical composition and biological activities of the essential oil from Moroccan endemic Oregano (*Origanum compactum* Benth). *Industrial Crops and Products,* 108: 729–737. doi:org/10.1016/ j.indcrop.2017.07.033.

[120] Mechergui, K., Jaouadi, W., Coelho, J.P., Khouja, M.L. (2016). Effect of harvest year on production, chemical composition and antioxidant activities of essential oil of oregano (*Origanum vulgare* subsp *glandulosum* (desf.) ietswaart) growing in North Africa. *Industrial Crops and Products* 90: 32–37. https://doi.org/10.1016/ j.indcrop.2016. 06.011.

[121] Asensio Clausia, M., Grosso Neslson, R., Juliani Rodolfo, H. (2015). Quality characters, chemical composition and biological activities of oregano (*Origanum spp.*) essential oils from central and southern Argentina. *Industrial Crops and Products,* 63, 203–213. doi:org/10.1016/j. indcrop.2014.09.056.

[122] Mechergui, K., Coelho, J.A., Serra, M.C., Lamine, S.B., Boukhchina, S., Khouja, M.L. (2010). Essential oils of *Origanum vulgare* L. sp. *glandulosum* (Desf.) Ietswaart from Tunisia: Chemical composition and antioxidant activity. *Journal of the Science of Food and Agriculture,* 90: 1745-1749. doi: 0.1002/jsfa.4011.

[123] Charai, M., Faid, M.., Chaouch, A. (1999). Essential oils from aromatic plants (*Thymus broussonetti* Boiss, *Origanum compactum* Benth, and *Citrus limon* (L) NL Burm) as natural antioxidants for olive oil. *Journal of Essential Oil Research,* 11 (4): 517–21. doi.org/10.1080 /10412905. 1999. 9701199.

[124] Ruben, O., Valeria, N., Ruben Grosso, N. (2014). Antioxidant activity of fractions from oregano essential oils obtained by molecular distillation. *Food Chemistry* 156: 212–219. https://doi.org/ 10. 1016 /j.foodchem.2014.01.087.

[125] Peñalvo, G.C., Robledo, V.R., Sánchez-Carnerero, C.C., Santander-Ortega, M.J., Castro-Vázquez, L., Victoria Lozano, M., Arroyo-Jiméne, M.M. (2016). Improving green enrichment of virgin olive oil by oregano. *Effects on Antioxidants. Food Chemistry,* 197: 509-515. doi:10.1016/j.foodchem.2015.11.002.

[126] Olmedo, R.H., Nepote, V., Grosso, N.R. (2013). Preservation of sensory and chemical properties in flavored cheese prepared with a cream cheese base using oregano and rosemary essential oils. *LWT–Food Science and Technology,* 53(2): 409–417. doi: 10.1016/j.lwt.2013.04.007.

[127] Lolos, M., Oreopoulou, V., Tzia, C. (1999). Oxidative stability of potato chips: effect of frying oil type, temperature and antioxidants. *Journal of Food Agriculture* 79 (11): 1524–8. doi:10.1002/(SICI)1097-0010(199908)79:11<1524::AID-JSFA401> 3.0.CO; 2-H.

[128] Kotsiou, K., Tasioula Margari, M., Kukurová, K., Ciesarová, Z. (2010). Impact of oregano and virgin olive oil phenolic compounds on acrylamide content in a model system and fresh potatoes. *Food Chemistry,* 123 (4): 1149–1155.https://doi.org /10.1016 /j. foodchem.2010.05.078

[129] Boroski, M., Giroux, H.J., Sabik, H., Petit, H.V., Jesui, V, Visentainer Matumoto-Pintro, P.T., Britten, M. (2019). Use of oregano extract and oregano essential oil as antioxidants in functional dairy beverage formulations. *LWT–Food Science and Technology,* 47:167-174. doi.org/ 10.1016/j.lwt.2011.12.018.

[130] Fasseas, M.K., Mountzouris, K.C., Tarantilis, P.A., Polissiou, M., Zervas, G. (2007). Antioxidant activity in meat treated with oregano and sage essential oils. *Food Chemistry,* 106 (3): 1188–1194. https://doi.org/10.1016/j.foodchem.2007.07.060.

[131] Hulankova, R., Borilova, G., Steinhauserova, I. (2013). Combined antimicrobial effect of oregano essential oil and caprylic acid in minced beef. *Meat Science,* 95 (2): 190–194. https:// doi. org/ 10. 1016 /j.meatsci.2013.05.003.

[132] Scollard, J., Francis Gillian. A., O'Beirne, D. (2013). Some conventional and latent anti-listerial effects of essential oils, herbs, carrot and cabbage in fresh-cut vegetable systems. *Postharvest Biology and Technology* 77: 87–93. https://doi.org/ 10.1016/ j.postharvbio. 2012.11.011.

[133] Al-Hijazeen, M., Lee, E.J., Mendonca, A., Ahn, D.U. (2016). Effect of oregano essential oil (*Origanum vulgare* subsp. hirtum) on the storage stability and quality parameters of ground chicken breast meat, *Antioxidants* (Basel) 5 (2) pii: E18. doi: 10.3390/antiox 5020018.

[134] Dutra, V.T., Castro, J.C., Menezes, J.L., Ramos, T.R., Nunes do Prado, I., Machinski, J.M., Graton Mikcha, J.M.., Alves de Abreu Filho., B. (2019). Bioactivity of oregano (*Origanum vulgare*) essential oil against Alicyclobacillus spp. *Industrial Crops and Products* 129: 345–349. https://doi.org/10.1016/ j.indcrop.2018. 12.025.

[135] Boroski, M., De Aguiar A.C., Boeing, J.S., Rotta, E.M., Wibby, C.L., Bonafe, E.G., De Souza, N.E., Visentainer, J.V. (2011). Enhancement of pasta antioxidant activity with oregano and carrot leaf. *Food Chemistry,* 125 (2): 696-700. doi.org/ 10.1016/j.foodchem.2010.09.068.

[136] Giannenas, I., Florou-Paneri, P., Botsoglou, N., Christaki, E., Spais, A.B. (2005). Effect of supplementing feed with oregano and/or α-tocopheryl acetate on growth of broiler chickens and oxidative stability of meat. *Journal of Animal and Feed Science,s* 14 (3): 521–535. doi:10.22358/jafs/67120/2005

[137] Kamel, C. (2000). A novel look at a classic approach of plant extracts. *Feed Mix,* 9 (6): 19-24.

[138] Cabuk, M., Bozkurt, M., Alcicek, A., Akbap, Y., Küçükyıllmaz, K. 2006. Effect of a herbal essential oil mixture on growth and internal organ weight of broilers from

young and old breeder flocks. *South African Journal of Animal Science,* 36 (2): 135–141. http://dx.doi.org/ 10.4314/ sajas.v36i2.3996.

[139] Lippens, M., Huyghebaert, G., Cerchiari, E. (2005). Effect of the use of coated plant extracts and organic acids as alternatives for antimicrobial growth promoters on the performance of broiler chickens. *European Poultry Science,* 6: 48–56. https://www.european- poultry-science.com/artikel.dll/m04-31mk_NjI1MDA.PDF.

[140] Khattak, F., Ronchi, A., Castelli, P., Sparks, N. (2014). Effects of natural blend of essential oil on growth performance blood biochemistry, cecal morphology, and carcass quality of broiler chickens. *Poultry Science,* 93 (1): 132–137. doi: 10.3382/ps.2013-03387.

[141] Peng, Q.Y., Li, J.D., Li, Z., Duanb, Z.Y., Wua, Y.P. (2016). Effects of dietary supplementation with oregano essential oil on growth performance, carcass traits and jejunal morphology in broiler chickens. *Animal Feed Science and Technology* 214: 148–153. doi:10.1016/j. anifeedsci. 2016.02.010

[142] Suchý, P., Strakova, E., Mas, N., Serman, V., Vecerek, V., Bedrica, L., Lukac, Z., Horvat, Z. (2010). The effect of a herbal additive on performance parameters in layers. *Tierarztliche Umschau,* 65: 74–78.

[143] Botsoglou, N.A., Florou-Paneri, P., Christaki, E., Fletouris, D.J., Spais, A.B. (2002). Effect of dietary oregano essential oil on performance of chickens and on iron-induced lipid oxidation of breast, thigh and abdominal fat tissues. *British Poultry Science,* 43: 223-230. doi:10.1080/00071660120121436.

[144] Lee, K.W., Everts, H., Kappert, H.J., Frehner, M., Losa, R., Beynen, A.C. (2003). Effects of dietary essential oil components on growth performance, digestive enzymes and lipid metabolism in female broiler chickens. *British Poultry Science,* 44 (3): 450-457. doi: 10.1080/ 0007166031000085508.

[145] Symeon, G.K., Zintilas, C., Demiris, N., Bizelis, L.A., Deligeorgis, S.G. (2010). Effects of oregano essential oil dietary supplementation on the feeding and drinking behaviour as well as the activity of broilers. *International Journal of Poultry Science,* 9(4): 401–405. doi: 10.3923/ijps. 2010.401.405.

[146] Basmacioğlu, M.H., Baysal, S., Misirlioğlu, Z., Polat, M., Yilmaz, H., Turan,, N. (2010). Effects of oregano essential oil with or without feed enzymes on growth performance, digestive enzyme, nutrient digestibility, lipid metabolism and immune response of broilers fed on wheatsoybean meal diets. *British Poulty Science,* 51(1):67–80. doi: 10.1080/00071660903573702.

[147] Jamroz, D., Wertelecki, T., Houszka M., Kamel, C. (2006). Influence of diet type on the inclusion of plant origin active substances on morphological and histochemical characteristics of the stomach and jejunum walls in chicken. *Journal of Animal Physiology and Animal Nutrition,* 90: 255–268. https://doi.org/10.1111/j.1439-0396.2005.00603.x.

[148] Theron, M. M, and Lues, J.F.R. (2007). Organic acids and meat preservation: a review. *Food Reviews International,* 23: 141–158. https://doi.org/10.1080/87559120701224964.

[149] Fonseca-Garcia, I., Escalera-Valente, F., Martinez-Gonzalez, S., Carmonagasca, C.A., Gutierrez-Arenas, D.A., Ávila-Ramos, F. (2017). Effect of oregano oil dietary supplementation on production parameters, height of intestinal villi and the antioxidant capacity in the breast of broiler. *Australian Journal of Veterinary Science,* 49: 83-89. https://scielo. Conicytcl/ pdf/ australjvs/v49n2/0719-8132-australjvs-49-02-00083.pdf.

[150] Janz, J.A.M., Morel, P.C.H., Wilkinson, B.H.P., Purchas, R.W. (2007=. Preliminary investigation of the effects of low-level dietary inclusion of fragrant essential oils and oleoresins on pig performance and pork quality. *Meat Science,* 75: 350–355. doi:10.1016/j.meatsci.2006.06.027.

[151] Jugl-Chizzola, U.E., Gabler, C., Hagmuller, W. Chizzola, R., Zitterl-Eglseer, K., Franz, C. (2006). Testing of the palatability of *Thymus vulgaris* L. and *Origanum vulgare* L. as flavouring feed additive for weaner pigs on the basis of a choice experiment. *Berliner und Münchener Tierärztliche Wochenschrift*, 119 (5-6): 238–243.

[152] Bilkei, G, and Gertenbach, W. (2001). Retrospective evaluation of the combined effect of high vitamin E and oregano phytogenic feed additives on the performance of "slow growing" fattening pigs. *Biologische Tiermedizin,* 18: 83–87.

[153] Kyriakis, S.C., Sarris, K., Lekkas, S., Tsinas, A.C., Giannakopoulos, C.G., Alexopolos, C., Saoulidis, K. In *Proceedings of the 15th Internat. Pig Vet. Soc.* (IPVS) Congress, Birmingham, UK, 1998, 106.

[154] Casey R Neill, M.S., Nelssen Jim. L., Tokach, Michael, D., Goodband Robert. D., DeRouchey, J.M., Dritz, S.S., Crystal Groesbeck, N., Kelly R Brown, M.S. (2006). Effects of oregano oil on growth performance of nursery Pigs. *Journal of Swine Health and Production,* (JSHAP), 14 (6): 312-316. https://www.aasv.org/shap/issues/v14n6/v14n6p312.pdf.

[155] Kulchaiyawat, C, and Honeyman, M. S. (2006). Effects of Oregano Supplemented Diets on Nursery Pig Performance. *Animal Industry Report*: AS 652, ASL R2156. https://lib.dr.iastate.edu/ cgi/viewcontent.cgi?article=1193 &context= ans _ air.

[156] Henn, J.D., Bertol, T.M., Fernandes de Mour, N., Coldebella, A., Rabenschlag de Brum, P.A., Casagrande1, M. (2010). Oregano essential oil as food additive for piglets: antimicrobial and antioxidant Potential. *Revista Brasilia De Zootecnica*, 39 (8): 1761-1767. http://www.scielo.br/ scielo.php?script=sci_arttext&pid=S1516-35982010 000800019.

[157] Walter, B.M, and Bilkei, G. (2004). Immunostimulatory effect of dietary oregano etheric oils on lymphocytes from growth-retarded, low-weight growing-finishing pigs and productivity. *Tijdschrift voor Diergeneeskunde,* 129: 178–181.

[158] Allan, P, and Bilkei, G. (2005). Oregano improves reproductive performance of sows. *Theriogenology,* 63: 716–721. doi.org/10.1016/j.theriogenology. 2003. 06.010.

[159] Amrik, B, and Bilkei,, G. (2004). Influence of farm application of oregano on performances of sows. *The Canadian Veterinary Journal,* 45: 674–677. https://www.ncbi.nlm.nih.gov/pmc/articles /PMC546446/.

[160] Tan, C.H., Wei, H., Sun, H., Ao, J., Long, G., Jiang, S., Peng, J. (2015). Effects of dietary supplementation of oregano essential oil to sows on oxidative stress status, lactation feed intake of sows, and piglet performance. *BioMed Research International,* 1:1–9. doi:10.1155/ 2015/ 525218.

[161] Busquet, M., Calsamiglia, S., Ferret, A., Kamel, C. (2006). Plant Extracts Affect *In Vitro* Rumen Microbial Fermentation. *Journal of Dairy Science,* 89: 761–771. doi: 10.3168/jds.S0022-0302(06)72137-3.

[162] Hristov, A.N., Lee, C., Cassidy, T., Heyler, K., Tekippe, J.A., Varga, G.A., Cort, B., Brandt, R.C. (2013). Effect of *Origanum vulgare* L. leaves on rumen fermentation, production, and milk fatty acid composition in lactating cows. *Journal of Dairy Science* 96: 1189–1202. https://doi.org/10.3168/jds.2012-5975.

[163] Lejonklev, J., Kidmose, U., Jensen, S., Petersen, M.A., Helwing, A.L., Mortensen, G., Weisbjerg M.R., Larsen, M.K., (2016). Effect of oregano and caraway essential oils on the production and flavor of cow milk. *Journal of Dairy Science* 99 (10): 7898–7903. doi:10.3168/jds.2016-10910.

In: Oregano: Properties, Uses and Health Benefits
Editor: Gema Nieto Martínez
ISBN: 978-1-53616-284-4

Chapter 8

THE APPLICATION OF OREGANO ESSENTIAL OIL AS A PREVENTIVE AGAINST ECTOPARASITIC PROTOZOAN DISEASE IN JUVENILE CHUM SALMON *ONCORHYNCHUS KETA*

Shinya Mizuno*
Salmon and Freshwater Fisheries Research Institute,
Hokkaido Research Organization, Eniwa, Hokkaido, Japan

ABSTRACT

Infections with the ectoparasitic protozoans *Ichthyobodo salmonis* and *Trichodina truttae* cause severe mortalities among juvenile chum salmon *Oncorhynchus keta* reared in hatcheries for the salmon stock enhancement program in Japan. This chapter first focused on dietary supplementation with oregano essential oil as a preventive against *I. salmonis* and *T. truttae* infections in juvenile chum salmon, then discussed the mechanism of control shown by the preventive measure, and finally characterized the susceptibility of various pathogens known to infect chum salmon to oregano essential oil as compared with other essential oils. Feeding juvenile chum salmon a diet supplemented with 0.02% oregano oil for at least 7 successive days prior to parasite exposure effectively controlled *I. salmonis* and *T. truttae* infection outbreaks. Among juvenile chum salmon reared in hatchery ponds, this method practically suppressed *I. salmonis* and *T. truttae* infections, and substantially reduced juvenile mortalities caused by the two protozoans. Dietary supplementation with carvacrol, the principal component of oregano essential oil, prevented *I. salmonis* and *T. truttae* infections. Carvacrol exterminated both of the protozoans from the body surface of juvenile salmon already infected with *I. salmonis* or *T. truttae*, and was detected in the skin of juveniles given feed supplemented with oregano oil. Of seven herb essential oils tested,

* Corresponding Author's E-mail: mizuno-shinya@hro.or.jp

only oregano oil intensively prevented infections of *I. salmonis* and *T. truttae* as well as the growth of other bacterial and fungal pathogens known to infect chum salmon. Together, these results demonstrate the feasibility of dietary supplementation with oregano essential oil as a preventive measure against ectoparasitic protozoan diseases in juvenile chum salmon; implicate the antiparasitic action of carvacrol as a possible mechanism of the prevention; and indicate the potential use of oregano oil as an antimicrobial against bacterial and fungal diseases in juvenile chum salmon.

Keywords: carvacrol, disease prevention, hatchery-reared fish, oregano essential oil, phytobiotics, protozoan infection

INTRODUCTION

Since the 1880s, Japan has conducted a hatchery-based stock-enhancement program for chum salmon *Oncorhynchus keta* to increase fishery returns (Kitada 2014). Infections by ectoparasitic protozoans often cause heavy mortalities among juvenile salmon in freshwater hatcheries. The flagellate *Ichthyobodo salmonis*, originally known as *Ichthyobodo necator*, and the ciliate *Trichodina truttae* can attach to the body surface of host juvenile salmon (Mizuno et al. 2016, 202, 2017a, 287, 2017b, 102; Urawa 1992a, 1569, 1992b, 31). Infection with *I. salmonis* causes disruption to epithelial cells and compromises osmoregulation in the juvenile fish, thereby reducing survival of the anadromous host in the marine environment (Urawa 1993, 107). Infection with *T. truttae* typically begins with severe scratching against hatchery pond walls, and can result in over 50% cumulative juvenile mortality in freshwater (Urawa 1992b, 32). Control of both *I. salmonis* and *T. truttae* outbreaks are therefore needed to decrease mortalities among hatchery-reared juvenile chum salmon.

In Japan, formalin was once used to eliminate *I. salmonis* and *T. truttae* on the body surface of juvenile chum salmon; however, this chemical has been prohibited in the hatchery stock enhancement program since 2003 because they are environmentally unsuitable. Moreover, no other fisheries drugs, such as antibiotics, antiprotozoans and anthelmintics, have been approved in Japan for the control of any parasites of salmonid species. Thus, salmon hatcheries presently use bath treatments with seawater (Khan 1991, 154) or diluted corn-vinegar (Urawa 2013, 215), which are not regarded as drugs in Japan, to control *I. salmonis* and *T. truttae* infections. Even so, severe body damage due to heavy infection by these parasites can cause mass mortality of juveniles even after the bath. Disinfection of rearing water by ultraviolet ray (UV) irradiation can prevent infections of both *I. salmonis* and *T. truttae* in juvenile chum salmon (Mizuno et al. 2019, 135), but hatchery managers are hesitant to purchase UV-disinfection equipment because of the high cost. Consequently, hatcheries require methods that are more feasible and cost-effective to prevent these two protozoans.

Several plant extracts have proven antipathogen properties for aquaculture purposes (Athanassopoulou, Pappas, and Bitchava 2009, 75; Chakraborty and Hancz 2011, 105; Citarasu 2010, 412; Murthy and Kiran 2013, 977; Ramudu and Dash 2013, 214; Reverter et al. 2014, 54; Syahidah et al. 2015, 32; Valladão, Gallani, and Pilarski 2014, 425). Natural extracts also have the advantage of inducing less drug resistance in various parasites, since their mechanisms of action are highly diverse (Blumenthal et al. 2000; Olusola, Emikpe, and Olaifa 2013). Dietary supplementation with oregano essential oil extracted from *Origanum* species has been shown to confer varying degrees of protection from various infections in fishes, such as parasitism by myxosporeans (Athanassopoulou et al. 2004, 221, 2016); by crustacean parasites (Athanassopoulou et al. 2016); and by pathogenic bacteria (Abdel-Latif and Khalil 2014, 253; Diler et al. 2017). However, the effects of dietary oregano supplementation on the prevention of ectoparasitic protozoans in salmonids are not yet known.

In this chapter, the first topic discussed dietary supplementation with oregano essential oil as a preventive measure against *I. salmonis* and *T. truttae* infections in juvenile chum salmon. The second topic considered the mechanism of the prevention measure on control of the two protozoans. These two topics reviewed an earlier work (Mizuno et al. 2018), and showed newly supplemental data. The third topic newly presented the superiority of oregano essential oil compared to six other essential oils as an antimicrobial against various pathogens known to infect chum salmon.

Prevention of Ectoparasitic Protozoans in Juvenile Chum Salmon through Dietary Supplementation with Oregano Essential Oil

In this topic, dietary supplementation with oregano essential oil extracted from *Origanum vulgare* was tested to determine an appropriate dose and feeding-treatment duration for the control of *I. salmonis* and *T. truttae* infections in hatchery-reared juvenile chum salmon. The feasibility of the preventive measure was verified in a salmon hatchery, as follows. The first part of the topic aimed to determine whether supplementation with 0, 0.01, 0.02, 0.05 or 0.10% oregano oil (% dry mass of diet) would best control *I. salmonis* and *T. truttae* infections in juvenile chum salmon. Uninfected juveniles were reared in small tanks with running spring water and fed an oregano-supplemented feed for 28 days; thereafter, the fish were exposed to both *I. salmonis* and *T. truttae* over a period of 24 days. Infection with either *I. salmonis* or *T. truttae* was least prevalent among fish that had been fed 0.02% oregano oil supplementation as a preventive measure, and these fish displayed the least mortalities as a result of infection with either protozoan (Mizuno et al. 2018, 534).

These results indicated that dietary supplementation with 0.02% oregano oil would be the most appropriate prescription for control of the two protozoans in juvenile chum salmon.

The second part of the topic investigated whether advanced feeding with 0.02% oregano oil for a period of 0, 7 or 14 days would be the best duration for achieving an antiparasitic effect against *I. salmonis* and *T. truttae* in juvenile chum salmon. Uninfected juveniles reared in small tanks with running spring water were given the supplemented feed for either 0, 7 or 14 successive days, prior to exposure to the protozoans. An antiparasitic effect against *I. salmonis* and *T. truttae* in the juveniles through the feeding treatment was observed in the order of 0 < 7 < 14 days (Figures 1, 2). This result demonstrated that at least seven successive days of feeding with the oregano-supplemented diet is needed for marked prevention of infections by the two protozoans in juvenile chum salmon. Infection with the gram-positive coccus *Lactococcus garvieae* was significantly prevented in adult rainbow trout *O. mykiss* through 8 weeks of dietary supplementation with 0.012-0.3% oregano oil extracted from *O. onites*, with 0.3% supplementation being the most effective diet treatment (Diler et al. 2017, 848). Infections with a myxozoan *Myxobolus* sp., the monogene *Diplectanum aequans*, and the copepod *Lernanthropus kroyeri* were prevented in juveniles of gilthead seabream *Sparus aurata*, sharpsnout seabream *Diplodus puntazzo*, and European seabass *Dicentrarchus labrax*, respectively, through dietary supplementation with 0.5-1.0% oregano oil extracted from *O. vulgare* (Athanassopoulou et al. 2004, 220). Thus, the effective concentration of oregano oil seems to vary depending on the fish species, the growth stage of the fish, the duration of the feeding treatment, and/or the component or origin of the oregano essential oil used.

The third part of the topic evaluated the practical use of dietary supplementation with 0.02% oregano oil through 52 days rearing of 800,000 juvenile chum salmon in hatchery ponds. The dietary oregano supplementation completely prevented infection by *I. salmonis* for 52 days and infection by *T. truttae* for 38 days, and according markedly reduced juvenile mortalities caused by the two protozoans (Mizuno et al. 2018, 535). Mild infections with *T. truttae* were observed from days 39 to 52, but never led to heavy mortalities among the oregano-supplemented juveniles. In contrast, fish given no dietary oregano (control group) showed high-intensity infections with *I. salmonis* and/or *T. truttae*; consequently, on day 12, these juveniles required a single bath treatment with corn vinegar to exterminate the protozoans. Nevertheless, high mortality occurred among these controls because *I. salmonis* was not entirely eradicated from the fish after the corn-vinegar bath. These results demonstrate the practical feasibility of the preventive measure against *I. salmonis* and *T. truttae* in large-scale juvenile chum salmon production. Even better, the prevention strategy improved the feed efficiency of the juveniles and ensured a healthier condition in terms of the metabolic, hematological, osmoregulatory and natural immunological parameters. Overall, these data reveal the safety of dietary oregano supplementation for juvenile chum salmon.

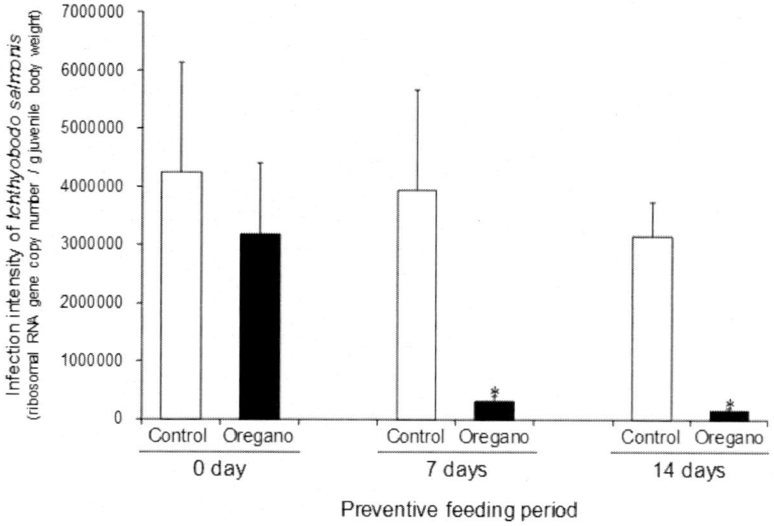

Figure 1. Effects of advance feeding with a diet supplemented with oregano essential oil on prevention of *Ichthyobodo salmonis* infection in juvenile chum salmon *Oncorhynchus keta*. Asterisks indicate significant differences in infection intensity of *I. salmonis* between the control group and oregano-supplemented group at each sampling time ($P < 0.05$: Nonparametric Mann-Whitney *U* test).

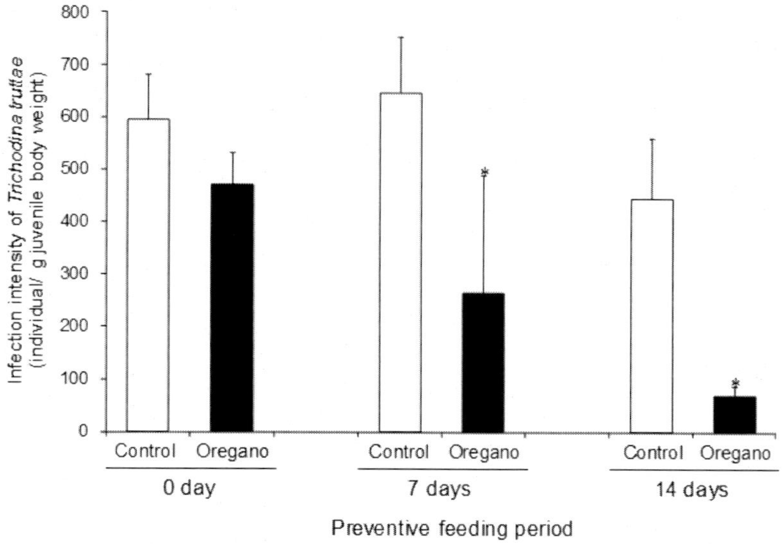

Figure 2. Effects of advance feeding with a diet supplemented with oregano essential oil on prevention of *Trichodina truttae* infection in juvenile chum salmon *Oncorhynchus keta*. Asterisks indicate significant differences in infection intensity of *T. truttae* between the control group and oregano-supplemented group at each sampling time ($P < 0.05$: Nonparametric Mann-Whitney *U* test).

Possible Mechanism of the Antiparasitic Effect of Oregano Supplementation in Juvenile Chum Salmon

The second topic examined which components of oregano essential oil are responsible for the antiparasitic effect and possible mechanism of the preventive measure on the control of *I. salmonis* and *T. truttae*. Oregano oil used in the present study consisted of 58.9% carvacrol, 15.6% *p*-cymene, 10.5% γ-terpinene, and 15.0% a combination of 17 other chemical compounds (% area of total ion chromatogram by gas chromatography/mass spectrometry). Thus, the first part analyzed the effect of feeding a diet variously supplemented with carvacrol, *p*-cymene and γ-terpinene on the control of *I. salmonis* and *T. truttae* outbreaks. Feed supplemented with 0.02% oregano oil and no other supplementation were prepared for positive and negative controls, respectively. Then, each of three major components was supplemented at the dose of the component contained in the oregano-supplemented diet. Infections of *I. salmonis* and *T. truttae* in the juvenile salmon were suppressed by dietary supplementation with either carvacrol or *p*-cymene (Figures 3, 4). In contrast, dietary supplementation with γ-terpinene prevented *T. truttae* infection only (Figure 4). Among the three components examined, carvacrol showed by far the most intensive antiparasitic effect on *I. salmonis* and *T. truttae*. These results suggest that the prevention capability depends on the antiparasitic action of three major components of oregano essential oil. An *in vitro* study reported that the antimicrobial action of oregano essential oil in relation to a food-poisoning bacterium depended on the activity of carvacrol (Mith et al. 2014, 414).

The second part tested exposure of the protozoans to carvacrol, *p*-cymene or γ-terpinene at the concentration of 0.5 g l^{-1} to identify the mechanism underlying the antiparasitic effect of the oregano oil. It is known that 0.5 g l^{-1} oregano oil can weakly exterminate both of *I. salmonis* or *T. truttae* from the body surface of juvenile salmon (Mizuno et al. 2018, 533). Sterilized spring water and 0.5 g l^{-1} oregano oil were used for treatments of negative and positive controls, respectively. Live juvenile salmon infected with *I. salmonis* and *T. truttae* were necessarily exposed to carvacrol, *p*-cymene or γ-terpinene, since no *in vitro* culture method has been established for either protozoan. The intensity of both *I. salmonis* and *T. truttae* infections in juvenile salmon decreased by each of carvacrol, *p*-cymene and γ-terpinene treatments (Figures 5, 6). Among the three components, carvacrol exterminated the most *I. salmonis* and *T. truttae*. These results suggest that three major components of oregano oil act directly on both *I. salmonis* and *T. truttae* through antiparasitic activity that is able to exterminate the protozoans from the body surface of juvenile chum salmon. In support of this supposition, *in vitro* treatment with oregano essential oil inhibited growth of the endoparasitic protozoan *Spironucleus vortens* isolated from the digestive tract of red discus *Symphysodon discus* (Puk and Guz 2014, 166).

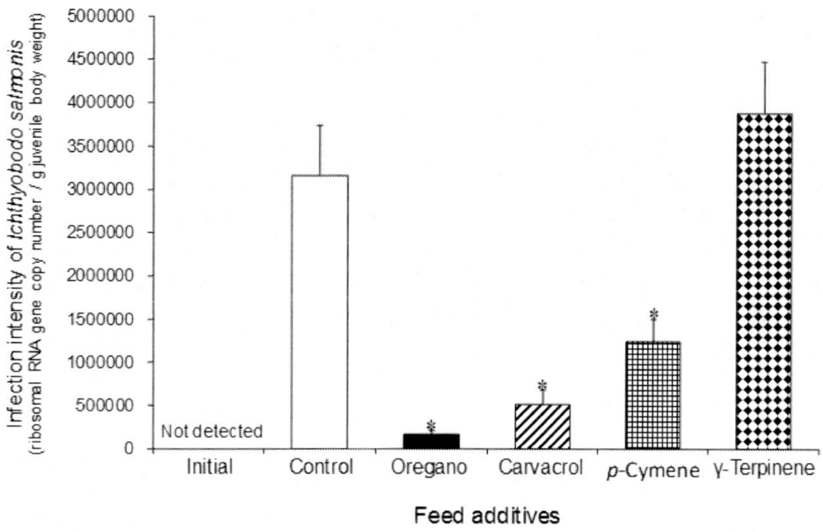

Figure 3. Effects of dietary supplementation with major components of oregano essential oil on prevention of *Ichthyobodo salmonis* infection in juvenile chum salmon *Oncorhynchus keta*. Asterisks indicate significant differences in the infection intensity of *I. salmonis* as compared with the control group ($P < 0.05$: Nonparametric Kruskal-Wallis test, followed by Mann-Whitney *U* test with the Bonferroni correction).

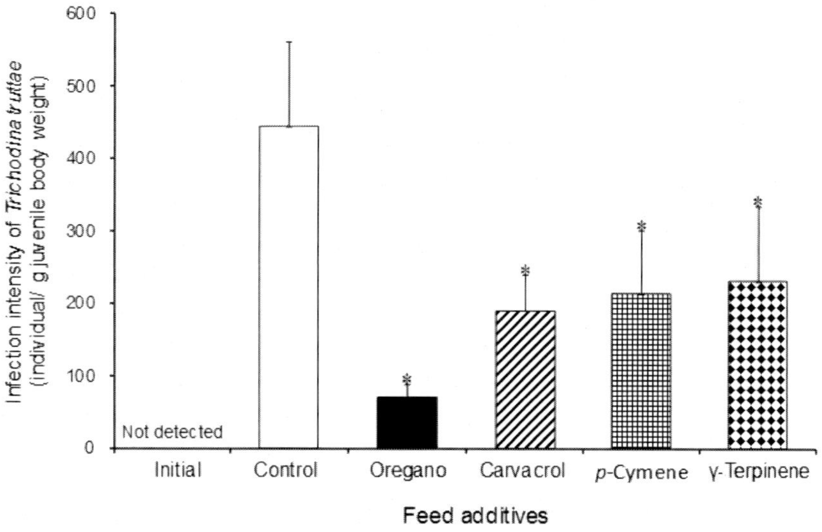

Figure 4. Effects of dietary supplementation with major components of oregano essential oil on prevention of *Trichodina truttae* infection in juvenile chum salmon *Oncorhynchus keta*. Asterisks indicate significant differences in infection intensity of *T. truttae* as compared with the control group ($P < 0.05$: Nonparametric Kruskal-Wallis test, followed by Mann-Whitney *U* test with the Bonferroni correction).

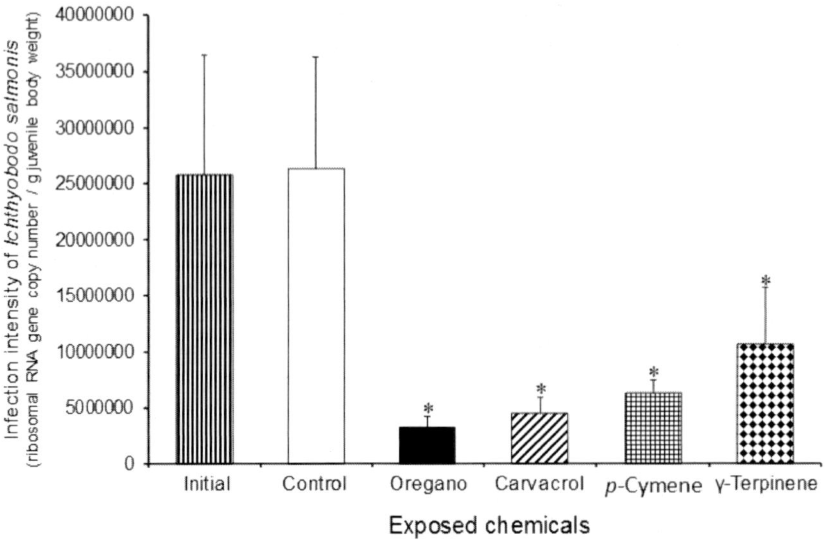

Figure 5. Effects of exposure to major components of oregano essential oil on extermination of *Ichthyobodo salmonis* from the body surface of juvenile chum salmon *Oncorhynchus keta*. Asterisks indicate significant differences in the infection intensity of *I. salmonis* as compared with the control group ($P < 0.05$: Nonparametric Kruskal-Wallis test, followed by Mann-Whitney *U* test with the Bonferroni correction).

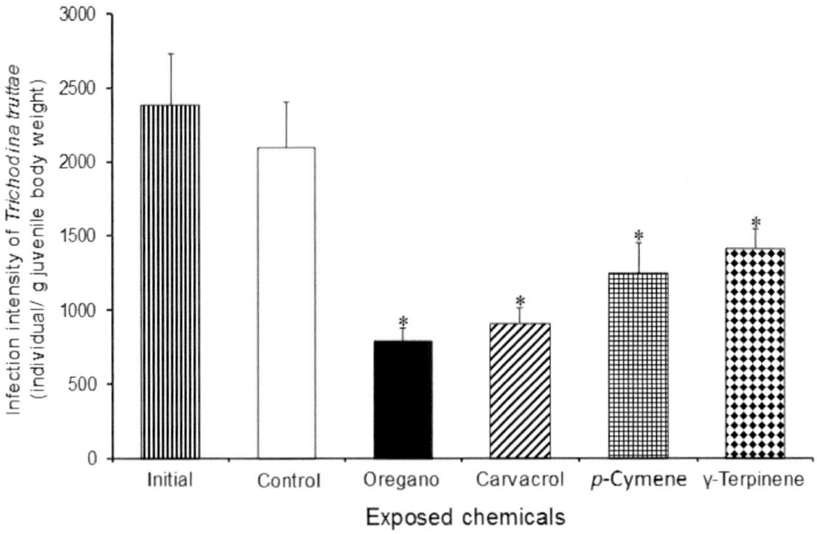

Figure 6. Effects of exposure to major components of oregano essential oil on extermination of *Trichodina truttae* from the body surface of juvenile chum salmon *Oncorhynchus keta*. Asterisks indicate significant differences in the infection intensity of *T. truttae* as compared with the control group ($P < 0.05$: Nonparametric Kruskal-Wallis test, followed by Mann-Whitney *U* test with the Bonferroni correction).

The third part investigated whether the supplemented feed could manifest in the presence of components of the essential oil on the body surface or skin of the juvenile salmon. Liquid chromatography-tandem mass spectrometry detected carvacrol in the skin of juveniles given the oregano-supplemented feed, while it was not detected in the control fish. These results suggest that carvacrol ended up on the body surface after the oregano essential oil was ingested by the juvenile salmon. Carvacrol was characterized by high permeability of the epithelial cell membrane (Cristani et al. 2007; Di Pasqua et al. 2007), which may contribute to the compound seeping through to the skin. Considering these overall results, a possible mechanism of the control of *I. salmonis* and *T. truttae* through dietary supplementation with the oregano oil was via carvacrol in the skin, which exerted an antiparasitic activity against *I. salmonis* and *T. truttae* on the fish's body surface. However, this topic does not provide direct evidence that carvacrol is transported from the internal body to the skin; further research is needed to prove this hypothesis.

Susceptibility of Pathogens Known to Infect Chum Salmon to Different Herb Essential Oils

Not only ectoparasitic protozoan diseases but also bacterial and fungal diseases cause serious mortalities of juveniles or embryos in seed production of chum salmon. Infection of *Flavobacterium psychrophilum* caused bacterial cold-water disease characterized by necrosis of the caudal peduncle in juvenile salmon (Misaka and Suzuki 2007). Infection of *F. branchiophilum* resulted in bacterial gill disease that caused decay of the gill epithelium and lessened the seawater adaptability of juvenile salmon (Wakabayashi 1980). Infection with *Saprolegnia diclina* induced growth of its hypha and resulted in suffocation of salmon embryos (Hatai 1980). Hence, the third topic examined the susceptibility of *I. salmonis*, *T. truttae*, *F. psychrophilum*, *F. branchiophilum* and *S. diclina* to seven different herb essential oils, including oregano oil, and then characterized the susceptibility to oregano essential oil shown by these fish pathogens as compared with six other essential oils.

Uninfected juvenile salmon were fed a diet supplemented with 0.02% essential oil of either oregano, Japanese mint, peppermint, spearmint, lavender, eucalyptus or fir tree for 14 days, and then exposed to *I. salmonis* and *T. truttae* for 28 days. Susceptibility of *I. salmonis* and *T. truttae* to the herb oils was evaluated by the infection intensity of each protozoan on juvenile salmon after transmission. Next, a patch test of 20 μl-each oil was conducted to examine *in vitro* susceptibility by *F. psychrophilum*, *F. branchiophilum* and *S. diclina*, which were cultured on laboratory dishes. Susceptibilities of bacterial and fungal pathogens were evaluated by the sizes of inhibition circles formed on the peripheries of the essential oils. The susceptibility of *I. salmonis* and *T. truttae* to these seven essential oils is shown in Figures 7 and 8, respectively. Figure 9 summarizes the susceptibility of *F. psychrophilum*, *F. branchiophilum* and *S. diclina* to the seven herb essential oils. Among these essential oils, oregano oil controlled intensive infections by *I. salmonis*, *T. truttae*, *F.*

psychrophilum, *F. branchiophilum* and *S. diclina*. Consequently, oregano essential oil was characterized as having the best antimicrobial activity among the various herbs.

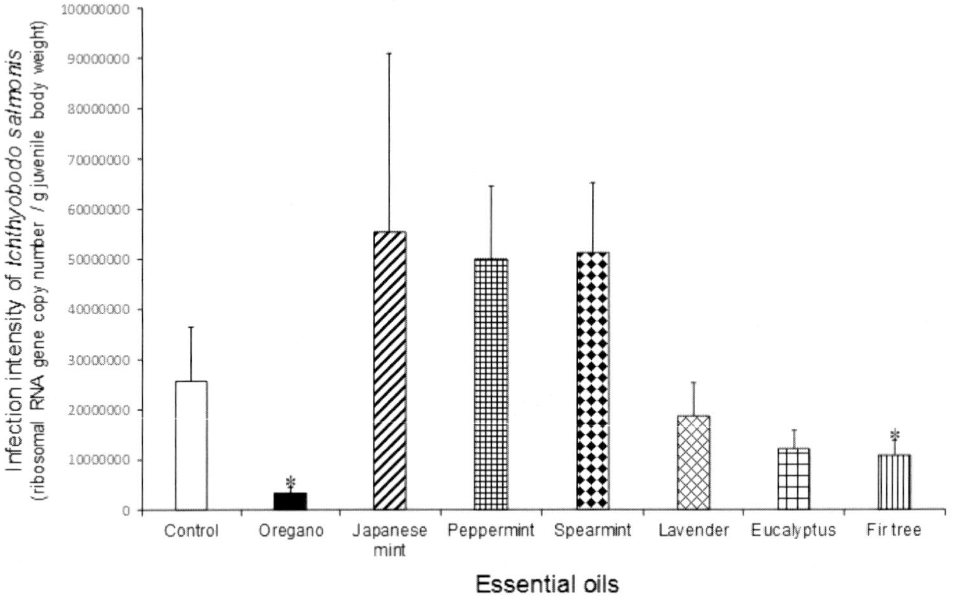

Figure 7. Susceptibility of *Ichthyobodo salmonis* to herb essential oils. Asterisks indicate significant differences in the infection intensity of *I. salmonis* as compared with the control group ($P < 0.05$: Nonparametric Kruskal-Wallis test, followed by Mann-Whitney U test with the Bonferroni correction).

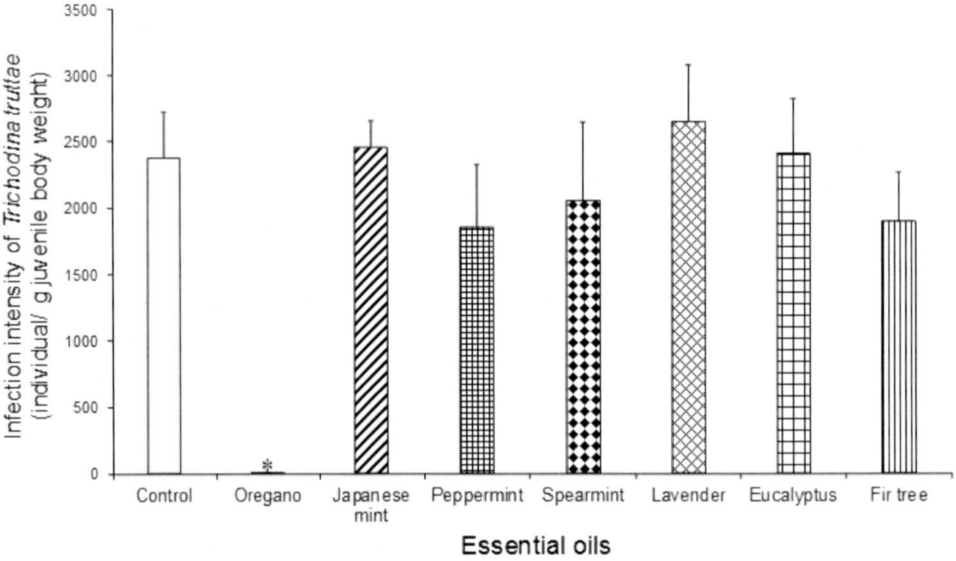

Figure 8. Susceptibility of *Trichodina truttae* to herb essential oils. Asterisk indicates significant difference in the infection intensity of *T. truttae* as compared with the control group ($P < 0.05$: Nonparametric Kruskal-Wallis test, followed by Mann-Whitney U test with the Bonferroni correction).

Herb essential oils	Diseases (Pathogens)		
	Bacterial cold-water disease (*Flavobacterium psychrophilum*)	Bacterial gill disease (*Flavobacterium branchiophilum*)	Saprolegniasis (*Saprolegnia diclina*)
Oregano	○	○	○
Japanese mint	●	●	□
Peppermint	□	□	●
Spearmint	●	●	●
Lavender	■	■	●
Eucalyptus	■	■	●
Fir tree	■	■	●

Figure 9. Susceptibility of bacterial and fungal pathogens known to infect chum salmon *Oncorhynchus keta* to herb essential oils. A patch test of 20 μl-each oil was conducted to examine *in vitro* susceptibility by pathogens, which were cultured on laboratory dishes (8.5 cm-diameter). Susceptibilities of pathogens were regarded as high (○), low(□), very low (●) and nothing (■) when the sizes of inhibition circles formed on the peripheries of essential oils were 8.5 cm, 3.0-4.0 cm, 1.0-2.0 cm, and 0 cm, respectively.

CONCLUSION

This chapter establishes dietary supplementation with oregano essential oil as a preventive measure for *I. salmonis* and *T. truttae* infections in hatchery-reared juvenile chum salmon. This method is now being practically applied in some Japanese salmon hatcheries; the method benefits hatcheries by removing the need for a specific protozoan control method during the rearing of juvenile salmon, thereby reducing labor and lightening the burden on hatchery managers. Widespread adoption of this preventive measure could contribute to the production of healthy juvenile salmon in hatcheries, thus ensuring a higher rate of fishery returns. Moreover, the intensive antimicrobial activity of oregano essential oil suggests its potential application for general, more extensive disease control in the hatchery program for chum salmon. A follow-up study of oregano essential oil as a fish-feed additive should elucidate the most appropriate dosages, treatment durations, and administration methods for preventing bacterial cold-water disease, bacterial gill disease, and saprolegniasis in chum salmon.

REFERENCES

Abdel-Latif, Hany M. R., and Riad H. Khalil. 2014. "Evaluation of two phytobiotics, *Spirulina platensis* and *Origanum vulgare* extract on growth, serum antioxidant activities and resistance of Nile tilapia." *International Journal of Fisheries and Aquatic Studies* 1:250–55.

Athanassopoulou, Fotini, Evdokia Karagouni, Eleni Dotsika, Basil Ragias, Panos Christofilloyanis, and Ioannis Vatsos. 2004. "Efficacy and toxicity of orally administrated anti-coccidial drugs for innovative treatments of *Myxobolus* sp. infection in *Puntazzo puntazzo*." *Diseases of Aquatic Organisms* 62:217–26.

Athanassopoulou, Fotini, Ioannis S. Pappas, and Konstantina Bitchava. 2009. "An overview of the treatments for parasitic disease in Mediterranean aquaculture." In *The Use of Veterinary Drugs and Vaccines in Mediterranean Aquaculture*, edited by Chris Rogers, and Bernardo Basurco, 65–83. Zaragoza: Ciheam Iams.

Athanassopoulou, Fotini, Mary Yiagnisis, M. Mante, Markos Kolygas, E. Gourzioti, and Yannis P. Kotzamanis. 2016. "Effects of dietary supplementation with oregano (*Origanum vulgare* Hirtum) and rosemary (*Rosmarinus officinalis*) essential oils on fish parasites in gilhead seabream (*Sparus aurata* L.) and European sea bass (*Dicentrarchus labrax* L.)." *Abstract of European Aquaculture Society 2016*. https://www.was.org/EasOnline/AbstractDetail.aspx?i=6773.

Blumenthal, Mark, Alicia Goldberg, Josef Brinckmann, Stephen Foster, and Varro E. Tyler. 2000. "Herbal Medicine." In *Expanded Commission E Monographs*, edited by Mark Blumenthal, Alicia Goldberg, and Josef Brinckmann, 293–96. Newton: Integrative Medicine Communications.

Chakraborty, Suman B., and Csaba Hancz. 2011. "Application of phytochemicals as immunostimulant, antipathogenic and antistress agents in finfish culture." *Reviews in Aquaculture* 3:103–19.

Citarasu, Thavasimuthu. 2010. "Herbal biomedicines: A new opportunity for aquaculture industry." *Aquaculture International* 18:403–14.

Cristani, Maria T., Manuela D'Arrigo, Giuseppina Mandalari, Francesco Castelli, Maria G. Sarpietro, Dorotea Micieli, Vincenza Venuti, Giuseppe Bisignano, Antonella Saija, and Domenico Trombetta. 2007. "Interaction of four monoterpenes contained in essential oils with model membranes: implications for their antibacterial activity." *Journal of Agricultural Food Chemistry* 55:6300–08.

Diler, Öznur, Öznur Gormez, Ibrahim Diler, and Secil Metin. 2017. "Effect of oregano (*Origanum onites* L.) essential oil on growth, lysozyme and antioxidant activity and resistance against *Lactococcus garvieae* in rainbow trout." *Aquaculture Nutrition* 23:844–51.

Di Pasqua, Rosangela, Gail Betts G., Nikki Hoskins, M. Edwards, Danilo Ercolini, and Gianluigi Mauriello. 2007. "Membrane toxicity of antimicrobial compounds from essential oils." *Journal of Agricultural Food Chemistry* 55:4863–70.

Hatai, Kishio. 1980. "Saprolegniasis in salmonids." *Fish Pathology* 14:199-206.

Khan, Rasul A. 1991. "Mortality in Atlantic salmon (*Salmo salar*) associated with trichodinid ciliates." *Journal of Wildlife Diseases* 27:153–55.

Kitada, Shuichi. 2014. "Japanese chum salmon stock enhancement: current perspective and future challenges." *Fisheries Science* 80:237–49.

Misaka, Naoyuki, and Kunio Suzuki. 2007. "Detection of *Flavobacteruim psychrophilum* in chum salmon *Oncorhynchus keta* and virulence of isolated strains to salmonid fishes." *Fish Pathology* 42:201–09.

Mith, Hasika, Rémi Duré, Véronique Delcenserie, Abdesselam Zhiri, Georges Daube, and Antoine Clinquart. 2014. "Antimicrobial activities of commercial essential oils and their components against food–borne pathogens and food spoilage bacteria." *Food Science & Nutrition* 2:403–16.

Mizuno, Shinya, Shigehiko Urawa, Mahito Miyamoto, Makoto Hatakeyama, Nobuhisa Koide, and Hiroshi Ueda. 2017a. "Quantitative analysis of *Ichthyobodo salmonis*, an ectoparasitic flagellate, infecting juvenile chum salmon *Oncorhynchus keta* in hatcheries." *Fisheries Science* 83:283–90.

Mizuno, Shinya, Shigehiko Urawa, Mahito Miyamoto, Makoto Hatakeyama, Nobuhisa Koide, and Hiroshi Ueda. 2019. "Experimental evidence on prevention of infection by the ectoparasitic protozoans *Ichthyobodo salmonis* and *Trichodina truttae* in juvenile chum salmon using ultraviolet disinfection of rearing water." *Journal of Fish Diseases* 42:129–40.

Mizuno, Shinya, Shigehiko Urawa, Mahito Miyamoto, Makoto Hatakeyama, Hayato Saneyoshi, Yoshitaka Sasaki, Nobuhisa Koide, and Hiroshi Ueda. 2016. "The epidemiology of the trichodinid ciliate *Trichodina truttae* on hatchery-reared and wild salmonid fish in Hokkaido." *Fish Pathology* 51:199–209.

Mizuno, Shinya, Shigehiko Urawa, Mahito Miyamoto, Makoto Hatakeyama, Yoshitaka Sasaki, Nobuhisa Koide, Shoichi Tada, and Hiroshi Ueda. 2018. "Effects of dietary supplementation with oregano essential oil on prevention of the ectoparasitic protozoans *Ichthyobodo salmonis* and *Trichodina truttae* in juvenile chum salmon *Oncorhynchus keta*." *Journal of Fish Biology* 93:528–39.

Mizuno, Shinya, Shigehiko Urawa, Mahito Miyamoto, Hayato Saneyoshi, Makoto Hatakeyama, Nobuhisa Koide, and Hiroshi Ueda. 2017b. "Epizootiology of the ectoparasitic protozoans, *Ichthyobodo salmonis* and *Trichodina truttae*, on wild chum salmon *Oncorhynchus keta*." *Diseases of Aquatic Organisms* 126:99–109.

Murthy, Shankar K., and B. R. Kiran. 2013. "Review on usage of medicinal plants in fish diseases." *International Journal of Pharmacy and Biological Sciences* 4:975–86.

Olusola, Sunday E., Benjamin O. Emikpe, and Flora, E. Olaifa. 2013. "The potentials of medicinal plants extracts as bio-antimicrobial in aquaculture." *International Journal of Medicinal Aromatic Plants* 3:404–12.

Puk, Krzysztof, and Leszek Guz. 2014. "Effects of medical plant extracts on the growth of the fish parasite *Spironucleus vortens*." *Medycyna Weterynaryina* 70:165–68.

Ramudu, Kurva R., and Gadadhar Dash. 2013. "A review on herbal drugs against harmful pathogens in aquaculture." *American Journal of Drug Discovery and Development* 3:209–19.

Reverter, Miriam, Nathalie Bontemps, David Lecchini, Bernard Banaigs, and Pierre Sasal. 2014. "Use of plant extracts in fish aquaculture as an alternative to chemotherapy: Current status and future perspectives." *Aquaculture* 433:50–61.

Syahidah, Ahmad, Che R. Saad, Hassan M. Daud, and Yasser M. Abdelhadi. 2015. "Status and potential of herbal applications in aquaculture: A review." *Iranian Journal of Fisheries Science* 14:27–44.

Urawa, Shigehiko. 1992a. "Epidermal responses of chum salmon (*Oncorhynchus keta*) fry to the ectoparasitic flagellate *Ichthyobodo necator*." *Canadian Journal of Zoology* 70:1567–75.

Urawa, Shigehiko. 1992b. "*Trichodina truttae* Mueller, 1937 (Ciliophora: Peritrichida) on juvenile chum salmon (*Oncorhynchus keta*): Pathogenicity and host-parasite interactions." *Fish Pathology* 27:29–37.

Urawa, Shigehiko. 1993. "Effects of *Ichthyobodo necator* infections on seawater survival of juvenile chum salmon (*Oncorhynchus keta*)." *Aquaculture* 110:101–10.

Urawa, Shigehiko. 2013. "Control of the parasitic flagellate *Ichthyobodo salmonis*, causative agent of marine mortalities of juvenile chum salmon." *North Pacific Anadromous Fish Commission Technical Report* 9:214–15.

Valladão, Gustavo M. R., Silvia U. Gallani, and Faviana Pilarski. 2014. "Phytotherapy as an alternative for treating fish disease." *Journal Veterinary Pharmacology and Therapeutics* 38:417–28.

Wakabayashi, Hisatsugu. 1980. "Bacterial gill disease of salmonid fish." *Fish Pathology* 14:185–89.

In: Oregano: Properties, Uses and Health Benefits
Editor: Gema Nieto Martínez
ISBN: 978-1-53616-284-4

Chapter 9

OREGANO: PROPERTIES AND USES IN THE NUTRITION OF BROILERS REARED UNDER HEAT STRESS

Mihaela Saracila**, Rodica Diana Criste, Tatiana Dumitra Panaite, Arabela Untea and Petru Alexandru Vlaicu

Laboratory of Chemistry and Nutrition Physiology,
National Research-Development Institute for Animal Biology
and Nutrition (INCDBNA- IBNA), Balotesti, Ilfov, Romania

ABSTRACT

In recent years, aromatic plants and the products derived from them have gained attention as phytogenic feed additives in animal nutrition, more so as in January 2006, the European Union banned the use of antibiotic growth promoters in animal feeds. Oregano (*Origanum vulgare L.),* sovarv in Romanian, is a perennial aromatic herb from the Lamiaceae family, which displays important antibacterial and antioxidant properties (particularly due to is phenolic compounds carvacrol and thymol) and a high content of trace elements (for example: Cu, Fe, Mn, Zn). The data on the chemical composition of *Origanum vulgare L.*, even the data on the same subspecies, are rather varied, being closely related to the climacteric conditions and the geographical areas of growth. Some authors studied the antimicrobial activity of the oils obtained from several oregano varieties and noticed that their efficacy depends on the location from where the plants have been harvested. Numerous studies show that oregano helps digestion and nutrient absorption, displays antibacterial properties and prevents imbalances in animal gut. These effects are more so important when young animals are reared under heat stress conditions, which bear upon the balance of the intestinal microflora. Due to these properties, oregano has been studied as phytoadditive in the diet formulations for broiler reared under heat stress (32°C).

* Corresponding Author's E-mail: mihaela.saracila@yahoo.com.

This chapter presents a review of findings regarding the chemical characterisation of oregano (as powder and essential oil) harvested from a culture (located at Livezeni, Mures County, latitude 46.55°N, longitude 24.63°E) of a Romanian producer of aromatic plants, with special emphasis on their impact on the microflora of the broiler reared under heat stress conditions.

Keywords: oregano, diet, broiler, antimicrobial, heat stress

INTRODUCTION

Since 2006, EU have banned the use of antibiotics as growth promoters in farm animals. Therefore, poultry breeders focus their efforts to control and remove pathogenic bacteria from feed, to ensure performance and to cut the economic losses, ensuring poultry products safety. In these conditions the interest for using "phytogenic compounds" from plants as alternatives increased [1]. The beneficial potential of the bioactive compounds was supported by the performance and heath state of the animals. The term of "phytogenic compound" refers to the parts (seeds, fruits, roots and leaves) of the different plants and spices (garlic, oregano, thyme, rosemary, coriander and cinnamon) or to essential oils [2]. Many beneficial properties of the phytogenic compounds derive from their bioactive molecules (carvacrol, thymol, cineol, linalool, anetol, allycin, capsaicin, allyl isothyocianat and piperine). The biological activity of these active compounds is well documented, as well as their antibacterial and antioxidant functions [2–4]. Their antiviral, antioxygenic, antiparasitic and insecticide properties were reported [4]. Currently the interest for the use of essential oils in animal feeding increased due to their high biological activity compared to the raw materials from which they were extracted. Aromatic plants, such as oregano, garlic, thyme, rosemary and sage are the most investigated in broiler feeding, as very rich essential oils sources. They are used either individually or in combination as fresh material or essential oils rich sources [5–7].

As mentioned above, oregano, a perennial aromatic herb belonging to the family of *Lamiaceae* [8], is the most studied for its phytochemical products and biological activity. Its name derives from the old Greek words "Oros" and "Ganos," which mean beauty of the mountains [9, 10]. *Origanum* genus, from the family of *Lamiaceae*, includes 38 species, 6 subspecies and 17 hybrids [11] widely spread in Europe, in the Mediterranean area, such as *Origanum vulgare L.*, *Origanum viride*, and *Origanum virens*. However, other species, such as *Origanum vulgare L. ssp.viride*, *Origanum vulgare L. ssp. hirtum*, *Origanum vulgare L. ssp. heracloticum*, *Origanum vulgare L. ssp. virens*, *Origanum vulgare L. ssp. Glandulosum*, *Origanum vulgare L. ssp. gracile* also are of scientific interest [12–14]. Oregano has been used even from the Antiquity. In the popular medicine, *O. vulgare* was used to cure breath disturbances, dyspepsia, painful menstruation, rheumatoid arthritis, scrofulosis and urinary tract disturbances [15]. As a medicinal plant, oregano is used due to the antimicrobial, anticoccidial, antifungal, anti-spasmolytic and antioxidant effects [16]. *Origanum* species are plants with ascendant or erect stems, subsessile or petiolate leaves and clustered flowers arranged in paniculate-corymbiform inflorescence [10]. Among *Origanum* species, *Origanum vulgare* grows to a height of about 20 cm, with woody stems and dark green leaves around 2 cm long. The plants protect the inclined soils, and are quite tolerant to cold and dryness [10].

The aerial parts of oregano *(Origani herba)* are used in therapeutic due to their high content of eessential oil and polyphenols. Regarding their therapeutic effects, the oregano aerial parts are well-known for their antioxidant [17–21], antibacterial, [18, 22], antifungal [23, 24], cytotoxic [25, 26], antiviral [27], immunomodulatory [28], antimutagenic [21, 29] and estrogen-like activities [30]. The aromatic plants, also known as herbs or spices, such as oregano, contain many bioactive compounds and have strong antibacterial, antiparasitic, cytotoxic and antioxidant activity [31–33]. Many oregano species grow only in the wild, but others, used as medicinal, culinary herbs, and garden plants, are cultivated. The essential oils from oregano have the highest potential as alternative to the use of antibiotics as growth promoters. The oregano essential oils can modify gut flora and reduce the microbial populations by supressing bacteria proliferation [34]. They are of great economic importance, not just for their use as spice, but also for their use in human and animal nutrition [10]. Oregano contains phenolic compounds (such as carvacrol), which have antimicrobial activity.

Oregano, whose the most popular Romanian name is *"sovarv,"* has also been used by the traditional medicine both for human and for animals. In Romania, *Origanum vulgare*, (fam. *Lamiaceae*), grows spontaneously in the Carpathians mounts, in bushes, near woods, on rocky land, in hay yards and orchards. The Romanian ancestor, "Dacians" people, used it as cure and as a dyestuff. It is increasingly appreciated for its various uses, and is cultivated on increasingly areas. For example, the volatile oils derived from *sovarv* had beneficial action on *Listeria monocytogenes* strain [35]. Moreover, the *in vitro* antioxidant activity of the *sovarv* essential oil and of its constituents (carvacrol, tymol) is similar or even better than that of α- tocopherol [35].

The aim of this chapter is to provide new experimental and solid scientific data on the effects of oregano as feed additive in broilers diet, reared under heat stress.

OREGANO-CHEMICAL CHARACTERIZATION

The data on the chemical composition of *Origanum vulgare L.*, are quite varied and are in close connection with the geographical area of growth, with the climacteric conditions, with the period of harvesting, method of extraction, storage conditions and with the analytical methods [36, 37]. The aerial parts of oregano (*Origani herba*) are used in therapeutics due to their high content of essential oil and polyphenols. According to the literature, the herbal product is also a source of sterols, terpenes, vitamin C, carotenoids and minerals [26, 38–42]. Carotenoids in oregano according to National Nutrient Database for Standard Reference Release (USDA, 2007) contain 4112 mcg β- carotene, 60 mcg β-cryptoxanthin and 826 mcg lutein and zeaxanthin. Chlorogenic acid, caffeic acid, ferulic acid, p-hydroxybenzoic acid, syringic acid, gallic acid, lithospermic acid, protocathehuic acid and origanoside have also been found in oregano aerial parts [25, 40, 41]. The aerial parts of *Origanum vulgare L.* are a source of flavones, such as glucosides of kempferol, quercetin, myricetin, apigenin, naringenin, luteolin, acacetin and taxifolin [12, 29, 38].

Table 1. Characterization of *Origanum vulgare* used in the experimental studies from IBNA (plant from a Romanian local producer) vs. those reported in different studies

Type	Origin	Quantified compounds	Reference
Powder (whole plant)	Livezeni, Targu Mures, Romania	*Chemical composition*: 91.29 g/100g dry matter; 5.26 g/100 g crude protein; 1.17 g/100 g crude fat; 37.58 g/100g crude fibre; 6.66 g/100g ash.	[46]
		Minerals: 0.46 g% Ca; 0.22% P; 8.46 mg/kg Cu; 400.11mg/kg Fe; 27.89 mg/kg Mn; 30.28 mg/kg Zn. *Amino acids:* 0.64% aspartic acid; 0.77% glutamic acid; 0.38% serine; 0.32% glycine; 0.46% threonine; 0.4% arginine; 0.42% alanine; 0.22% tyrosine; 0.38% valine; 0.32% phenylalanine; 0.29% isoleucine; 0.56% leucine; 0.33% lysine.	Unpublished results (Saracila et al.)
Leaves	Ecopharm Hellas S.A. Kilkis, Greece	*Chemical composition*: 906 g/kg dry matter; 157g/kg crude protein; 52 g/kg crude fat; 99 g/kg ash.	[47]
	Rauischholzhausen, Germany	*Chemical composition*: 90.00% dry matter; 11.1% crude protein; 4.04% crude fat; 2.0 mg/g Ca; 19.5% P.	[48]
Powder	Local market, India	*Chemical composition*: 9.06% crude protein; 17.43% crude fiber.	[45]
Herb	Local market, Poland	*Minerals:* 0.35 mg/g Al; 0.026 mg/g Ba; 16.3 mg/g Ca; 0.41 mg/g Fe; 13.4 mg/g K; 2.92 mg/g Mg; 0.05 mg/g Mn; 0.07 mg/g Na; 2.07 mg/g P; 2.22mg/g S; 0.020 mg/g Sr; 0.017 mg/g Zn.	[44]
	Jirny, Prague-East, Czech	*Polyphenols*: 2540 mg GA/100 g DM total phenolic content, 4189 mg AA/100 g DM DPPH	[49]
	Local market from India	*Chemical composition and polyphenols content*: 9.06% Protein; 17.43% Fiber; 87.80 mg GAE/100g DW total phenol content	[45]
	Local market, Konya, Turkey	*Minerals:* 1043 mg/kg Ca, 159 mg/kg Fe, 19625 mg/kg K, 7.43 mg/kg Cr, 79.8 mg/kg Ba	[50]

Where: GA- gallic acid; GAE- Equivalent gallic acid; DW- dry weight; DM- dry matter; AA- ascorbic acid; DPPH- 2,2-diphenyl-1-picrylhydrazyl; Ca- calcium; P- phosphorus; Mg- magnesium; Cu- copper; Na- sodium; Mn- manganasse; Sr- strontium; Zn- zinc; Fe-iron; K- potassium; Cr- chromium; Ba- barium; S-sulfur.

The plant exhibits high oil concentrations (1.1–8.2%, v/w, depending on its habitat), about 10 times higher than its relative species (*O. vulgare subsp vulgare*, *O. vulgare subsp viridulum*, *O. vulgare subsp gracile*, *O. vulgare subsp viride*) [43]. The oregano plant contains antioxidants (8%) and tannins (2%) [44]. It also has high levels of polyphenols, which give it high antioxidant capacity [45].

Table 1 shows a selection of literature data on the characteristics of the oregano plants. Table 1 data show a great variety of values, which can be explained mainly by the subspecies, by the geographic origin, soil, by the part of the plant that was used, and by the drying technology.

In the oregano powder from plants harvested from Romania, was determined [46] a low level of crude protein (5.26%), but a high concentration of crude fibre (37.58%). Also in oregano plants purchased from a local market in India, dried, grounded, packed in sterilized plastic bags and treated in microwave at 915 MHz for 1 min, was reported [45] a higher concentration of protein (9.06%) and a lower crude fibre (17.43%). In contrast, a researcher team [47] reported higher concentrations of crude protein (15.7%) and fat (5.2%) in oregano plants harvested in Greece. According to others authors [9], oregano also has a relatively modest energy and fat content (66 kcal/100 g and 2 g fat/100 g, respectively). The chemical analysis of oregano plant (Table 1) harvested from Romania, showed rather large amounts of essential amino acids, such as glutamic acid (0.77%), aspartic acid (0.64%) and leucine (0.56%).

Plant materials can be a valuable source of many micronutrients present in herbs [41]. Aromatic and rich taste oregano is also high in minerals [44], such as K, Ca, Mg, P, Zn, Mn, Fe, Cu, S, Cl, I and Se, whereas its Na content is low [9]. As shown in Table 1, oregano plant from Romania has high levels of Fe (400.11 mg/kg), Mn (27.89 mg/kg), Zn (30.28 mg/kg) and Ca (0.46 g%). Similar concentrations of Fe (410 mg/kg) and P (0.207 g%) were reported by [44] in oregano plants purchased from a local market in Poland. Unlike these results, the Ca concentrations were 64.56% higher, in the oregano plants grown in Romania (Table 1). Analysing the oregano plants purchased from a local market in Konya, Turkey, it was reported [50] higher levels of Ca (1043 mg/kg), Fe (159 mg/kg), K (19625 mg/kg), Cr (7.43 mg/kg) and Ba (79.8 mg/kg), which are important structural components of tissues with cellular function and could influence the water and acid-base balance. This rich mineral composition (both micro- and macro-elements) explain the beneficial effect of oregano on the body, taken into consideration that minerals are of critical importance in the diet, even though they comprise only 4–6% of the human body. Essential trace elements are Zn, Fe, Si, Mn, Cu, F, I and Cr. The major minerals serve as structural components of tissues and function in cellular and basal metabolism, water and acid-base balance [51–53].

Table 2. Major constituents of *Origanum vulgare* used in the experimental studies from IBNA (essential oil as commercial product and plant from a Romanian local producer) vs. those reported in different studies

Type	Origin	Sampling period	Extraction method details	Compounds detection method	Compounds and their concentrations in the essential oil	Reference
PLANT	Livezeni, Targu Mures, Romania	ND	ND	GC-MS	Sabinene (56.57%); eucalyptol (12.27%)	[61]
	Poland	mid August, 2007	ND	GC-MS	Sabinene (20.13%); Germacrene D (17.22%)	[62]
	Qassim, Saudi Arabia	ND	ND	GC-MS	Carvacrol (72.32%); trans-caryophyllene (6.22%); 1,3-pentadiene trimethyl (5.32%)	[63]
ESSENTIAL OIL	China commercial product	ND	Liquid-solid extraction	GC -MS	Carvacrol (59.08%); p-cymene (20.75%); γ-terpinene (4.45%)	[61]
	Santar´em, Ribatejo, Portugal	summer 2008	hydrodistillation for 3 h (Clevenger system)	GC-MS	Carvacrol (14.5%); β-Fenchyl alcohol (12.8%); thymol (12.6%); γ -Terpinene (11.6%)	[15]
	Greek oregano	ND	ND	GC-MS	Carvacrol (77.9%); p-Cymene (5.4%); γ-Terpinene (4.6%); Thymol (3%)	[10]
	Noshahr, Mazandaran province, Iran	July, 2012.	hydrodistillation (Clevenger type apparatus)	GC -MS	Thymol (37.129%); carvacrol (9.573%); gama-Terpinene (9.668%); Carvacrol, methyl ether (6.88%); cis-alpha-bisabolene (6.80%)	[64]
	Sicilian commercial plant, Italy	ND	hydrodistillation (apparatus 'Quick Fit' 1011)	GC -MS and GC-FID	Thymol (32.4%); Carvacrol (16.7%); p-cimene (11.5%); gama-terpinene (10.4%)	[65]
	Commercial oil, Belgrade, Serbia	ND	ND	GC -MS	Carvacrol (33.51%); caryophyllene (10.29%); spathulenol (8.44%); p-cimene (6.68%) thymol (5.67%)	[66]
	Commercial oil from Guinness Chemical Ltd., Portlaoise, Ireland	ND	ND	GC -MS	Carvacrol (68.5%) Thymoquinone (12.1%) p-Cymene (7.8%)	[67]
	Bari, Italy	ND	steam extraction	GC -MS	a-Pinene (5.1%); Cymene (25%); Eucalyptol (2.8%)	[68]

Type	Origin	Sampling period	Extraction method details	Compounds detection method	Compounds and their concentrations in the essential oil	Reference
	Faisalabad, Pakistan.	July-August 2008	hydro-distillation for 3 h using a Clevenger-type apparatus and dried over anhydrous sodium sulfate	GC -MS and GC-FID	Thymol (21.6%); carvacrol (18.8%); o-cymene (13.5%); a-terpineol (8.57%); a- pinene (3.2%)	[69]
	Concórdia, state of Santa Catarina, Brazil	October, 2009 - April, 2010	steam-distillation of the aerial part	GC -MS and GC-FID	γ-Terpinene (31.68, 1056); (Z)-β -Ocimene (16.03, 1038); (E)-β -Ocimene (11.68, 1047); o-Cymene (11.43, 1022)	[70]
	Green City, Glasgow, UK	2001	distilled using a Clevenger-type apparatus	GC -MS	γ-terpinene (170), 1,8-cineole (60) and an unidentified terpene	[6]
	Hadjeb Elayoun, Tunisia	ND	water distillation	GC -MS	Carvacrol (69.55%); cymol (10.57%)	[71]

ND= not described; GC-MS = gas-cromatography/mass spectrometry; GC-FID= gas chromatography/flame ionisation detector.

Although abundant chemical compounds have been isolated from oregano, the most important group, from a commercial and practical point of view, refers to its volatile oils basically composed of terpenoids [9]. The essential oils, or the volatile oils, are aromatic oily liquids extracted from various parts of the plants, such as the flowers, buds, seeds, leaves, stems, bark, wood, fruits and roots [54]. They are water steam-volatile distilled or organic-solvent (ethanol, methanol, toluene, or other organic solvents) extracts and have been used habitually for millennia in several areas worldwide. However, only a few essential oils have useful antibacterial properties. The most used are thymol, trans-cinnamaldhyde, carvacrol and eugenol [55].

The herbs of *Origanum* genus are rich in essential oils and contain large amounts of phenols, lipids, fatty acids, flavonoids and anthocyanins [49]. Flavonoids and phenolic acids from oregano have been reported with antioxidant properties [56]. These compounds can be extracted using different polar solvents like water, methanol and ethanol to obtain antioxidant-rich extracts. The antioxidant activity of the herbs depends on many factors, including the type of herbs, the methods and conditions of cultivation, harvesting, post-harvesting processing and subsequent processing [57]. The oregano plant was reported to have antioxidant activity [58]. The phenolic compounds, flavonoids [59] and phenolic acids, protect the dietary oil against oxidation [60].

Table 2 shows the major constituents of *Origanum vulgare* from plant and essential oil used in our feeding trials versus those reported in different studies. The major volatile compounds quantified determined in the oregano plants grown at Livezeni, Romania (Table 2), are sabinene (56.57%) and eucalyptol (12.27%). A research who evaluated the chemical composition of the oregano plants depending on the stage of development at harvesting reported high levels of sabinene, 20.13%, respectively [72]. These authors showed that the essential oil obtained from blooming flowers has no carvacrol. They also concluded that the developmental stage of the plant at harvesting is of major importance for the chemical composition, the best moment being the stage of full bloom.

The carvacrol percentage in the oregano essential oil is highly dependent on the *Origanum* species, the extraction method, storage conditions, and laboratory method analysis [73]. These primary components could be present in different proportions depending on the species, on the climate and growing conditions [74]. As the Table 2 shows, the literature data on major volatile compounds of oregano is varied.

The composition of oregano essential oil in individual components is variable [10]. Oregano essential oil usually contains large amounts of various compounds such as terpenes, alcohols, acetones, phenols, acids, aldehydes and esters [75]. These substances play a protective role against bacterial, fungal or insect attacks. Consequently, the essential oregano oils are safe mixtures of natural oils [76].

The monoterpene phenols: thymol and carvacrol, together with γ -terpinene and p-cymene are the main components in many essential oils of *Laminaceae* family plant. Thymol and carvacrol are biosynthesized by aromatization of γ -terpinene to p-cymene followed by hydroxylation of p-cymene [77]. Carvacrol (2-methyl-5-(1-methlethyl) phenol) is a hydrophobic phenolic compound synthesized from p-cymene and α-terpinene [78]. Carvacrol, thymol, γ -terpinene, and linalool are known to possess strong antioxidant properties [79, 80] and carvacrol and thymol also exhibit antibacterial activity against several bacteria [81–84]. These compounds can interact with some cellular structures causing the inhibition of the cell growth or cell death [85], are responsible for the driving force of protons, electron flow, active transport, and coagulation of cell contents [86, 87].

The other essential oil compounds also show variable concentrations in the samples analysed. The analysis conducted in Romania (Table 2), revealed high concentrations of two monoterpene hydrocarbons, p-cymene (20.75%) and γ-terpinene (4.45%), which support the strong antioxidant properties of the oregano oil [88], and which account for about 5-7% of its total [89]. These results are in agreement with those reported in other study [90], in which has been identified large amounts of p-cymene and γ-terpinene in the essential oregano oil. It was analysed the chemical composition of the essential oregano oil, and reported 0.9% α-pinene, 1.2% β-pinene, 0.1% α-phellandrene, 4.0% p-cymene, 1.5% limonene, 5.6% γ-terpinene, 1.5% linalool, 0.1% camphor and 5.4% caryophyllene oxide [22].

The essential oregano oil used in the experimental diets formulated for broilers reared under heat stress, also contained other volatile compounds: 1.33% α-pinene, 0.21% α-phellandrene; 1.10% limonene; 1.19% caryophyllene oxide (Table 8). In another study [47], it was analysed the essential oregano oil and reported 0.22% α-pinene; 0.08% α-phellandrene; 0.19% limonene; 0.29% caryophyllene oxide.

STUDIES REGARDING THE USE OF OREGANO IN BROILER DIETS

Effect of the Dietary Oregano on Broilers Reared under Normal Environmental Temperatures

The replacement of antibacterial growth promoters with other efficient, safe, and natural substances is a crucial point for the poultry industry, especially in broiler-meat production [10]. Many natural compounds used as alternatives to antibiotics in animal feed have shown positive effects on growth performance and on different health parameters [2, 91, 92]. Since poultry adjust strongly their feed intake according to the demand of energy, feed conversion ratio is therefore a very sensitive parameter in responses to growth promoters [93]. Natural feed ingredients have shown beneficial impacts on the cell wall of the gastrointestinal tract, intestinal functions, the overall productivity of birds, meat quality and storage safety [94]. Some studies [95–97] show essential oils to be a promising alternative to growth promoter antibiotics (e.g., avilamycin) in improving chicken production. Table 3 shows some effects of essential oils on physiological actions.

Table 3. Effects of essential oils on animal physiology [98]

Effect	Physiological action
Intensification of taste	Impulses to central nervous system
Increased secretion of digestive juices	Improved digestion
Increased activity of digestive enzymes	Improved nutrient digestion and absorption
Inhibition of oxidative processes	Reduced level of peroxides in the gut intestinal tract
Inhibition of growth of bacteria and fungi in feed and gut intestinal tract	Reduction of toxins

The mechanisms by which the phytobiotics exert their benefits on the gut remain unclear, but possible mechanisms might be proposed as follows: (i) modulating the cellular membrane of microbes; (ii) membrane disruption of the pathogens, (iii) increasing the hydrophobicity of the microbial species which may influence the surface characteristics of microbial cells and thereby affect the virulence properties of the microbes, (iv) stimulating the growth of favourable bacteria such as lactobacilli and bifidobacteria in the gut, (v) acting as an immunostimulatory substance and (vi) protecting the intestinal tissue from microbial attack [99, 100].

Based on the chemical characterisation of oregano, so far, some encouraging experimental results were reported for broilers [101]. Furthermore, the combination of the potential effects of the dietary supplementation with oregano oil, beneficial in terms of production and harmful in terms of welfare, suggests that it is important to investigate its potential consequences on the feeding behaviour of farm animals. Oregano can be added to the feed as dried plant, as essential oil (alone or in mixture with other plant essential oils), or used as a source of carvacrol and thymol [10]. Oregano oil is generally recognized as safe by the United States Food and Drug Administration and has beneficial effects on the intestinal microflora [102], feed utilization [103, 104], and digestive enzymes stimulation [105].

The literature review shows a great variability on the effectiveness of different doses of dietary plant inclusion. Thus, supplementation with oregano (essential oil or powder) was shown to improve growth performance of poultry [97, 106] Also, it was reported [106] that the gradual introduction of the oregano plant and its oil into diets reduced the average daily fed intake and significantly improved the feed conversion ratio of chicks compared to the control group that received a conventional diet formulation. This is due to the capacity of aromatic compounds and essential oils to act along the animal digestive tract to improve appetite, bacterial modulation, and is able to induce a number of benefits on well being [107]. In other study, other authors [108] showed that the bodyweight, average daily weight gain and feed conversion ratio improved in the broilers treated with dry oregano (5 g/kg) as unique supplement, or in combination with α-tocopheryl acetate. Essential oil from oregano (*Origanum vulgare L.*), mixed in different portions with essential oil from clove (*Syzgium aromaticum*) and anise (*Pimpinella anisum L.*) could be used in broiler nutrition as a potential natural growth promoter for poultry [16].

Other studies have shown significant improvements on the bioproductive parameters for broilers along with the inclusion of oregano oil in diets [109]. It was reported [97] that adding oregano essential oil (*Origanum genus*) at 300 and 600 mg/kg in broiler chicken feed increased average daily gain. According to the authors, this result may be related to increased villus height and decreased crypt depth in the jejunum of broiler chicken. In addition, the administration of 600 mg/kg of feed of oregano essential oil improved the percentage of thigh muscle and decreased abdominal fat percentage in broiler chickens (1-42 days). Feeding broilers with diet containing oregano essential oil (250 mg/kg) increased body weight and gain compared with the control containing no antibacterial or anticoccidial additives [110]. Other authors [111] investigated the effects of different essential oils (oregano, anise, fennel, black cumin), included in Ross 308 broiler (1-42 days) diets at levels of 125 and 250 mg/kg, on growth performance. They reported higher body weights and weight gain when 250 mg/kg oregano essential oil was added to broiler diet compared to those fed with other oils or to chickens not treated with essential oils, both at the end of the breeding stage and during the growth stages. The lowest feed conversion ratio was recorded at chickens with oregano essential oil included in amount of 250 ppm. The oregano essential oil leads to the improvement of nutritional and bioproductive indexes in broiler chickens as compared to the use of other essential oils. Another researcher team [112] showed that supplementation of broiler Ross 308 diets with 600 and 1200 mg/kg oregano essential oil significantly improved feed conversion ratio compared with the control in either grower or overall experimental periods. Recently, the use of Mexican oregano oil (0.4 g/kg) in chicken diets improved feed efficiency rate, body weight and high-density lipoproteins in broiler chickens [113].

However, several studies [102, 114] reported that oregano had no significant effect on animal performance. It was also observed no effect of oregano (different levels of dried oregano leaves) on Cobb 500 broiler performance during the starter phase [115]. They compared two levels of inclusion of 2.5 to 20 g/kg of oregano leaves with 55 mg/kg penicillin and noticed that diets supplemented with oregano leaves did not influence the final weight (kg), the feed conversion ratio (kg feed/kg gain) or the mortality rate. The authors concluded that a higher level of oregano have to be included into the diets to obtain stronger positive results from. In the same way, it was observed that the performance of birds fed with dietary 50 and 100 mg of oregano essential oil /kg feed was unaffected by the experimental diets [88]. Similar finding has also been reported by other researchers, who were found that the levels of 150 and 300 mg/kg dietary oregano essential oil did not improve performance in chickens [116]. This finding is very similar to another study [117] who investigated the effect of a product (Biostrong 510, Delacon, Steyregg, Austria), consisting in a mixture of essential oils with thymol and anethole as lead active components and phytoadditives including herbs and spices on the growth performance and ileal digestibility of nutrients of Cobb 500 broilers.

On the other hand, oregano (*Origanum vulgare*) exerted *in vitro* antimicrobial and bactericidal action [100]. Oregano essential oil is very active against moulds especially aflatoxigenic strains and foodborne bacteria such as *Aspergillus niger*, *Aspergillus flavus*, *Aspergillus ochraceus*, *Staphylococcus aureus*, *Salmonella typhimurium*, *Campylohacter jejuni* and *Clostridiurn sporogenes* [118]. Several authors showed that oregano has the potential to enhance broiler performance and to reduce the bacterial populations from the gastrointestinal tract, such as *Clostridium perfringens* and *Escherichia coli* [108, 112].

Other authors [119] investigated the essential oregano oil inclusion on intestinal properties (the number of *Escherichia coli* and Lactobacilli) in Ross 308 broilers diet. The supplementation of experimental diets with oregano oil resulted in a significant decrease ($P \leq 0.05$) of the *E. coli* populations compared to the control diet, but for the total number of Lactobacilli was not different between the treatments. Other studies too, determined the inhibitory effects of essential oils against pathogens such as *C. perfringens* or *E. coli* [120]. The reduction of the number of pathogenic bacteria in the intestine increased the intestinal absorption capacity.

Effect of Using Oregano in the Diet of Broilers Reared under Heat Stress (Own Studies)

Broilers may be exposed to a variety of stressors during transport from the production farms to the processing facilities, including thermal challenges of the microenvironment, acceleration, vibration, motion, impacts, fasting, withdrawal of water, social disruption, and noise [121, 122]. Under stressful conditions, young animals suffer from changes in the composition and activity of the gut microbiota [123, 124]. As part of this complex combination of factors, thermal stress, in particular heat stress, plays a major role, which causes major economic losses to the poultry industry. The ideal temperature for poultry is 25- 30°C for optimum body weight and 15-27°C for feed efficiency. The gastrointestinal tract is particularly responsive to stressors such as heat stress, which modify the normal and protective microbiota [125] and decrease the integrity of the intestinal epithelium [126], impairing the productive performance of animals.

Along with stressor factor, diet and age have also a major influence on the composition of the gut bacterial community of broilers [93]. Different natural agents are used to minimize the harmful effects of heat stress on performance of broilers. At present, oregano (*Origanum vulgare L.*) is one of the many plants that are used as supplements in animal's diets for its above-mentioned beneficial activity, but there are not many studies on its effect on broilers reared under heat stress conditions. For this reason, a project entitled "Efficient feeding solutions for the preservation of gut health in broiler reared under heat stress," run by IBNA (National Institute for Biology and Animal Nutrition), Balotesti, Romania, studied the effects of several phytoadditives (plants and essential oils), added to the diets of broilers reared under heat stress (32°C) on performance and gut health. Oregano was among the investigated plants used as powder as well as essential oil.

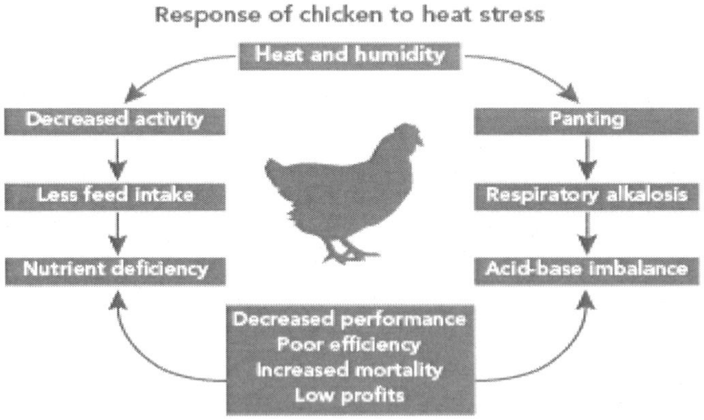

Source: https://www.viv.net/articles/blog/heat-stress-an-integrated-approach.

Figure 1. Response of chicken to heat stress.

The plant cultivated by a Romanian producer of medicinal herbs in Livezeni, Romania (46.55°N latitude, 24.63°E longitude) was harvested at late developmental stage. The landscape from the area of harvesting is hilly, fragmented by long valleys and high hills, with a temperate climate (warm summer and cold winters) and a layer of black, brown acid, colluvial soils, cernosiom and regosols. The average annual rainfall reaches 663 mm. The harvested plant was *Origani herba* (consisting of stems, branched stems, leaves and inflorescence). The plant material was conditioned by drying in thin layers, for three weeks, in darkness, at an environmental temperature of 20°C. from about 2.5 kg fresh plant material, resulting 1 kg of dried oregano. After drying, plant material was ground to produce the oregano powder which was included as such into the feed formulation.

Data on the chemical composition of the oregano powder used in our study are presented in Table 1 and 2 mentioned above.

The effect of oregano powder was evaluated in a study [46], carried out on 64, day-old Cobb 500, chicks, weighed individually and housed in an experimental hall where temperature was increased and maintained at 32°C and 23h light regimen. During the starter phase (1-14 days), all chicks received a commercial diet without oregano supplementation. Heat stress did not influence the performance of broiler during this phase [46].

Table 4. Formulation and composition of the broiler chicken diet [46]

Ingredient	**Grower phase (14 – 35 days)**	
	Control diet	**Oregano powder diet**
Corn, %	59.8	56
Soybean meal, %	28.2	28.83
Gluten, %	5	5
Plant oil, %	3.3	4.47
Lysine, %	0.24	0.23
Methionine, %	0.22	0.23
Choline, %	0.05	0.05
Calcium carbonate, %	0.54	0.53
Monocalcium phosphate, %	1.33	1.33
Salt, %	0.32	0.33
Premix, %	1	1
Oregano powder, %	-	2
Total	**100**	**100**
*Chemical composition determined**		
Dry matter, %	87.29	87.61
Crude protein, %	21.15	21.22
Ether extractives, %	5.37	6.35
Crude fibre, %	3.42	4.02
Ash, %	5.50	4.90

1kg premix for group C (in both stages) contains: = 1100000 UI/kg vit. A; 200000 UI/kg vit. D3; 2700 UI/kg vit. E; 300 mg/kg Vit. K; 200 mg/kg Vit. B1; 400 mg/kg Vit. B2; 1485 mg/kg pantothenic acid; 2700 mg/kg nicotinic acid; 300 mg/kg Vit. B6; 4 mg/kg Vit. B7; 100 mg/kg Vit. B9; 1.8 mg/kg Vit. B12; 2000 mg/kg Vit. C; 8000 mg/kg manganese; 8000 mg/kg iron; 500 mg/kg copper; 6000 mg/kg zinc; 37 mg/kg cobalt; 152 mg/kg iodine; 18 mg/kg selenium; 50 g sodium monensin /kg.

*Chemical composition on dry matter (DM) basis.

This paper presented the investigations carried out during grower phase (14-35 days). Chicks were weighed, assigned to two groups (32 chicks/group) and housed in the same experimental hall, where the temperature was maintained at 32°C, with 36% humidity and 23h light regimen throughout entire experimental period. The chicks had free access to the water and feed. Compared to the diet formulation for the control group (control diet), a commercial one, the formulations for the experimental group included 2% dry oregano powder (oregano powder diet) (Table 4). Broiler performance (bodyweight, weight gain, feed intake and feed conversion ratio) were monitored throughout the experimental period. At the end of the feeding trial, 6 chicks from each group were slaughtered and samples of intestinal content were collected for bacteriological assessment (determination of the *Enterobacteriaceae*, *E. coli* and Lactic acid bacteria).

The results of the chemical analysis of the oregano powder diet revealed a high level of crude fibre (Table 4). Therefore, the compound feeds used during the grower phase, which included 2% dry oregano had high levels of crude fibre, because as it can be seen in Table 1, oregano had a high level of crude fibre, respectively, 37.58 g/100g.

Table 5. Effect of the dietary oregano powder on broiler performance (14-35 days) [46]

Parameters	Period (days)	Control diet	Oregano powder diet	SEM	p-value
Bodyweight (g)	14	412	392.083	4.831	0.2568
	35	2016.923	1876.667	29.748	0.0820
Average daily feed intake (g/chick/day)	14-35	106.523^{a}	102.433^{b}	1.286	0.0141
Average daily weight gain (g/chick/day)	14-35	73.714	70.207	1.813	0.3808
Feed conversion ratio (g feed/g gain)	14-35	1.538	1.569	0.042	0.7393

Where: $^{a-b}$ Mean values within a row having different superscripts are significantly different, using the least significant difference test (P<0.05). SEM: standard error of the mean.

Table 5 shows the effect of the dietary oregano powder on broiler performance (14-35 days). Under thermal stress condition, oregano diet decreased slightly broiler weight and average weight gain and significantly decreased daily average feed intake. However, the feed conversion was not affected. No mortalities were recorded in any of the two groups throughout the experimental weeks under heat stress. Similarly, other authors [106] reported that graded amounts of oregano and its essential oil reduced the daily feed intake of broilers and significantly improved feed conversion compared with that of control birds. By contrast, investigating different levels of dietary oregano (2.5-7.5 g/kg feed), it was demonstrated that the bodyweight, average daily weight gain and feed conversion ratio improved in the broilers treated with 5 g/kg dry oregano administrated alone or in combination with α-tocopheryl acetate [108]. However, oregano effects were higher at 5.0 and 7.5 g/kg, than at 2.5 and 10.0 g/kg [108].

Table 6 data show a significant ($P \leq 0.05$) decrease of ileal populations of *Enterobacteriaceae* colony-forming units in the group fed diet with 2% oregano than in control group. Very important is the fact that oregano powder diet increased significantly ($P \leq 0.05$) the number of lactic acid bacteria which are known for preserving the balance of the gut microbiota.

Table 6. Effect of the dietary oregano powder on the ileal microbial population of broilers (lg_{10} CFU*/g wet digesta) [46]

Parameters	Control diet	Oregano powder diet	SEM	p-value
Enterobacteriaceae, lg_{10}	7.252^{a}	7.205^{b}	0.009	0.0941
Escherichia coli, lg_{10}	5.600^{a}	5.613^{a}	0.089	0.6935
Lactic acid bacteria, lg_{10}	6.312^{a}	6.806^{b}	0.109	0.0115

Where: *CFU- colony forming units;

$^{a\text{-}b}$ Mean values within a row having different superscripts are significantly different, using the least significant difference test (P<0.05). SEM: standard error of the mean.

Table 7. Formulation and composition of the broiler chicken diet [127]

Ingredients	Grower phase (14 – 35 days)		Finisher phase (35 – 42 days)	
	Control diet	Oregano essential oil diet	Control diet	Oregano essential oil diet
Corn, %	62	62	60.45	60.45
Soybean meal, %	26.58	26.57	25.54	25.53
Oil %	2.5	2.5	3.72	3.72
Oregano Oil, %	-	*0.01*	-	*0.01*
Gluten %	4	4	6	6
Methionine, %	0.26	0.26	0.25	0.25
Lysine, %	0.48	0.48	0.2	0.2
Carbonate, %	1.4	1.4	1.33	1.33
Monocalcium phosphate, %	1.36	1.36	1.13	1.13
Salt, %	0.37	0.37	0.33	0.33
Choline, %	0.05	0.05	0.05	0.05
Vitamin-mineral premix* with coccidiostat, %	1	-	-	-
Vitamin-mineral premix without coccidiostat, %	-	1	1	1
Total	100	100	100	100
Chemical composition - calculated				
Dry matter, %	87.70	87.92	89.60	90.53
Organic matter, %	82.17	82.86	84.81	85.50
Crude protein, %	20.51	21.77	19.40	19.07
Ether extractives, %	4.13	4.30	5.59	5.65
Fibre, %	3.49	3.81	3.53	3.98
Ash, %	5.53	5.06	4.79	5.03
Nitrogen-free extractives, %	54.04	52.98	56.29	56.80
Calcium, mg/kg DM	0.84	0.85	0.85	0.84
Phosphorus, mg/kg DM	0.84	0.75	0.85	0.88

*1kg premix vitamin-mineral contains: = 1.350.000 IU/kg vit. A; 300.000 IU/kg vit. D3; 2700 IU/kg vit. E; 200 mg/kg Vit. K; 200 mg/kg Vit. B1; 480 mg/kg Vit. B2; 1485 mg/kg pantothenic acid; 2700 mg/kg nicotinic acid; 300 mg/kg Vit. B6; 4 mg/kg Vit. B7; 100 mg/kg Vit. B9; 1.8 mg/kg Vit. B12; 2500 mg/kg Vit. C; 7190 mg/kg manganese; 6000 mg/kg iron; 600 mg/kg copper; 6000 mg/kg zinc; 50 mg/kg cobalt; 114 mg/kg iodine; 18 mg/kg selenium; 50 g sodium monensin /kg.

The results are in agreement with other author's results which showed that the supplementation of experimental broilers with 300 and 600 mg/kg, essential oregano oil, under thermoneutral conditions, significantly lowered the viable counts of caecal *E. coli* compared with both the control and with the 1200 mg/kg essential oregano oil supplemented group [112].

A second feeding experiment on Cobb 500 broiler chicks, reared under heat stress, evaluated the effect of the oregano (*Origanum vulgare L.*) essential oil on broiler performance and balance of the intestinal microflora. The study used 64, 1-day-old Cobb 500 chicks, weighed individually and housed in an experimental hall with high constant temperature (32°C), humidity 36% and 23 h light regimen. During the starter phase (1-14 days), all chicks received a commercial diet formulation with corn and soybean meal as basic ingredients and the results show that the stress temperature produced did not affect the broiler performance. In this paper we presented the investigations carried out during grower (14-35 days) and finisher phase (35-42 days). Unlike the control group, the diet for the experimental group (oregano essential oil diet) included 0.01% oregano essential oil (Table 7).

The essential oregano oil was purchased from China, Jiangxi Xuesong Natural Medicinal Oil Co., Ltd., and was analysed for its profile of volatile compounds (Table 8). The chicks had free access to the water and feed. Throughout the experimental period from 14 to 42 days, body weight gain was recorded weekly and feed intake was recorded daily. Six broilers/ group were slaughtered in the end of the experiment (42 days), and samples of caecal and intestinal content were collected for bacteriological examination.

Table 8. Volatile compounds identified in oregano essential oil [61]

Compounds	CAS number	Essential oil (%)
α-Pinene	80-56-8	1.33
Camphene	79-92-5	
Sabinene	3387-41-5	
β-Pinene	127-91-3	1.79
β-Myrcene	123-35-3	
α-Phellandrene	99-83-2	0.21
p-Cymene	99-87-6	20.75
Limonene	138-86-3	1.10
Eucalyptol (1,8-Cineole)	470-82-6	
E-β-Ocimene	3779-61-1	
γ-terpinene	99-85-4	4.45
cis-Sabinene hydrate	15826-82-1	
α-Terpinolene	586-62-9	0.98
Linalool	78-70-6	1.19
Camphor	76-22-2	0.14
Estragole	140-67-0	0.85
Carvacrol	499-75-2	59.08
Caryophyllene	87-44-5	6.95
Germacrene D	23986-74-5	
Caryophyllene oxide	1139-30-6	1.19

Where CAS- Chemical Abstract Service.

Table 9 shows the volatile profile of oregano essential oil used in this study, data published in a previous paper of this research team [61]. The GC/MS profile of oregano essential oil revealed the presence of 13 identified molecules belonging to different chemical classes: carvacrol (59.08%), as principal constituent and an oxygenated monoterpene, which according to some authors [128], forms 81.9% of the oil. These data are in agreement with the data of other authors who studied the composition of oregano essential oil purchased from Guangzhou, China and identified carvacrol as major constituent [129].

Other volatile compounds have also been identified in the composition of the oregano essential oil used in the experimental diet formulations: 1.33% α-pinene, 0.21% α-phellandrene; 1.10% limonene; 1.19% caryophyllene oxide (Table 8).

Previous analyses of the authors of the present study on oregano and other phytochemicals (blueberry, nettle extract) showed that the oregano and blueberry extracts have about the same concentration of polyphenols (564.10 mg gallic acid equivalent/100 mL, respectively, 570.02 mg gallic acid equivalent/100 mL), but the oregano extract has almost two times more flavonoids (396.49 mg equivalent catechin/100 mL vs. 204.26 mg equivalent catechin/100 mL for blueberry extract). The oregano alcoholic extract displayed the strongest reducing power (80.8 mM FeSO4 equivalent /100mL; the nettle alcoholic extract had the lowest reducing power (13 mM FeSO4 equivalent /100mL, while the blueberry alcoholic extract also had a strong reducing power (49 FeSO4 equivalent /100mL. Analysing the antioxidant capacity and phenolic content of six *Labiatae* spices (oregano, sage, thyme, rosemary, mint, sweet basil), it was indicated that the total antioxidant capacity and phenolic content decreased in the following order: oregano > sage >thyme > rosemary > mint > sweet basil [130]. Oregano exhibited the most powerful antioxidant capacity among the five *Labiatae* spices, over 3-fold greater than sweet basil. In a comparative screening of three medicinal plants oregano, lavender and lemon balm, other researchers [131] also showed that oregano and lavender extracts present the most effective antioxidant capacity in scavenging DPPH radicals. The oregano alcoholic extract inhibited the superoxide anion. This anion, which resulted from enzymatic processes, is not very aggressive, but it can generate, in the presence of water, the most aggressive free radical, the hydroxyl radical. The hydroxyl radical is highly unstable and, in order to be stabilized, it can take a hydrogen atom from various organic molecules (lipids, proteins, nucleic acids), generating chain reactions (radical mechanism) of oxidation in those molecules. The nitric oxide is synthesized in cells under the action of nitric oxide synthase enzyme and has the ability of reacting very rapidly with the superoxide anion to form peroxinitrite (ONOO-), which is an oxidant with similar properties with the hydroxyl radical. The nettle extract showed the strongest power of inhibition against to the nitric oxide (57.47%) vs. oregano (54.79%) and blueberry extract (10.73%). Oregano and blueberry extracts had good inhibition power against the hydrogen peroxide (30.92%, respectively, 20.23%), but the nettle alcoholic extract was the best (32.77%).

Table 9 shows the effect of dietary oregano essential oil on broiler performance (14-42 days). The results published by some authors [127] showed that dietary supplementation with oregano essential oil (0.01%) had an increasing effect on growth performance of broilers reared under heat stress (32° C). The final weight and the average daily weight gain of the broilers treated with 0.01% oregano oil was different from that of control group and from those obtained in the first feeding experiment in which entire oregano plant was used.

Table 9. Effect of the dietary oregano essential oil on broiler performance (14-42 days) [127]

Parameter	Control diet	Oregano essential oil diet	SEM	p-value
Initial weight (g)	318.96	301.18	5.989	0.544
Final weight (g)	1873.21	2128.46	5.161	0.167
Average daily weight gain (g)	51.88	60.79	1.683	0.139
Average daily fed intake (g feed/broiler/day)	80.05	88.54	2.804	0.650
Feed conversion ratio (kg feed/kg gain)	2.18	2.33	0.122	0.759

SEM: standard error of the mean.

In another study [110] it was investigated the effect of oregano essential oil 250 mg /kg of diet (*Origanum vulgare L., ssp. hirtum*) in broiler diets, alone or in combination with vitamin C (200 mg/kg) under heat stress conditions (38 °C). The authors showed an increased average daily gain, bodyweight and a reduced feed efficiency ($P<0.05$) in the birds fed with diets including vitamin C and oregano essential oil (alone or in combination), compared to those fed the basal diet. Average daily feed intake was not significantly influenced by dietary oregano essential oil and vitamin C ($P>0.05$). Other researchers [132] investigated the effects of adding dietary oregano (*Origanum syriacum*) essential oil (100, 300, 600 mg/kg) to improve performance parameters and improve intestinal histology and microflora of broilers both at normal temperature (22°C) and under heat-stress conditions (36°C). The study found that adding oregano essential oil into the diet provided a similar effect to that of the antibiotic, even at the 600 mg/kg dose. Under thermoneutral conditions, it was reported [133] also the effect of two levels (0.005 and 0.01% in feed) of oregano oil on broiler performance and found that, during the first and second weeks of age, both doses had a significant effect on body weight gain compared with birds reared on a control (antibiotic free) diet. The results are in contradiction with other reports [134, 135] on the use of oregano in chicken diets for which the authors found no difference on the average body weight and feed conversion.

Improvements in growth indices and production was explained through the significant effect of oregano on the gut structure [136]. The authors investigated the effect of oregano oil on the fasted broiler intestinal morphology and observed a significant increase of crypt depth and villi height in the ileum after nine hours fasting, which could be indirectly correlated with the increase of intestinal permeability.

Numerous microbiological analysis on the gut was done in the broiler chickens. The two main sites of microbial activity are the crop and the caecum [137], although microbe-host interactions elsewhere in the digestive tract may have important consequences for health [138]. The antimicrobial properties of essential oils and extracts can be dose-dependent bacteriostatic and/or bactericidal [93]. Due to the hydroxyl group present in the structure of phenolic compounds from oregano oil, carvacrol is one of the most active plants extract against pathogens [139].

Table 10. The effect of *Origanum vulgare L.* essential oil in the diet of broilers (14-42d) on intestinal microbiota composition (lg_{10} CFU*/g wet intestinal digesta) [61]

Parameters	Control diet	Oregano essential oil diet	SEM	p-value
Enterobacteriaceae, lg_{10}	7.349^a	7.337^b	0.009	<0.0001
E. coli, lg_{10}	6.070^a	5.994^b	0.014	<0.0001
Staphylococci, lg_{10}	5.886^a	5.863^b	0.006	<0.0001
Lactobacilli, lg_{10}	6.406^a	6.978^b	0.082	<0.0001
Salmonella spp.	Absent	Absent	-	-

Where: *CFU- colony forming units; $^{a-b}$ Mean values within a row having different superscripts are significantly different by the least significant difference test (P<0.05); SEM: standard error of the mean.

Table 11. The effect of *Origanum vulgare L.* essential oil in the diet of broilers (14-42d) on caecal microbiota composition (lg_{10} CFU*/g wet caecal digesta) [61]

Parameters	Control diet	Oregano essential oil diet	SEM	p-value
Enterobacteriaceae, lg_{10}	11.360^a	11.331^b	0.009	<0.0001
E. coli, lg_{10}	10.106^a	10.086^b	0.007	<0.0001
Staphylococci, lg_{10}	8.804^a	8.775^b	0.008	<0.0001
Lactobacilli, lg_{10}	11.257^a	11.284^b	0.012	<0.0001
Salmonella spp.	Absent	Absent	-	-

Where: *CFU- colony forming units; $^{a-b}$ Mean values within a row having different superscripts are significantly different by the least significant difference test (P<0.05).; SEM: standard error of the mean.

The results of previously described IBNA experiment showed that the total *Enterobacteriaceae*, *E. coli* and *Staphylococci* count was significantly ($P \leq 0.05$) lower both in the intestinal and caecal microbiota of the experimental groups than in control group, while the lactobacilli count was significantly ($P \leq 0.05$) higher in oregano diet group than in control diet group (Table 10, 11). Oregano oil exert bactericidal effect due to the chemical composition rich in phenolic compounds which may cause damage in bacterial envelope a key element in the life of bacteria and many studies demonstrated this effect. A group of researchers [140] isolated band patterns from different chicken gut regions exposed to serious bacterial challenges, including the duodenum, jejunum, and ileum, relative to the caecum and colon at different ages and observed that the birds fed the oregano essential oil diets displayed a minor shift (62.7%) between these fore and hind gut compartments versus the control basal diet (without additives) group (53.7%). It was showed that the addition of oregano aqueous extract to broiler chickens improved body weight up to 36 d of age and increased total serum IgG [141]. *Lactobacilli spp.* numbers were elevated in the ileum and caecum in all groups supplemented with aqueous extract, while *Staphylococcus spp.* count was consistently lower in intestinal tracts from the aqueous extract supplemented birds. A significant lower number of *Escherichia coli* and *Clostridium perfringens* was found in broilers receiving dietary oregano oil compared to control diet [119, 120]. The total number of lactobacilli was not different between the treatments [119]. The reduction of the number of pathogenic bacteria in the intestine increased the intestinal absorption capacity [120].

With regard to the caecal microbiota, the results (Table 11) revealed that the inclusion of oregano (*Origanum vulgare L.*) oil (oregano essential oil diet) in broilers diet reduced the total number of *Enterobacteriaceae, E. coli and Staphylococci*, which was significantly ($P \leq 0.05$) lower compared to the control group, while the total number of lactobacilli was significantly ($P \leq 0.05$) higher in oregano diet group compared to the control diet group. Another group of researchers [112] evaluated the effect of the inclusion of oregano oil (*Origanum vulgare L.*) in diets for Ross 308 broilers reared under heat stress (34°C) and reported also a strong antibacterial effect of the oregano oil against caecal *E. coli*. Instead, others [5] pointed out the potentially adverse effects induced by the dietary essential oils on the healthy intestinal bacteria. These authors reported that the inclusion of oregano oil in broilers diet showed a strong bactericidal effect against isolated lactobacilli in manure samples. No populations of *Salmonella spp.* were identified in caecum microflora.

Acknowledgments

This work was supported by a grant of the Romanian Ministry of Education and Research (Project PN 19 09 0102).

Thank you to Dr. Ionelia Taranu, Head of Laboratory of Biology, from National Research-Development Institute for Animal Biology and Nutrition (INCDBNA- IBNA), Balotesti, Romania for the manuscript corrections.

Conclusion

The biological activity of volatile plant metabolites is the property that can find application in animal nutrition. Oregano, as powder or essential oil, contains a variety of functional bioactive compounds with antioxidant and antimicrobial activity and might be a promising feed additive in boh normal and heat stress conditions. The experimental results presented in this chapter demonstrated overall that, under heat stress, the dietary oregano (powder or essential oil) given to broiler chicks had a favourable action in maintaining the health of the intestinal tract, by preserving the balance of the populations of microorganisms colonizing the small intestine and the caecum. Moreover, oregano essential oil has a positive effect not only on the instestinal health but also on broiler performance under heat sress conditions and it is more efficient than the oregano plant. Further research is required, to determine the optimal level of oregano inclusion (as powder or essential oil) in broiler diets, which alleviates the adverse effects of the heat stress on broiler performance and on gut microflora balance. However, because oregano is used frecquently and appreciated as spice in human nutrition, this bears upon its use in animal feeding and also its dietary inclusion might increase the feeding cost.

REFERENCES

[1] Masoud Jafari, 2012. "Utilization of poultry by-product meal in diets for broiler chickens." *African Journal of Agricultural Reseearch*. 7 (9): 1425–1430. doi: https://doi.org/10.5897/AJAR11.1558.

[2] Windisch, W., Schedle, K., Plitzner, C. and Kroismayr, A. 2008. "Use of phytogenic products as feed additives for swine and poultry." *Journal of Animal Science*. 86 (suppl_14): E140–E148. doi: https://doi.org/10.2527/jas.2007-0459.

[3] Ruberto, G., Tiziana Baratta, M., Sari, M. and Kaâbeche, M. 2002. "Chemical composition and antioxidant activity of essential oils from Algerian Origanum glandulosum Desf." *Flavour and Fragrance Journal*. 17 (4): 251–254. doi: https://doi.org/10.1002/ffj.1101.

[4] Burt, S. 2004. "Essential oils: their antibacterial properties and potential applications in foods—a review." *International Journal of Food Microbiology*. 94 (3): 223–253. doi: https://doi.org/https://doi.org/10.1016/j.ijfoodmicro.2004.03.022.

[5] Horošová, K., Bujňáková, D. and Kmeť, V. 2006. "Effect of oregano essential oil on chicken Lactobacilli and E. coli." *Folia Microbiologica*. 51 (4): 278–280. doi: https://doi.org/10.1007/BF02931812.

[6] Cross, D. E., McDevitt, R. M., Hillman, K. and Acamovic, T. 2007. "The effect of herbs and their associated essential oils on performance, dietary digestibility and gut microflora in chickens from 7 to 28 days of age." *British Poultry Science*. 48 (4): 496–506. doi: https://doi.org/10.1080/00071660701463221.

[7] Puvača, N., Stanačev, V., Glamočič, D., Levič, J., Perič, L., Stanačev, V. and Milič, D. 2013. "Beneficial effects of phytoadditives in broiler nutrition." *World's Poultry Science Journal*. 69 (1): 27–34. doi: https://doi.org/10.1017/S0043933913000032.

[8] Cosge, B., Turker, A., Ipek, A. and Gurbuz, B. 2009. Chemical Compositions and Antibacterial Activities of the Essential Oils from Aerial Parts and Corollas of

Origanum acutidens (Hand.-Mazz.) Ietswaart, an Endemic Species to Turkey. *Molecules*.

[9] Kintzios, S. E. 2012. "Oregano." *Handbook of Herbs and Spices: Second Edition*. 2: 417–436. doi: https://doi.org/10.1533/9780857095688.417.

[10] Giannenas, I., Bonos, E., Skoufos, I., Tzora, A., Stylianaki, I., Lazari, D., Tsinas, A., Christaki, E. and Florou-Paneri, P. 2018. "Effect of herbal feed additives on performance parameters, intestinal microbiota, intestinal morphology and meat lipid oxidation of broiler chickens." *British Poultry Science*. 59 (5): 545–553. doi: https://doi.org/10.1080/00071668.2018.1483577.

[11] Martino, L. De, Feo, V. De, Formisano, C., Mignola, E. and Senatore, F. 2009. "Chemical composition and antimicrobial activity of the essential oils from three chemotypes of origanum vulgare l. ssp. hirtum (Link) ietswaart growing wild in campania (Southern Italy)." *Molecules*. 14 (8): 2735–2746. doi: https://doi.org/10.3390/molecules14082735.

[12] Teuscher, E., Anton, R. and Lobstein, A. 2005. *Plantes aromatiques*. [*Aromatic Plantes*]. Ed Tec & Doc.

[13] Béjaoui, A., Chaabane, H., Jemli, M., Boulila, A. and Boussaid, M. 2013. "Essential oil composition and antibacterial activity of Origanum vulgare subsp. glandulosum Desf. at different phenological stages." *Journal of medicinal food*. 16 (12): 1115–1120. doi: https://doi.org/10.1089/jmf.2013.0079.

[14] Lukas, B., Schmiderer, C. and Novak, J. 2015. "Essential oil diversity of European Origanum vulgare L. (Lamiaceae)." *Phytochemistry*. 119: 32–40. doi: https://doi.org/https://doi.org/10.1016/j.phytochem.2015.09.008.

[15] Teixeira, B., Marques, A., Ramos, C., Serrano, C., Matos, O., Neng, N. R., Nogueira, J. M. F., Saraiva, J. A. and Nunes, M. L. 2013. "Chemical composition and bioactivity of different oregano (Origanum vulgare) extracts and essential oil." *Journal of the Science of Food and Agriculture*. 93 (11): 2707–2714. doi: https://doi.org/10.1002/jsfa.6089.

[16] Ertas, O. N., Güler, T., Çiftçi, M., Dalkiliç, B. and Gülcihan Simsek, Ü. 2005. "The effect of an essential oil mix derived from oregano, clove and anise on broiler performance." *International Journal of Poultry Science*. 4 (11): 879–884. doi: https://doi.org/10.3923/ijps.2005.879.884.

[17] Cervato, G., Carabelli, M., Gervasio, S., Cittera, A., Cazzola, R. and Cestaro, B. 2000. "Antioxbdant Properties of Oregano (Origanum Vulgare) Leaf Extracts." *Journal of Food Biochemistry*. 24 (6): 453–465. doi: https://doi.org/10.1111/j.1745-4514.2000.tb00715.x.

[18] Chun, S. S., Vattem, D. A., Lin, Y. T. and Shetty, K. 2005. "Phenolic antioxidants from clonal oregano (Origanum vulgare) with antimicrobial activity against Helicobacter pylori." *Process Biochemistry*. 40 (2): 809–816. doi: https://doi.org/https://doi.org/10.1016/j.procbio.2004.02.018.

[19] Chishti, S., Kaloo, Z. A. and Sultan, P. 2013. "Medicinal importance of genus Rheum : A review." *Journal of Pharmacognosy and Phytotherapy*. 5 (10): 170–177. doi: https://doi.org/10.5897/JPP2013.0285.

[20] Skotti, E., Anastasaki, E., Kanellou, G., Polissiou, M. and Tarantilis, P. A. 2014. "Total phenolic content, antioxidant activity and toxicity of aqueous extracts from selected Greek medicinal and aromatic plants." *Industrial Crops and Products*. 53: 46–54. doi: https://doi.org/10.1016/j.indcrop.2013.12.013.

[21] Gupta, C. and Prakash, D. 2014. "Nutraceuticals for geriatrics." *Journal of traditional and complementary medicine*. 5 (1): 5–14. doi: https://doi.org/10.1016/j.jtcme.2014.10.004.

[22] Ličina, B. Z., Stefanović, O. D., Vasić, S. M., Radojević, I. D., Dekić, M. S. and Čomić, L. R. 2013. "Biological activities of the extracts from wild growing Origanum vulgare L." *Food Control*. 33 (2): 498–504. doi: https://doi.org/https://doi.org/10.1016/j.foodcont.2013.03.020.

[23] Kocić-Tanackov, S., Dimić, G., Tanackov, I., Pejin, D., Mojović, L. and Pejin, J. 2012. "The inhibitory effect of oregano extract on the growth of Aspergillus spp. and on sterigmatocystin biosynthesis." *LWT - Food Science and Technology*. 49 (1): 14–20. doi: https://doi.org/10.1016/j.lwt.2012.04.013.

[24] Fonseca, A. O. S., Pereira, D. I. B., Botton, S. A., Pötter, L., Sallis, E. S. V., Júnior, S. F. V., Filho, F. S. M., Zambrano, C. G., Maroneze, B. P., Valente, J. S. S., Baptista, C. T., Braga, C. Q., Ben, V. D. and Meireles, M. C. A. 2015. "Treatment of experimental pythiosis with essential oils of Origanum vulgare and Mentha piperita singly, in association and in combination with immunotherapy." *Veterinary Microbiology*. 178 (3): 265–269. doi: https://doi.org/https://doi.org/10.1016/j.vetmic.2015.05.023.

[25] Chia-Hua, L., Tzung-Han, C. and Hsiou-Yu, D. 2010. "Inhibition of melanogensis by a novel origanoside from Origanum vulgare." *Journal of Dermatological Science*. 57 (3): 170–177. doi: https://doi.org/https://doi.org/10.1016/j.jdermsci.2009.12.009.

[26] Marrelli, M., Cristaldi, B., Menichini, F. and Conforti, F. 2015. "Inhibitory effects of wild dietary plants on lipid peroxidation and on the proliferation of human cancer cells." *Food and Chemical Toxicology*. 86: 16–24. doi: https://doi.org/https://doi.org/10.1016/j.fct.2015.09.011.

[27] Zhang, X. L., Guo, Y. S., Wang, C. H., Li, G. Q., Xu, J. J., Chung, H. Y., Ye, W. C., Li, Y. L. and Wang, G. C. 2014. "Phenolic compounds from Origanum vulgare and their antioxidant and antiviral activities." *Food Chemistry*. 152: 300–306. doi: https://doi.org/https://doi.org/10.1016/j.foodchem.2013.11.153.

[28] Orhan, I. E., Mesaik, M. A., Jabeen, A. and Kan, Y. 2016. "Immunomodulatory properties of various natural compounds and essential oils through modulation of

human cellular immune response." *Industrial Crops and Products*. 81: 117–122. doi: https://doi.org/https://doi.org/10.1016/j.indcrop.2015.11.088.

[29] Gulluce, M., Karadayi, M., Guvenalp, Z., Ozbek, H., Arasoglu, T. and Baris, O. 2012. "Isolation of some active compounds from Origanum vulgare L. ssp. vulgare and determination of their genotoxic potentials." *Food Chemistry*. 130 (2): 248–253. doi: https://doi.org/10.1016/j.foodchem.2011.07.024.

[30] Bagheri Ziari, S., Naji, T. and Hosseinzadeh Sahafi, H. 2015. "Comparison of the effects of Origanum vulgare with LHRH-A2 and 17β-estradiol on the ultrastructure of gonadotroph cells and ovarian oogenesis in immature Trichogaster trichopterus." *Animal Reproduction Science*. 161: 32–39. doi: https://doi.org/https://doi.org/10.1016/j.anireprosci.2015.07.009.

[31] Sivropoulou, A., Papanikolaou, E., Nikolaou, C., Kokkini, S., Lanaras, T. and Arsenakis, M. 1996. "Antimicrobial and Cytotoxic Activities of Origanum Essential Oils." *Journal of Agricultural and Food Chemistry*. 44 (5): 1202–1205. doi: https://doi.org/10.1021/jf950540t.

[32] Christaki, E., Bonos, E., Giannenas, I. and Florou-Paneri, P. 2012. Aromatic Plants as a Source of Bioactive Compounds. *Agriculture*.

[33] Giannenas, I., Bonos, E., Christaki, E. and Florou-paneri, P. 2013. "Essential Oils and their Application in Animal Nutrition." *Med Aromat Plants*. 2 (6): 1–12. doi: https://doi.org/10.4172/2167-0412.1000140.

[34] Papatsiros, V. 2013. "Alternatives to antibiotics for farm animals." *CAB Reviews: Perspectives in Agriculture, Veterinary Science, Nutrition and Natural Resources*. 8 (032). doi: https://doi.org/10.1079/PAVSNNR20138032.

[35] Hancianu, M., Cioanca, O., Aprotosoaie, A. C. and Miro, A. 2014. *Plante medicinale de la A la Z*. Polirom.

[36] Russo, M., Galletti, G. C., Bocchini, P. and Carnacini, A. 1998. "Essential Oil Chemical Composition of Wild Populations of Italian Oregano Spice (Origanum vulgare ssp. hirtum (Link) Ietswaart): A Preliminary Evaluation of Their Use in Chemotaxonomy by Cluster Analysis. 1. Inflorescences." *Journal of Agricultural and Food Chemistry*. 46 (9): 3741–3746. doi: https://doi.org/10.1021/jf980087w.

[37] Ortega-Ramirez, L. A., Rodriguez-Garcia, I., Silva-Espinoza, B. A. and Ayala-Zavala, J. F. 2015. *Oregano (Origanum spp.) oils*. Elsevier Inc.

[38] Koukoulitsa, C., Karioti, A., Bergonzi, M. C., Pescitelli, G., Di Bari, L. and Skaltsa, H. 2006. "Polar Constituents from the Aerial Parts of Origanum vulgare L. Ssp. hirtum Growing Wild in Greece." *Journal of Agricultural and Food Chemistry*. 54 (15): 5388–5392. doi: https://doi.org/10.1021/jf061477i.

[39] Baranauskienė, R., Venskutonis, P. R., Dambrauskienė, E. and Viškelis, P. 2013. "Harvesting time influences the yield and oil composition of Origanum vulgare L. ssp. vulgare and ssp. hirtum." *Industrial Crops & Products*. 49 (Complete): 43–51. doi: https://doi.org/10.1016/j.indcrop.2013.04.024.

[40] Martins, N., Barros, L., Santos-Buelga, C., Henriques, M., Silva, S. and Ferreira, I. C. F. R. 2014. "Decoction, infusion and hydroalcoholic extract of Origanum vulgare L.: Different performances regarding bioactivity and phenolic compounds." *Food Chemistry*. 158: 73–80. doi: https://doi.org/https://doi.org/10.1016/j.foodchem. 2014.02.099.

[41] Vallverdu-Queralt, Regueiro, A., Alvarenga, J., Rinaldi, J. F., Martinez-Huelamo, M., Leal, L. N. and Lamuela-Raventos, R. M. 2015. "Characterization of the phenolic and antioxidant profiles of selected culinary herbs and spices: caraway, turmeric, dill, marjoram and nutmeg." *Food Science and Technology*. 35: 189–195.

[42] Antal, D., Citu, C., Ardelean, F., Dehelean, C., Vlaia, L., Soica, C., Vlaia, V., Biris, M. and Sas, I. 2015. "Metallome of Origanum Vulgare : the Unknown Side of a Medicinal and Aromatic Plant Used Worldwide." 63 (August).

[43] Sotiropoulou, D. E. and Karamanos, A. J. 2010. "Field studies of nitrogen application on growth and yield of Greek oregano (Origanum vulgare ssp. hirtum (Link) Ietswaart)." *Industrial Crops and Products*. 32 (3): 450–457. doi: https://doi.org/https://doi.org/10.1016/j.indcrop.2010.06.014.

[44] Zagula, G., Fabisiak, A., Bajcar, M., Czernicka, M, Saletnik, B. and Puchalski, C. 2016. "Mineral components analysis of selected dried herbs." 5 (2): 121–124.

[45] Dhillon, G. K., Kaur, A. and Ahluwalia, P. 2013. "Effect of Oregano Herb on Dough Rheology and Bread Quality." 4 (1): 17–26. doi: https://doi.org/10.19070/2326-3350-130008.

[46] Criste, R. D., Panaite, T. D., Tabuc, C., Saracila, M., Soica, C. and Olteanu, M. 2017. "Effect of Oregano and Rosehip Supplementson Broiler (14-35 Days) Performance, Carcass and Internal Organs Development and Gut Health." *Agrolife Scientific Journal*. 6 (1): 75–83.

[47] Bampidis, V. A., Christodoulou, V., Florou-Paneri, P., Christaki, E., Spais, A. B. and Chatzopoulou, P. S. 2005. "Effect of dietary dried oregano leaves supplementation on performance and carcass characteristics of growing lambs." *Animal Feed Science and Technology*. 121 (3–4): 285–295. doi: https://doi.org/ 10.1016/j.anifeedsci. 2005.02.002.

[48] Yousif, S. D. 2014. "Influence of Oregano (Origanum vulgare L.), Fennel (Foeniculum vulgare L.) and Hop cones (Humulus lupulus L.) on biogas and methane production.": 1–106.

[49] Kourimská, L., Ešlerová, K. and Khatri, Y. 2016. "The effect of storage on quality of herbs genus Origanum." *Potravinarstvo*. 10 (1): 207–214. doi: https://doi.org/10. 5219/608.

[50] Özcan, M. 2004. "Mineral contents of some plants used as condiments in Turkey." *Food Chemistry*. 84 (3): 437–440. doi: https://doi.org/10.1016/S0308-8146(03) 00263-2.

[51] Nielsen, F. H. 1984. "Ultratrace Elements in Nutrition." *Annual Review of Nutrition.* 4 (1): 21–41. doi: https://doi.org/10.1146/annurev.nu.04.070184.000321.

[52] Smith, K. 1988. *Trace Minerals in Foods.* Taylor & Francis.

[53] Macrae, R., Robinson, R. K. and Sadler, M. J. 1993. *Encyclopaedia of Food Science, Food Technology, and Nutrition: Malt-pesticides and herbicides.* Academic Press.

[54] Miguel, M. G. 2010. "Antioxidant activity of medicinal and aromatic plants. A review." *Flavour and Fragrance Journal.* 25 (5): 291–312. doi: https://doi.org/10.1002/ffj.1961.

[55] Mehdi, Y., Létourneau-Montminy, M. P., Gaucher, M. Lou, Chorfi, Y., Suresh, G., Rouissi, T., Brar, S. K., Côté, C., Ramirez, A. A. and Godbout, S. 2018. "Use of antibiotics in broiler production: Global impacts and alternatives." *Animal Nutrition.* 4 (2): 170–178. doi: https://doi.org/10.1016/j.aninu.2018.03.002.

[56] Leyva-López, N., Gutierrez-Grijalva, P. E., Ambriz-Perez, L. D. and Heredia, B. J. 2016. Flavonoids as Cytokine Modulators: A Possible Therapy for Inflammation-Related Diseases. *International Journal of Molecular Sciences.*

[57] Škrovánková, S., Mišurcová, L. and Machů, L. 2012. Chapter Three - Antioxidant Activity and Protecting Health Effects of Common Medicinal Plants. J. B. T. -A. in F. and N. R. Henry, ed. Academic Press. 75–139.

[58] Puertas-Mejía, M., Hillebrand, S., Stashenko, E. and Winterhalter, P. 2002. "In vitro radical scavenging activity of essential oils from Columbian plants and fractions from oregano (Origanum vulgare L.) essential oil." *Flavour and Fragrance Journal.* 17 (5): 380–384. doi: https://doi.org/10.1002/ffj.1110.

[59] El-Desoky, S. K., Kawashty, S. A. and Sharaf, M. 2008. "Two new flavonoids from Origanum vulgare AU - Hawas, Usama W." *Natural Product Research.* 22 (17): 1540–1543. doi: https://doi.org/10.1080/14786410600898987.

[60] Exarchou, V., Nenadis, N., Tsimidou, M., Gerothanassis, I. P., Troganis, A. and Boskou, D. 2002. "Antioxidant Activities and Phenolic Composition of Extracts from Greek Oregano, Greek Sage, and Summer Savory." *Journal of Agricultural and Food Chemistry.* 50 (19): 5294–5299. doi: https://doi.org/10.1021/jf020408a.

[61] Turcu, R., Tabuc, C., Vlaicu, Pa., Panaite, T., Buleandra, M. and Saracila, M. 2018. "Effect of the Dietary Oregano (Origanum Vulgare L.) Powder and Oil on the Performance, Carcass and Organs Development of Broilers Reared Under Heat Stress (32°C)." *Scientific Papers-Animal Science Series: Lucrări Ştiinţifice-Seria Zootehnie.* 69 (1): 69–207.

[62] Nurzyńska-wierdak, R. and Nata 2009. "Herb yield and chemical composition of common oregano (Origanum vulgare L.) essential oil according to the plant's developmental stage." *Herba Polonica.* 55 (3): 55–62.

[63] Al-Turki, A. I., El-Ziney, M. G. and Abdel-Salam, A. M. 2008. "Chemical and anti-bacterial characterization of aqueous extracts of oregano, marjoram, sage and

licorice and their application in milk and labneh." *Journal of Food, Agriculture and Environment*. 6 (1): 39–44.

[64] Vazirian, M., Mohammadi, M., Farzaei, M., Amin, G. and Amanzadeh, Y. 2015. "Chemical composition and antioxidant activity of Origanum vulgare subsp. vulgare essential oil from Iran." *Research Journal of Pharmacognosy*. 2 (1): 41–46.

[65] Baratta, M. T., Dorman, H. J. D., Deans, S. G., Biondi, D. M. and Ruberto, G. 1998. "Chemical Composition, Antimicrobial and Antioxidative Activity of Laurel, Sage, Rosemary, Oregano and Coriander Essential Oils." *Journal of Essential Oil Research*. 10 (6): 618–627. doi: https://doi.org/10.1080/10412905.1998.9700989.

[66] Dimitrijević, S. I., Mihajlovski, K. R., Antonović, D. G., Milanović-Stevanović, M. R. and Mijin, D. Ž. 2007. "A study of the synergistic antilisterial effects of a sub-lethal dose of lactic acid and essential oils from Thymus vulgaris L., Rosmarinus officinalis L. and Origanum vulgare L." *Food Chemistry*. 104 (2): 774–782. doi: https://doi.org/10.1016/j.foodchem.2006.12.028.

[67] Gutierrez, J., Barry-Ryan, C. and Bourke, P. 2008. "The antimicrobial efficacy of plant essential oil combinations and interactions with food ingredients." *International Journal of Food Microbiology*. 124 (1): 91–97. doi: https://doi.org/10.1016/j.ijfoodmicro.2008.02.028.

[68] Rosato, A., Vitali, C., Piarulli, M., Mazzotta, M., Argentieri, M. P. and Mallamaci, R. 2009. "In vitro synergic efficacy of the combination of Nystatin with the essential oils of Origanum vulgare and Pelargonium graveolens against some Candida species." *Phytomedicine*. 16 (10): 972–975. doi: https://doi.org/10.1016/j.phymed.2009.02.011.

[69] Hussain, A. I., Anwar, F. and Rasheed, S. 2011. "chemotherapeutic properties of the essential oils from two Origanum species growing in." *Ultrasonics*. (August 2008).

[70] Silveira, S. M. da, Cunha Júnior, A., Scheuermann, G. N., Secchi, F. L. and Vieira, C. R. W. 2012. "Chemical composition and antimicrobial activity of essential oils from selected herbs cultivated in the South of Brazil against food spoilage and foodborne pathogens." *Ciência Rural*. 42 (7): 1300–1306. doi: https://doi.org/10.1590/S0103-84782012000700026.

[71] Mathlouthi, N., Bouzaienne, T., Oueslati, I., Recoquillay, F., Hamdi, M., Urdaci, M. and Bergaoui, R. 2012. "Use of rosemary, oregano, and a commercial blend of essential oils in broiler chickens: In vitro antimicrobial activities and effects on growth performance." *Journal of Animal Science*. 90 (3): 813–823. doi: https://doi.org/10.2527/jas.2010-3646.

[72] Nurzyńska-Wierdak, R., Bogucka-Kocka, A., Sowa, I. and Szymczak, G. 2012. "The composition of essential oil from three ecotypes of origanum vulgare L. SSP. Vulgare cultivated in Poland." *Farmacia*. 60 (4): 571–577.

[73] Barros-Velazquez, J. 2015. *Antimicrobial Food Packaging*. Elsevier Science.

[74] Ávila Sosa Sánchez, R., Portillo-Ruiz, M. C., Viramontes-Ramos, S., Muñoz-Castellanos, L. N. and Nevárez-Moorillón, G. V. 2015. "Effect of Mexican Oregano (Lippia berlandieri Schauer) Essential Oil Fractions on the Growth of Aspergillus spp. in a Bread Model System." *Journal of Food Processing and Preservation*. 39 (6): 776–783. doi: https://doi.org/10.1111/jfpp.12287.

[75] Negi, P. S. 2012. "Plant extracts for the control of bacterial growth: Efficacy, stability and safety issues for food application." *International Journal of Food Microbiology*. 156 (1): 7–17. doi: https://doi.org/https://doi.org/10.1016/j.ijfood micro.2012.03.006.

[76] Brenes, A. and Roura, E. 2010. "Essential oils in poultry nutrition: Main effects and modes of action." *Animal Feed Science and Technology*. 158 (1–2): 1–14. doi: https://doi.org/10.1016/j.anifeedsci.2010.03.007.

[77] Nhu-Trang, T. T., Casabianca, H. and Grenier-Loustalot, M. F. 2006. "Deuterium/hydrogen ratio analysis of thymol, carvacrol, γ-terpinene and p-cymene in thyme, savory and oregano essential oils by gas chromatography–pyrolysis–isotope ratio mass spectrometry." *Journal of Chromatography A*. 1132 (1): 219–227. doi: https://doi.org/https://doi.org/10.1016/j.chroma.2006.07.088.

[78] Poulose, A. J. and Croteau, R. 1978. "Biosynthesis of aromatic monoterpenes: Conversion of γ-terpinene to p-cymene and thymol in Thymus vulgaris L." *Archives of Biochemistry and Biophysics*. 187 (2): 307–314. doi: https://doi.org/ https://doi.org/10.1016/0003-9861(78)90039-5.

[79] Ruberto, G. and Baratta, M. T. 2000. "Antioxidant activity of selected essential oil components in two lipid model systems." *Food Chemistry*. 69 (2): 167–174. doi: https://doi.org/https://doi.org/10.1016/S0308-8146(99)00247-2.

[80] Safaei-Ghomi, J., Ebrahimabadi, A. H., Djafari-Bidgoli, Z. and Batooli, H. 2009. "GC/MS analysis and in vitro antioxidant activity of essential oil and methanol extracts of Thymus caramanicus Jalas and its main constituent carvacrol." *Food Chemistry*. 115 (4): 1524–1528. doi: https://doi.org/https://doi.org/10.1016/ j.foodchem.2009.01.051.

[81] Aligiannis, N., Kalpoutzakis, E., Mitaku, S. and Chinou, I. B. 2001. "Composition and Antimicrobial Activity of the Essential Oils of Two Origanum Species." *Journal of Agricultural and Food Chemistry*. 49 (9): 4168–4170. doi: https://doi. org/10.1021/jf001494m.

[82] Faleiro, L., Miguel, G., Gomes, S., Costa, L., Venâncio, F., Teixeira, A., Figueiredo, A. C., Barroso, J. G. and Pedro, L. G. 2005. "Antibacterial and Antioxidant Activities of Essential Oils Isolated from Thymbra capitata L. (Cav.) and Origanum vulgare L." *Journal of Agricultural and Food Chemistry*. 53 (21): 8162–8168. doi: https://doi.org/10.1021/jf0510079.

[83] Rodríguez-Meizoso, I., Marin, F. R., Herrero, M., Señorans, F. J., Reglero, G., Cifuentes, A. and Ibáñez, E. 2006. "Subcritical water extraction of nutraceuticals

with antioxidant activity from oregano. Chemical and functional characterization." *Journal of Pharmaceutical and Biomedical Analysis*. 41 (5): 1560–1565. doi: https://doi.org/https://doi.org/10.1016/j.jpba.2006.01.018.

[84] Simitzis, P. E., Deligeorgis, S. G., Bizelis, J. A., Dardamani, A., Theodosiou, I. and Fegeros, K. 2008. "Effect of dietary oregano oil supplementation on lamb meat characteristics." *Meat Science*. 79 (2): 217–223. doi: https://doi.org/https://doi.org/10.1016/j.meatsci.2007.09.005.

[85] Lorenzo, S., Francesca, P., Chiara, M., Giulia, T., Eleonora, B., Fausto, G. and Rosalba, L. 2014. "Characterization of oregano (Origanum vulgare) essential oil and definition of its antimicrobial activity against Listeria monocytogenes and Escherichia coli in vitro system and on foodstuff surfaces." *African Journal of Microbiology Research*. 8 (29): 2746–2753. doi: https://doi.org/10.5897/AJMR2014.6677.

[86] Denyer, S. P. 1995. "Mechanisms of action of antibacterial biocides." *International Biodeterioration & Biodegradation*. 36 (3–4): 227–245. doi: https://doi.org/10.1016/0964-8305(96)00015-7.

[87] Pauli, A. 2001. "Antimicrobial properties of essential oil constituents." *International Journal of Aromatherapy*. 11 (3): 126–133. doi: https://doi.org/https://doi.org/10.1016/S0962-4562(01)80048-5.

[88] Botsoglou, N. A., Florou-Paneri, P., Christaki, E., Fletouris, D. J. and Spais, A. B. 2002. "Effect of dietary oregano essential oil on performance of chickens and on iron-induced lipid oxidation of breast, thigh and abdominal fat tissues." *British Poultry Science*. 43 (2): 223–230. doi: https://doi.org/10.1080/00071660120121436.

[89] Adam, K., Sivropoulou, A., Kokkini, S., Lanaras, T. and Arsenakis, M. 1998. "Antifungal Activities of Origanum vulgare subsp. hirtum, Mentha spicata, Lavandula angustifolia, and Salvia fruticosa Essential Oils against Human Pathogenic Fungi." *Journal of Agricultural and Food Chemistry*. 46 (5): 1739–1745. doi: https://doi.org/10.1021/jf9708296.

[90] Kokkini, S., Karousou, R., Hanlidou, E. and Lanaras, T. 2004. "Essential oil composition of Greek (Origanum vulgare ssp. hirtum) and Turkish (O. onites) oregano: A tool for their distinction." *Journal of Essential Oil Research*. 16 (4): 334–338.

[91] Jamroz, D., Wertelecki, T., Houszka, M. and Kamel, C. 2006. "Influence of diet type on the inclusion of plant origin active substances on morphological and histochemical characteristics of the stomach and jejunum walls in chicken." *Journal of Animal Physiology and Animal Nutrition*. 90 (5-6): 255–268. doi: https://doi.org/10.1111/j.1439-0396.2005.00603.x.

[92] Steiner, T. 2009. *Phytogenics in Animal Nutrition: Natural Concepts to Optimize Gut Health and Performance*. Nottingham University Press.

[93] Wallace, R. J., Oleszek, W., Franz, C., Hahn, I., Baser, K. H. C., Mathe, A. and Teichmann, K. 2010. "Dietary plant bioactives for poultry health and productivity." *British Poultry Science*. 51 (4): 461–487. doi: https://doi.org/10.1080/00071668.2010.506908.

[94] Alagawany, M., Abd El-Hack, M. E., Farag, M. R., Shaheen, H. M., Abdel-Latif, M. A., Noreldin, A. E. and Patra, A. K. 2018. "The usefulness of oregano and its derivatives in poultry nutrition." *World's Poultry Science Journal*. 74 (3): 463–473. doi: https://doi.org/10.1017/S0043933918000454.

[95] Khattak, F., Ronchi, A., Castelli, P. and Sparks, N. 2013. "Effects of natural blend of essential oil on growth performance, blood biochemistry, cecal morphology, and carcass quality of broiler chickens." *Poultry Science*. 93 (1): 132–137. doi: https://doi.org/10.3382/ps.2013-03387.

[96] Pirgozliev, V., Bravo, D., Mirza, M. W. and Rose, S. P. 2015. "Growth performance and endogenous losses of broilers fed wheat-based diets with and without essential oils and xylanase supplementation." *Poultry Science*. 94 (6): 1227–1232. doi: https://doi.org/10.3382/ps/peu017.

[97] Peng, Q. Y., Li, J. D., Li, Z., Duan, Z. Y. and Wu, Y. P. 2016. "Effects of dietary supplementation with oregano essential oil on growth performance, carcass traits and jejunal morphology in broiler chickens." *Animal Feed Science and Technology*. 214: 148–153. doi: https://doi.org/10.1016/j.anifeedsci.2016.02.010.

[98] Günther, K. D. 1990. "Gewürzstoffe können die Leistung erhöhen [Spices can increase performance." *Kraftfutter. Concentrated feed*. 73: 469–474].

[99] Vidanarachchi, J. K., Mikkelsen, L. L., Sims, I., Iji, P. a and Choct, M. 2005. "Phytobiotics : alternatives to antibiotic growth promoters in monogastric animal feeds." *Recent Advances in Animal Nutrition in Australia*. 15 (Kamel 2001): 131–144.

[100] Windisch, W. and Kroismayr, A. 2007. "Natural phytobiotics for health of young piglets and poultry. Mechanisms and application." *Growth (Lakeland)*. 85: 643–644.

[101] Giannenas, I. A., Florou-Paneri, P., Botsoglou, N. A., Christaki, E. and Spais, A. B. 2005. "Effect of supplementing feed with oregano and/or α-tocopheryl acetate on growth of broiler chickens and oxidative stability of meat." *Journal of Animal and Feed Sciences*. 14 (3): 521–535. doi: https://doi.org/10.22358/jafs/67120/2005.

[102] Jang, I. S., Ko, Y. H., Kang, S. Y. and Lee, C. Y. 2007. "Effect of a commercial essential oil on growth performance, digestive enzyme activity and intestinal microflora population in broiler chickens." *Animal Feed Science and Technology*. 134 (3): 304–315. doi: https://doi.org/https://doi.org/10.1016/j.anifeedsci.2006.06.009.

[103] Lee, K. W., Everts, H., Kappert, H. J., Frehner, M., Losa, R. and Beynen, A. C. 2003. "Effects of dietary essential oil components on growth performance, digestive

enzymes and lipid metabolism in female broiler chickens." *British Poultry Science*. 44 (3): 450–457. doi: https://doi.org/10.1080/0007166031000085508.

[104] Lewis, M. R., Rose, S. P., Mackenzie, A. M. and Tucker, L. A. 2003. "Effects of dietary inclusion of plant extracts on the growth performance of male broiler chickens." *British Poultry Science*. 44 (sup1): 43–44. doi: https://doi.org/10.1080/713655281.

[105] Hashemipour, H., Khaksar, V., Rubio, L. A., Veldkamp, T. and van Krimpen, M. M. 2016. "Effect of feed supplementation with a thymol plus carvacrol mixture, in combination or not with an NSP-degrading enzyme, on productive and physiological parameters of broilers fed on wheat-based diets." *Animal Feed Science and Technology*. 211: 117–131. doi: https://doi.org/https://doi.org/10.1016/j.anifeedsci.2015.09.023.

[106] Halle, I., Thomann, R. and Bauermann, U. 2004. "Effects of a graded supplementation of herbs and essential oils in broiler feed on growth and carcass traits." *Landbauforshung ....*: 292–294.

[107] Kamel, C. 2001. "Tracing modes of action and the roles of plant extracts in non-ruminants": 2001: 135-150.

[108] Giannenas, I. A., Florou-Paneri, P., Papazahariadou, M., Botsoglou, N. A., Christaki, E. and Spais, A. B. 2004. "Effect of diet supplementation with ground oregano on performance of broiler chickens challenged with Eimeria tenella." *Archiv fur Geflugelkunde*. 68 (6): 247–252. doi: https://doi.org/10.1007/978-3-319-46709-2.

[109] Bozkurt, M., Küçükyılmaz, K., Çatlı, A. U. and Çınar, M. 2009. "The effect of single or combined dietary supplementation of prebiotics, organic acid and probiotics on performance and slaughter characteristics of broilers." *South African Journal of Animal Science*. 39: 197–205.

[110] Ghazi, S., Amjadian, T. and Norouzi, S. 2015. "Single and combined effects of vitamin C and oregano essential oil in diet, on growth performance, and blood parameters of broiler chicks reared under heat stress condition." *International Journal of Biometeorology*. 59 (8): 1019–1024. doi: https://doi.org/10.1007/s00484-014-0915-4.

[111] Stef, L., Simiz, E., Marcu, A., Stef, D., Gherasim, V., Pet, I., Pătruică, S., Ahmadi, M., Manciu, A. and Julean, C. 2018. "The Effect of Essential Oils on the Bioproductive Performance of Broilers." 51 (1): 43–49.

[112] Roofchaee, A., Rani, M.. and Ebrahimzadeh, M. A. 2011. "Effect of dietary oregano (Origanum vulgare L.) essential oil on growth performance, cecal microflora and serum antioxidant activity of broiler chickens." *African Journal of Biotechnology*. 10 (32): 6177–6183. doi: https://doi.org/10.5897/AJB10.2596.

[113] Zamora, G. M., Meléndez, L. A. D., Hume, M. E. and Vázquez, R. S. 2017. "Performance, blood parameters, and carcass yield of broiler chickens supplemented

with Mexican oregano oil." *Revista Brasileira de Zootecnia*. 46 (6): 515–520. doi: https://doi.org/10.1590/S1806-92902017000600006.

[114] Lee, K. W., Everts, H., Kappert, H. J., Yeom, K. H. and Beynen, A. C. 2003. "Dietary Carvacrol Lowers Body Weight Gain but Improves Feed Conversion in Female Broiler Chickens." *Journal of Applied Poultry Research*. 12 (4): 394–399. doi: https://doi.org/10.1093/japr/12.4.394.

[115] Karimi, A., Yan, F., Coto, C., Park, J. H., Min, Y., Lu, C., Gidden, J. A., Lay, J. O. and Waldroup, P. W. 2010. "Effects of level and source of oregano leaf in starter diets for broiler chicks." *Journal of Applied Poultry Research*. 19 (2): 137–145. doi: https://doi.org/10.3382/japr.2009-00088.

[116] Basmacioğlu, H., Tokuşoğlu, Ö. and Ergül, M. 2004. "The effect of oregano and rosemary essential oils or alpha-tocopheryl acetate on performance and lipid oxidation of meat enriched with n-3 PUFA'S in broilers." *South African Journal of Animal Sciences*. 34 (3): 197–210.

[117] Amad, A. A., Männer, K., Wendler, K. R., Neumann, K. and Zentek, J. 2011. "Effects of a phytogenic feed additive on growth performance and ileal nutrient digestibility in broiler chickens." *Poultry Science*. 90 (12): 2811–2816. doi: https://doi.org/10.3382/ps.2011-01515.

[118] Paster, N., Juven, B. J., Shaaya, E., Menasherov, M., Nitzan, R., Weisslowicz, H. and Ravid, U. 1990. "Inhibitory effect of oregano and thyme essential oils on moulds and foodborne bacteria." *Letters in Applied Microbiology*. 11 (1): 33–37. doi: https://doi.org/10.1111/j.1472-765X.1990.tb00130.x.

[119] Mohiti-Asli, M. and Ghanaatparast-Rashti, M. 2015. "Dietary oregano essential oil alleviates experimentally induced coccidiosis in broilers." *Preventive Veterinary Medicine*. 120 (2): 195–202. doi: https://doi.org/10.1016/j.prevetmed.2015.03.014.

[120] Zeng, Z., Zhang, S., Wang, H. and Piao, X. 2015. "Essential oil and aromatic plants as feed additives in non-ruminant nutrition: A review." *Journal of Animal Science and Biotechnology*. 6 (1). doi: https://doi.org/10.1186/s40104-015-0004-5.

[121] Mitchell, M. A. and Kettlewell, P. J. 1998. "Physiological stress and welfare of broiler chickens in transit: solutions not problems!" *Poultry Science*. 77 (12): 1803–1814. doi: https://doi.org/10.1093/ps/77.12.1803.

[122] Warriss, P. D., Pagazaurtundua, A. and Brown, S. N. 2005. "Relationship between maximum daily temperature and mortality of broiler chickens during transport and lairage." *British Poultry Science*. 46 (6): 647–651. doi: https://doi.org/10.1080/00071660500393868.

[123] Suzuki, K., Harasawa, R., Yoshitake, Y. and Mitsuoka, T. 1983. "Effects of crowding and heat stress on intestinal flora, body weight gain, and feed efficiency of growing rats and chicks." *Nihon juigaku zasshi. The Japanese journal of veterinary science*. 45 (3): 331—338. doi: https://doi.org/10.1292/jvms1939.45.331.

[124] Fuller, R. 1999. "Probiotics for farm animals." *Probiotics : a critical review*.

[125] Bailey, M. T., Lubach, G. R. and Coe, C. L. 2004. "Prenatal stress alters bacterial colonization of the gut in infant monkeys." *Journal of pediatric gastroenterology and nutrition*. 38 (4): 414—421. doi: https://doi.org/10.1097/00005176-200404 000-00009.

[126] Lambert, G. P. 2009. "Stress-induced gastrointestinal barrier dysfunction and its inflammatory effects." *Journal of Animal Science*. 87 (suppl_14): E101–E108. doi: https://doi.org/10.2527/jas.2008-1339.

[127] Vlaicu, Pa., Panaite, D. T., Olteanu, M., Turcu, P. R., Saracila, M. and Criste, R. D. 2018. "Effect of the Dietary Oregano (Origanum Vulgare L.) Powder and Oil on the Performance, Carcass and Organs Development of Broilers Reared Under Heat Stress (32°C)." *Scientific Papers-Animal Science Series: Lucrări Ştiinţifice-Seria Zootehnie*. 69: 69–207.

[128] Bakkali, F., Averbeck, S., Averbeck, D. and Idaomar, M. 2008. "Biological effects of essential oils – A review." *Food and Chemical Toxicology*. 46 (2): 446–475. doi: https://doi.org/https://doi.org/10.1016/j.fct.2007.09.106.

[129] Cheng, C., Zou, Y. and Peng, J. 2018. "Oregano Essential Oil Attenuates RAW264.7 Cells from Lipopolysaccharide-Induced Inflammatory Response through Regulating NADPH Oxidase Activation-Driven Oxidative Stress." *Molecules (Basel, Switzerland)*. 23 (8): 1857. doi: https://doi.org/10.3390/molecules23081857.

[130] Shan, B., Cai, Y. Z., Sun, M. and Corke, H. 2005. "Antioxidant capacity of 26 spice extracts and characterization of their phenolic constituents." *Journal of Agricultural and Food Chemistry*. 53 (20): 7749–7759. doi: https://doi.org/10.1021/jf051513y.

[131] Spiridon, I., Colceru, S., Anghel, N., Teaca, C. A., Bodirlau, R. and Armatu, A. 2011. "Antioxidant capacity and total phenolic contents of oregano (Origanum vulgare), lavender (Lavandula angustifolia) and lemon balm (Melissa officinalis) from Romania." *Natural Product Research*. 25 (17): 1657–1661. doi: https://doi.org/10.1080/14786419.2010.521502.

[132] Tekce, E. and Gül, M. 2016. "Effects of Origanum syriacum essential oil added in different levels to the diet of broilers under heat stress on performance and intestinal histology." *European Poultry Science*. 80 (October). doi: https://doi.org/10.1399/eps.2016.157.

[133] Galal, A. A. A. el-G., El-Araby El-Sayed, I., Hassanin, O. and Omar, A. el-S. 2014. "ositive Impact of Oregano Essential Oil on Growth Performance, Humoral Immune Responses and Chicken Interferon Alpha Signalling Pathway in Broilers." 892 (October 2013): 880–892. doi: https://doi.org/10.1002/da.22291.

[134] Barreto, M. S. R., Menten, J. F. M., Racanicci, A. M. C., Pereira, P. W. Z. and Rizzo, P. V 2008. "Plant extracts used as growth promoters in broilers." *Brazilian Journal of Poultry Science*. 10: 109–115.

[135] Marcinčák, S., Cabadaj, R., Popelka, P. and Šoltýsová, L. 2008. "Antioxidative effect of oregano supplemented to broilers on oxidative stability of poultry meat." *Slovenian Veterinary Research*. 45 (2): 61–66.

[136] Gilani, S., Howarth, G. S., Nattrass, G., Kitessa, S. M., Barekatain, R., Forder, R. E. A., Tran, C. D. and Hughes, R. J. 2018. "Gene expression and morphological changes in the intestinal mucosa associated with increased permeability induced by short-term fasting in chickens." *Journal of Animal Physiology and Animal Nutrition*. 102 (2): e653–e661. doi: https://doi.org/10.1111/jpn.12808.

[137] Smith, H. W. 1965. "The development of the flora of the alimentary tract in young animals." *The Journal of Pathology and Bacteriology*. 90 (2): 495–513. doi: https://doi.org/10.1002/path.1700900218.

[138] Lan, Y., Verstegen, M. W. A., Tamminga, S. and Williams, B. A. 2005. "The role of the commensal gut microbial community in broiler chickens." *World's Poultry Science Journal*. 61 (1): 95–104. doi: https://doi.org/doi: 10.1079/WPS200445.

[139] Zinoviadou, K. G., Koutsoumanis, K. P. and Biliaderis, C. G. 2009. "Physico-chemical properties of whey protein isolate films containing oregano oil and their antimicrobial action against spoilage flora of fresh beef." *Meat Science*. 82 (3): 338–345. doi: https://doi.org/https://doi.org/10.1016/j.meatsci.2009.02.004.

[140] Betancourt, L., Rodriguez, F., Phandanouvong, V., Ariza-Nieto, C., Hume, M., Nisbet, D., Afanador-Téllez, G., Van Kley, A. M. and Nalian, A. 2014. "Effect of Origanum chemotypes on broiler intestinal bacteria." *Poultry Science*. 93 (10): 2526–2535. doi: https://doi.org/10.3382/ps.2014-03944.

[141] Franciosini, M. P., Casagrande-Proietti, P., Forte, C., Beghelli, D., Acuti, G., Zanichelli, D., Dal Bosco, A., Castellini, C. and Trabalza-Marinucci, M. 2016. "Effects of oregano (Origanum vulgare L.) and rosemary (Rosmarinus officinalis L.) aqueous extracts on broiler performance, immune function and intestinal microbial population." *Journal of Applied Animal Research*. 44 (1): 474–479. doi: https://doi.org/10.1080/09712119.2015.1091322.

In: Oregano: Properties, Uses and Health Benefits
Editor: Gema Nieto Martínez
ISBN: 978-1-53616-284-4

Chapter 10

ANTIMICROBIAL AND ANTIOXIDANT ACTIVITY OF OREGANO ESSENTIAL OIL BY ESR (ELECTRON SPIN RESONANCE)

Gema Nieto[1,2,*], Amaury Taboada-Rodríguez[1], Mogens L. Andersen[2] and Leif H. Skibsted[2]

[1]Department of Food Technology, Nutrition and Food Science, Veterinary Faculty, University of Murcia, Murcia, Spain

[2] Food Chemistry, Department of Food Science, University of Copenhagen, Frederiksberg C, Denmark

ABSTRACT

The aim of this study was to study the antioxidant activity and the antimicrobial activity against Salmonella, of the essential oil of oregano (EOs) and the posterior addition at doses of 0.05% (O_1) and 0.4% (O_2) in pork patties. For that 3 batches of pork burgers (minced to 5 mm and 2% salt) were prepared: the control group C, Level1 (0.05% EOs), and Level2 (0.4% EOs). The burgers were packed with modified atmosphere (70% O_2: 20% CO_2: 10% N_2) and stored for a maximum of 6 days at 4°C in natural lighting conditions. The total Salmonella counts was determined using Brilliant green agar medium (BGA), 37°C, 48h. A validated PCR identification protocol from the EU ''Food PCR'' for Salmonella, was used both for the confirmation of presumptive colonies and for determining presence or absence of the pathogen. In addition, the antioxidant activity of the essential oil in a model system (Fenton reaction), and in burgers with ESR (electron spin resonance) evaluated by free radical formation during heating at 55°C and its binding to PBN (α-fenil-N-tert-butilnitrona) on days 0, 3 and 6 of storage was studied. The results showed that O showed antimicrobial effect and prooxidat effect at phenol concentration ≥

* Corresponding Author's E-mail: gnieto@um.es.

12 mg GAE/L. In patties O1, the radical formation after 3 hours of heating at 55°C was significantly lower ($P < 0.05\%$) than in control samples (C) and O_2 throughout the storage. In general, all patties inoculated and stored in modified atmosphere, the results showed that Salmonella spp. survived after 9 days of storage. However, in treated patties with 0.4% of O the growth of Salmonella was significantly lower ($P < 0.05\%$) than control meat from day 3 of storage. The results indicate that the use of 0.05% essential oil of oregano, as a natural antioxidant in pork burgers, being a good strategy of conservation.

Keywords: oregano, antioxidant, antimicrobial, functional, meat

INTRODUCTION

Nowadays, consumers are demanding foods free of chemical additives. Therefore, the search of new methodologies and new ingredients is an interesting strategy in order to produce meat products. In this sense, the use of natural preservatives, such as essential oils, could be a new method of preserving food using natural additives (Nieto et al., 2010, 2011).

Oregano is an aromatic shrub grown in many parts of the world. The fresh and dried leaves are frequently used in traditional Mediterranean cuisine as an additive. Its essential oil is a rich source of biologically active compounds with antioxidant and antimicrobial activity.

In general, many essential oils from spices have gained interest for the researchers. Especially the case of essential oil from rosemary that is listed in the FDA: U.S. Food and Drug Administration, and in the EFSA (European Food Safety Authority) as a food preservative. Therefore, there is an increased interest for essential oils as natural alternatives.

Another important aspect is that natural extracts are considered as GRAS (generally recognized as safe), and they have shown synergism with other methods of preservation.

Among the numerous properties of oregano, the antioxidant activity is hightlighted because it can delay or inhibit lipid oxidation. When oregano essential oil is added into food, it could minimize rancidity; retard the formation of toxic oxidation products, and as a consequence of this to maintain nutritional quality.

In meat and meat products, lipid oxidation is a major cause of deterioration of quality (Nieto et al., 2010, 2011). Chelating agents and synthetic and natural antioxidants are the most effective inhibitors of lipid oxidation. In this sense, the use of oregano essential oil (OE) to preserve meat products could be a good alternative to the use of artificial antioxidants.

Previous studies have shown the application of oregano in meat and meat products, with good properties to inhibit lipid oxidation in meat patties (Nieto et al., 2013), to reduce rancidity in minced beef (Hulankova et al., 2013), wildebeest meat (Shange et al., 2019) in lamb burgers (Fernandes et al., 2017) and in cooked sheep sausages (Fernandes et al., 2018).

In contrast, a previous study reported that the use of inadequate doses of oregano could show a pro-oxidant behavior under certain conditions (Nieto et al., 2011). This prooxidant effect could damage important molecules, such as, proteins, carbohydrates or DNA (Aruoma et al., 1997). Therefore, the importance of evaluating the exact doses of essential oil with prooxidant effect is high. Before using a natural extract or essential oil, the prooxidant potential should be tested. In this sense, in order to evaluate the prooxidant effect of essential oils, a reliable method is necessary, which is not easy because lipid oxidation is a phenomenon that produces free radicals of short life that are difficult to determine. The determination of these free radicals is difficult; therefore the technique used in this study (ESR: electronic spin resonance) is necessary to detec radicals. Previous studies have reported that ESR has been applied in different food models as an indicator of the first stages of lipid oxidation (Monahan et al., 1993; Thomsen et al., 2000; Bolumar et al., 2011).

In addition, these lipid radicals are reactive species and their detection limit is below the detection limit of ESR that was established in 10^9-10^8 M (Andersen and Skibsted 2002). The technique "spin trap" is based on the reaction of radicals with diamagnetic compounds, known as "spin adducts," which accumulate at a concentration detectable by ESR (>10^7-10^6 M). The detection of these radicals is an indirect detection of the radicals involved in lipid oxidation. The results of TBARS (Monahan et al., 1993), peroxide values (Carlsen et al., 2003), rancimad (Velasco et al., 2004) and sensory analysis (Thomsen et al., 2000) are consistent with the results obtained by ESR. Therefore, the study of radical formation after addition of essential oil into meat using ESR is a preliminary assay in order to know the exact concentration of the essential oil with antioxidant effect.

Regarding antimicrobial effect, essential oils have reported antiviral, antifungal and antibacterial activities; therefore, they can be alternatives to standard antimicrobial products (Ferreira et al., 2010; Giatrakou, Ntzimani, & Savvaidis, 2010). In this sense, several mechanisms are associated with the antimicrobial properties of essential oil: Ghosh et al., (2014) explained that the disolution of the cytoplasmic membrane in the hydrophobic domain could be the main reason for the antimicrobial capacity of the essential oils. Moreover, other authors reported that other mechanism is the denaturation of proteins (Dorman and Deans (2000) and Hammer et al., (1999).

In general, Dorman and Deans (2000) and Hammer et al., (1999) reported that main phenolic compounds in essential oils with antibacterial properties are carvacrol, eugenol, and thymol (from various plant origins). In addition, they showed a different behaviour against Gram-negative or Gram-positive bacteria. Moreover, diferent studies have shown that properties of essential oils were able to inhibit growth of Staphylococcus aureus and Listeria monocytogenes (Liang et al., 2012), Zygosaccharomyces bailli (Chang et al., 2012) and Bacillus cereus (Ghosh et al., 2014).

The objectives of this work were: to develop a model oxidation system (Fenton reaction) to study both antioxidant and prooxidant activities of oregano essential oil using electronic resonance spectroscopy-ESR-; to establish the minimum essential oil concentration with antioxidant and pro-oxidant effect; evaluate the antioxidant capacity of oregano essential oil in pork burgers during storage under usual marketing conditions using ESR and to study the antimicrobial activity of essential oil against *Salmonella* inoculated in pork patties.

Material And Methods

Oregano Essential Oil

The essential oil of oregano (*Origanum vulgare* L) with a density of 0.938 g/ml at 20°C was obtained by steam extraction of leaves. Between the 32 components identified in the oregano essential oil, accounting for 89.5% of the oil, the major components were carvacrol (61.21%), p-cymene (15.12%) and γ-terpinene (4.80%), terpinolene (3.63%), β-caryophyllene (2.62%), and α-pinene (2.34%).

Total Phenolics Compounds

The amount of total phenolics in essential oils was determined according to the Folin–Ciocalteu method. Samples (200 µl, two replicates) were mixed with 1.0 ml of Folin–Ciocalteu's reagent (diluted 1:10 with water) and 0.8 ml of a 7.5% solution of sodium carbonate was added. The absorption at 765 nm was measured after 30 min with a Cary 3 UV–vis spectrophotometer (Varian Techtron Pty. Ltd., Mulgrave, Victoria, Australia). The total phenolic content is expressed as gallic acid equivalents (GAE) in mg/l of essential oil.

Fenton Reaction by ESR

The effect of oregano essential oil on the formation of short-lived radicals was tested in a model system based on the iron chemistry in the Fenton reaction A total of 4 mL of 0.0032 M POBN (α- (4-pyridyl-1-oxide) -N-tert-butrynitrone) in a 1M aqueous solution of ethanol was mixed with 20 µL of a solution of $FeSO_4$ (0.022 M) and 50 µL of oregano essential oil (according to Graversen et al., 2008). For reference, 50 µL of Mili Q water was replaced by the essential oil. The reaction was initiated by the addition of 80 µL H_2O_2 (0.024 M), and mixed for 30 s. Subsequently, 50 µl were transferred to ESR micropipettes

(Brand, Wertheim, Germany) and the spectrum was recorded after 2 minutes in a Miniscope MS 200 ESR spectrometer (Magnettech, Berlin, Germany) with the following parameters: microwave power, 4 mW; scanning width, 7.5 mT; Sweep time, 4 min; width modulation, 0.12 mT; amplitude, 500; and constant time, 0.3 s.

The addition of 1-hydroxyethyl radicals to the spin trap POBN produces stable spin adducts, CH_3-CHOH/POBN, which are detectable by ESR (Rødtjer et al., 2006).

Reaction. 1. $Fe^{3+} + H_2O_2 \rightarrow \cdot OH + OH^- + Fe^{3+}$
Reaction. 2. $CH_3CH_2OH + \cdot OH \rightarrow CH_3 \cdot CHOH + H_2O$
Reaction. 3 $CH_3CH_2OH + POBN \rightarrow CH_3 \cdot CHOH/POBN$

The degree of inhibition (IESR) was calculated from the height of the central peak of the signal of POBN adducts spin by the following formula:

$$I_{ESR} = [1 - (\text{Peak height}_{sample}/\text{Peak height}_{reference})] \times 100\%$$

Elaboration of Burgers

Fresh, semi-boneless pork meat shoulders (Boston butts) were purchased from a local meat supplier. Upon arrival, the Boston butts were processed in a cool room at ~6°C to yield one single batch of meat. Fat and lean tissues were manually separated and the connective tissue discarded. Fat and lean meat were grounded separately with a meat grinder (Braher International, San Sebastian, Spain) using 5 mm orifice plates, and then mixed for 10 min using an RM-60 Mixer (Mainca, Granollers, Spain). Meat batter with target fat percentage of 30% was obtained by mixing fat and lean meat after determination of fat percentage in each by HFT-2000 fat analyzer (Data Support Co., Inc., Encino, CA, USA).

Seven lots of 2 kg meat batter, each prepared in duplicate, were prepared. Pork patties were prepared from six lots of meat batter (each 2 kg) with oregano (O) essential oils added at two different levels: 0.05% or 0.4%. A lot (2 kg) without addition of essential oil was used for preparation of control (C) pork patties. Twenty pork patties (100 g each) were prepared using a conventional burger-maker before being packaged in polystyrene trays (B5-37, AERpack, Spain). The trays were overwrapped with oxygen-permeable polyvinyl chloride (PVC) film (650 $cm^3\ m^{-2}\ h^{-1}$ at 23°C) for storage under aerobic conditions (AE). The pork patties were stored in a cabinet illuminated with white fluorescent light (620 lx) simulating retail display conditions at 4°C for up to 6 days.

Determination of the Generation of Radicals during the Storage of Burgers by Means of ESR

The ESR measurements were made in a JEOL FR 30 ESR spectrophotometer (JEOL Ltd., Tokyo, Japan) at room temperature. N-t-butyl- a-phenyl nitrone (PBN) (Sigma Aldrich Chemie, Steinheim, Germany) was used as a spin trap. Based on the method by Carlsen, Andersen, and Skibsted (2001), meat (4 g) was cut in small pieces, suspended in 28.5 ml of 50 mM MES buffer pH 5.7 and 1.5 ml of 400 mM PBN dissolved in ethanol was added. This solution was homogenised at 13,500 rpm for 30 s using an Ultra Turrax T25 homogeniser (Jane and Kunkel IKA-Labortechnick, Staufen, Germany). Then, 4 ml of this solution was transferred to 10 ml glass tubes with screw caps and incubated at 55 C for 3 h. This solution was filtered through filter paper before being transferred to a quartz capillary tube and into the ESR cavity for measurement.

The operational settings for the ESR equipment were: Microwave power 16 mW, sweep width 50.00 Gauss, sweep time 2 min, modulation width 1.25 Gauss, time constant 0.3 s. The height of first peak of the centerfield duplet relative to the height of the builtin Mn (II)-standard was calculated and used to quantify the relative concentrations of radical spin adducts in the meat samples. A solution of TEMPO (2,2,6,6-tetramethylpiperidin-1-yloxy, Aldrich, Steinheim, Germany) (2 lM) was measured and the height of the centerfield peak was compared to the height of the manganese peak for day-to-day corrections. The reported values are the average of two measurements for each of the two independent incubation extracts.

Antimicrobial Activity

The bacterial cells of *Salmonella* spp. were pelleted by centrifugation at 5000 g for 15 min at 5°C, washed twice in 10 ml of 0.1 M phosphate buffered saline (PBS), pH 7.0, and diluted to 1.0×10^8 cfu/ml in PBS for the inoculation of burgers samples. Cell counts were determined by serial dilution and subsequent enumeration on tryptone soy agar (Oxoid).

Burgers contamination with *Salmonella* spp. was performed at a level close to 100 ufc/g/cm^2. Analyses were performed on days 0, 3, 6 and 9 of storage. 3 hamburgers were analyzed for each day of control. The samples used in the microbiological analysis were homogenized with a Masticator (IUL Instruments GmbH, Königswinter, Germany) and diluted in peptone water (Merck. 64271, Darmstadt, Germany). The total Salmonella counts were determined using Brilliant green agar medium (BGA), 37ºC, 48h (ISO 6579, 2002). The plates were incubated in a culture oven ST 6120 (Heraeus SA, Boadilla, Madrid, Spain). Specific PCR-based Salmonella confirmation was performed. Colonies of *Salmonella spp.* were picked from BGA (Brilliant Green Agar) plates and suspended in 30 μl of sterile distilled water. The conditions used for PCR are shown in Table 1.

Table 1. PCR conditions

	Sequences	PCR conditions
Salmonella	139(5'-GTGAAATTATCGCCACGTTCGGGCAA -3') 141 (5'- TCATCGCACCGTCAAAGGAACC -3')	94°C 1min, 30°cycles 94°C 30s, 64 C 30s, 72°C 1min, final extension 5 min at 72°C.

RESULTS AND DISCUSSION

Phenolics Compunds

Results of present study reported that the concentration of total phenolic compounds in the essential oil of oregano is 785.92 mg GAE/g. While in USDA database reported the total phenolic content of this herb at 3789 mg GAE per 100 g product (Haytowitz & Bhagwat, 2010). Skendi, Irakli & Chatzopoulou (2017) reported a value of 5500 mg GAE per 100 g oregano. The differences between this study and found previous references is due to that the levels in essential oil are very low, and are not comparable to what is normally found in plant extracts of e.g., rosemary extract as would be expected. Jongberg et al., (2012) reported that phenolic compounds are hydrophilic and scacerly soluble in essential oils.

The main compounds identified in the different essential oil of Origanum (OEO) are carvacrol and thymol, which are responsible for the characteristic odour and the antimicrobial and antioxidant activity. Previous reports from different oregano species have shown that the most common flavonoids found in oregano are flavones, flavonols, flavanones and flavanols. Such as the study reported by Skendi, Irakli & Chatzopoulou (2017) that analysed the phenolic content in *Origanum vulgare ssp hirtum* L. and detected phenolic acids and their derivatives, flavonoids and monoterpenes, specifically the most abundant compounds were naringenin, rutin, carvacrol, kaempferol, rosmarinic acid, caffeic acid, luteolin, epigallocatechine and epicatechin. Specifically, regarding oregano essential oil, Asensio et al., (2015) studied the composition of four oregano-types from Argentina, and showed that they are rich in diterpenoids, triterpenoids, sesquiterpenoids, being trans-sabinene hydrate the most abundant compound in the essential oils (Asensio et al., 2015).

The different composition between different authors is due to the variability between different oregano species, because the concentration of phenolic compounds in oregano depends on several factors like temperature, geographical localization, weather, soil conditions, harvesting time, water, among others and also depend on the oregano chemotypes within the same species (Croteau, Kutchan & Lewis, 2015). Moreover, different results also depend on the different solvent extraction used; there are different species of oregano and different solvent extraction that produces different profile of bioactive compounds.

Fenton Reaction Model System with ESR Detection of POBN Spin Adducts

The Fenton model system used to assess the protective properties of plant extracts (including also adverse prooxidative effects) is based on the basic Fenton assay. Antioxidative potential of oregano eesential oil was quantified by indirectly measuring their ability to scavenge 1-hydroxyethyl radicals ($CH_3 \cdot CHOH$), which result from the interaction of ethanol with the highly reactive hydroxyl radical ($\cdot OH$) generated by Fenton chemistry. The $CH_3 \cdot CHOH$ species was trapped by POBN producing a spin adduct, the formation was monitored using ESR spectroscopy. Antioxidants, present after the addition of small amounts of plant extracts to the Fenton mixture, compete for $CH_3 \cdot CHOH$ and $\cdot OH$, and the level of detectable POBN spin adducts decreases according to the radical scavenging activity of the different extracts.

Antioxidants added in small amounts to the Fenton mixture compete for CH_3-CHOH and -OH, therefore the detectable levels of spin POBN adducts decrease in accordance with the capacity of the antioxidants components to capture the radicals (Figure 1). In this sense, the intensity of the signal corresponding to the spin adducts POBN is proportional to the concentration of formed radicals. Figure 1 shows that the oregano essential oil reduces the formation of spin adducts at a concentration <12 mg GAE/L, however, from this concentration the effect is the opposite, increasing the formation of spin adducts and causing an effect prooxidant A maximum intensity of spin adducts formation of 140% is observed at a concentration of 13 mg GAE/L of essential oil (Figure 1). The results show that oregano essential oil can have prooxidant effects in systems that contain small amounts of iron (II). This effect is likely to be caused by the ability of the flavonoids to reduce Fe^3 + to Fe^2 + (Rødtjer et al., 2006), thus increasing the formation of hydroxyl radicals by the Fenton reaction.

The antioxidant properties of oregano have been extensively documented *in vivo* and *in vitro*. Since the antioxidant mechanisms of oregano essential oils is based on its ability to donate a hydrogen, to quench free radicals by donation of an electron and its ability to delocalize the unpaired electron within the aromatic structure of the phenolic constituents (Fernández-Pachón et al., 2008).

The antioxidative activity of plant extracts is commonly ascribed to their radical scavenging and to metal-ion chelation, and the antioxidant activity of essential oils has mainly been ascribed to their reducing properties playing important roles in scavenging radicals or decomposing peroxides (Brewer, 2011). Chelation of prooxidative transition metal ions is consideredless important, as metal chelating activity requires the presence of vicinal OH-groups absent in most terpenes to coordinate the metal ions (Perron & Brumaghim, 2009).

These compounds can donate hydrogen atoms to free radicals and convert them to more stable non-radical products. The antioxidant effect is the result of various possible mechanisms of action involving transition-metal chelating activity, singlet-oxygen-quenching capacity, and free-radical scavenging activity.

As can be observed in Figure 1, the total phenolics in essential of oregano, expressed as mg gallic acid equivalents (GAE) per L, determined according to the Folin-Ciocalteu method and evaluated using ESR acting as prooxidant is 12 mg gallic acid equivalents (GAE) per L.

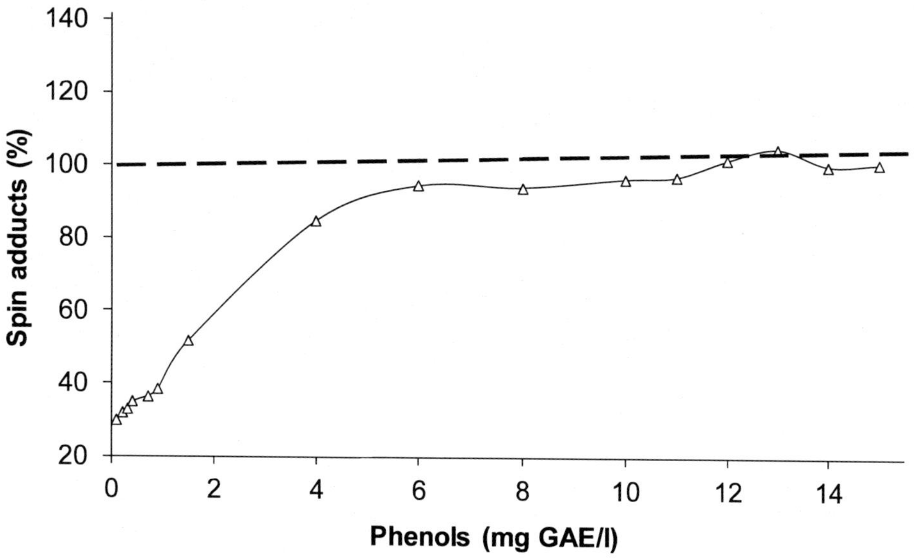

Figure 1. The effects of oregano essential oils on the formation of POBN spin adducts in the Fenton assay. The level of spin adducts formed in a control experiment without addition of oregano essential oil are equal to 100%.

This prooxidant effect has been previously shown in the Fenton reaction with natural extracts such garlic added in pressurized chicken meat and subsequently packed in freezing (Mariutti et al., 2008), distilled leaf of rosemary and thyme (Nieto et al., 2011), cherry pulp (Rødtjer et al., 2006), with a secondary metabolite of terpenoid origin from Olea europea, such as oleuropein (Mazziotti et al., 2006), with and with. In this sense, Cao et al., (1997) used the ORAC measure to conclude that flavonoids can change from antioxidants to pro-oxidants depending on the concentration. Therefore, oregano essential oil properties vary depending on the concentration. Therefore, the potential prooxidant properties of the essential oil suggest that precautions must be taken prior to its use as an antioxidant in foods.

Generation of Radicals during the Storage of Meat

After studying the properties of the essential oil in a model system, this section studies the behavior of the essential oil added in pork burgers packed in aerobic conditions for 9 days.

PBN adducts-spin formation occurs by the addition of radical species to the PBN molecule at the carbon of the alpha position attached to the nitronil group. Figure 2 shows as expected, that during the heating of the burgers with PBN the formation of free radicals takes place, which react with radicals forming spin adducts, which can be detected by REE, since they accumulate at a detectable concentration and in different measure depending on the sample: greater number of free radicals in C, followed by O_1 and finally lower level in O_2. The nature of the radicals trapped by the PBN is a subject still under study, since different radicals involved in lipid oxidation are indirectly detected by electronic spin resonance with PBN (Andersen et al. 2005).

The spin REE method used in this work detects the amount of radicals formed during 3 h of meat incubation; therefore, it provides a measure of the oxidative damage of the system. In order to explore the main mechanism of oxidation in the burgers and the supposed protection by the addition of the oregano essential oil, the formation of radicals was monitored during the storage at 4°C for 9 days of the samples C, O_1 and O_2.

Figure 2 shows that the different concentration levels of lipid radicals obtained from day 1 of storage indicated that the heating increased the oxidation to a different extent depending on the addition of the essential oil and the oil concentration, being higher in C and showing significant differences ($P < 0.05$) between C, O_1 and O_2.

On the other hand, on day 9 of storage, the levels of radicals decreased in O_1 burgers. The explanation for this effect is because when increasing the storage period, the concentration of radicals is lower at day 3 and 6 than at day 0, because the samples have less fresh lipids to feed the oxidation cycle and therefore, have less tendency to form radicals.

Regarding the effect of the addition of oregano essential oil, Figure 2 shows that the relative concentration of radicals is significant ($P < 0.05$) higher in control meat and in O1 and O2, showing significant differences between C, O1 and O2 throughout storage. It is interesting to note the low tendency to form radicals of samples O2, showing an antioxidant effect that dependent of the dose. Effect previously shown by Yang et al., (1993), who observed that the antioxidant activity of several garlic compounds and garlic extracts was dose dependent.

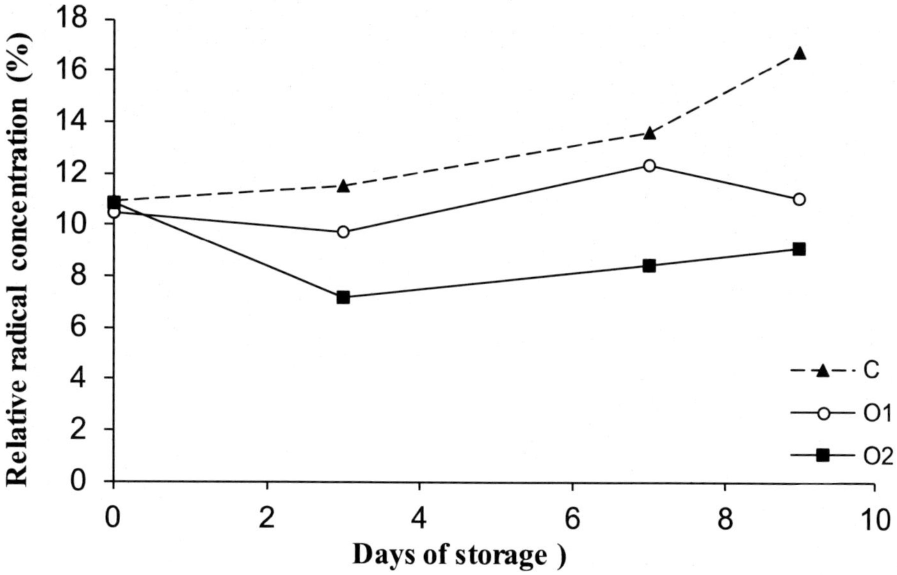

Figura 2. Relative radical concentration in burguers Control (C), O_1 (0,04% oregano essential oil) y O_2 (0,5% oregano esential oil) evaluated by ESR.

Focusing on published works with meat, several studies have shown the effect of oregano in preventing oxidation in meat. For example, Nieto et al., (2013) reported that 0.05 - 0.4% oregano essential oil reduced protein oxidation in pork patties for 12 days at 4 °C. Shange et al., (2019) reported that 1% oregano essential oil reduced lipid oxidation in black wildebeest meat storaged for 9 days at 3°C.

Other studies showed the diferent form application of oregano, such as its inclusión into packaging film. Paparella et al., (2016) studied the incorporation of 4% oregano essential oil in combination of chitosan based film and Oussalah et al., (2004) studied the oregano essential oil incorporation in bioactive packaging systems.

Antimicrobial Activity

The antimicrobial effects of oregano *essential oil* at 0.05 and 0.4%, on *Salmonella spp.* in pork burgers during storage at 4°C, are shown in Table 2. The initial populations of *Salmonella* spp. (2.55 log cfu/g) in control samples (*C*) were increased ($P < 0.05$) and reached a value of 2.70 log cfu/g by the end of storage. In contrast, the populations of *Salmonella* spp. in *EO*s samples at the two levels (R_1, O_1 and R_2, O_2) were decreased during the storage.

Table 2. Average total viable count of *Salmonella* spp. in burgers made with two levels of rosemary and oregano essential oils (Level 1: $O_1 = 0.05\%$ *EOs*), and (Level 2: $O_2 = 0.4\%$ *EOs*) at 0, 3, 6 and 9 days under retail conditions

		Day 0	Day 3	Day 6	Day 9
O	C	2.57 ± 0.05	2.48 ± 0.21[a]	2.57 ± 0.14[a]	2.60 ± 0.21[a]
	O_1	2.50 ± 0.09	2.51 ± 0.24[a]	2.44 ± 0.05[a]	2.40 ± 0.12[a]
	O_2	2.55 ± 0.15	2.37 ± 0.15[b]	1.98 ± 0.01[b]	1.79 ± 0.19[b]

M ± SD: mean ± standard deviation. C: control.

[a, b, c:] different letters within a same column (different EOs treatment) differ significantly (P < 0.05).

The addition of oregano essential oils at 0.05% in minced pork meat did not show any antibacterial activity against Salmonella. Treatment of pork burger meat with oregano *EO* at 0.4% showed lower antimicrobial ($P < 0.05$) activity against *Salmonella* than those of the treatments rosemary *EO* at 0.4% from day 3 of storage at 4°. Among the examined treatments, the addition of oregano *EO* at 0.4% proved the most efficient treatments to control *Salmonella* in minced pork meat. The level 0.4% of the essential oils studied showed a bactericidal effect against the pathogen.

This effect was dose dependent, and the higher level of essential oils showed a greater effect (P < 0.05) anti-pathogen. Among the examinated treatments, O at 0.4% proved the most efficient treatments to control Salmonella in pork burgers, since it showed a bacteriostatic effect against the pathogen. The results pointed to the possibility of using essentials oil of oregano at 0.4% to preserve raw meat products.

In the same line that our results, the antibacterial activity of oregano *EO* against *Salmonella* was previously found in vitro experiments or in other food tests. In vitro experiments, the inhibitory activity of the oregano *EO* against *Salmonella* was proved by using the disc diffusion method (Chorianopoulos et al., 2004) or on agar plates (Seydim et al., 2006) at various concentrations (0.2% to 4%). Peñalver et al., (2005) used the broth microdilution method and estimated that the MIC (minimum inhibitory activity) of oregano *EO* against *S. Enteritidis* was 0.25% (v/v).

And the study of Koutsoumanis et al., (1999) whose showed that the addition of oregano essential oil to taramasalad resulted in a decline in the number of *S. enteritidis* cells immediately after inoculation with increased death rate. According to our results, a reduction of *Salmonella* was observed and its death rate depended on the pH, the storage temperature and the essential oil concentration.

The antimicrobial effect of oregano essential oil shown in this study is due to the compounds presents in the oil. Between the 32 components in the essential oil of oregano, representing 89.5% of the total, the major components of oregano essential oil are carvacrol (61.21%), p-cymene (15.12%) and γ-terpinene (4.80%), terpinolene (3.63%), β-caryophillene (2.62%) and α-terpinene (2.34%). (Viuda-Martos et al., 2007).

Furthermore, antimicrobial activities of the *EOs* are difficult to correlate to a specific compound due to their complexity and variability. Nevertheless, some researchers reported that there is a relationship between the chemical composition of the most abundant components in the *EOs* and the antimicrobial activity (Farag et al., 1989). For example, α/β-pinene (monoterpene hydrocarbons abundant in *O EO*) is well-known chemicals having antimicrobial potentials (Pattnaik et al., 1997). On the other hand, based on a report, α/β-pinene (monoterpene hydrocarbons abundant in *O EO*) had slight activity against a panel of microorganisms. As a result of these findings, the higher antimicrobial activities of oregano *EO* could be attributed to its particular chemotype characterised by its complexity with oxygenated-hydrocarbons as dominant components and the presence of equivalent amounts of monoterpene hydrocarbons and sesquiterpene hydrocarbons.

Moreover, many reports mentioned that carvacrol and their precursors (p-cymene and γ-terpinene) are biologically and functionally closely associated (Ultee et al., 2002). In that context, p-cymene was abundant in the *EO* of *O* (15.12%). Meanwhile, oregano essential oil contains a moderately higher level of γ-terpinene (4.80% and 0.18%, respectively).

Previous study by Hulankova, Borilova & Steinhauserova (2013) reported that 0.2% oregano essential oil exhibited antimicrobial activity in miced beef inoculated with *Listeria monocytogenes* for 10 days at 3ºC, while colour and sensory quality were maintained.

Regarding the PCR analysis, all the colonies of *Salmonella spp.* isolates were confirmed by the Salmonella-specific PCR-based methodology. The primer set used for specific amplification of Salmonella genomic DNA fragments has been previously published (Rahn et al., 1992). For positive samples, an amplified fragment of 284 bp of *invA* gene was clearly visualized in a horizontal agarose gel electrophoresis stained with ethidium bromide.

CONCLUSION

This study showed that essential oil of common food spices, particularly oregano at 0.4% are capable inhibiting pathogenetic microorganism in pork burgers. In contrast, the addition of essential oils at 0.05% did not show any antibacterial activity against *Salmonella*. Of the various essential levels, the 0.4% of oregano was of particular promise as it exhibited strong effects against *Salmonella*.

Electronic spin resonance has proven to be a simple technique to study the antioxidant and prooxidant activity of oregano essential oil, establishing the concentration of phenolic compounds with prooxidant activity of oregano essential oil in a value greater than or equal to 12 mg GAE/L of essential oil.

In the pork burgers analyzed, the essential oil of oregano added to 0.4% and 0.05% exerted antioxidant action. Taking into account the results obtained of antibacterial and antioxidant activity, the incorporation of oregano essential oil in 0.05% could be considered as natural antioxidant and antimicrobial in pork burgers and a safe alternative to standard synthetic products.

Therefore, the addition of oregano essential in meat processing is a strategy that incorporates natural antioxidants to enhance the nutritional and health benefits of meat; and the application of essential oil to eliminate or minimize the formation of carcinogens for chemical safety of cooked and processed meats.

References

Adame-Gallegos, J. R., Andrade-Ochoa, S., Nevarez-Moorillon, G. V. (2016). Potential use of Mexicano regano essential oil against parasite, fungal and bacterial pathogens. *Journal of essential oil bearing plants, 19:* 553-567.

Aherne, S., Kerry, J., O'Brien, N. (2007). Effects of plant extracts on antioxidant status and oxidant-induced stress in Caco-2 cells. *Brithis Journal of Nutrition, 97:* 321-328.

Ahmad Shah, M., Don Bosco, S. J., Ahmad Mir, S. (2014). Plant extracts as natural antioxidants in meat and meat products. *Meat Science, 98(1):* 21-33.

Almeida, A. P., Rodríguez-Rojo, S., Serra, A. T., Vila-Real, H., Simplicio, A. L., Delgadilho, I., da Costa, S. B., da Costa, L. B., Nogueira, I. D., Duarte, C. M. M. (2013). Microencapsulation of oregano essential oil in starch-based materials using supercritical fluid technology. *Innovative food science & emerging technologies, 20:* 140-145.

Alves-Silva, J. M., Zuzarte, M., Marques, C., Salgueiro, L., Guirão, H. (2016). Protective effects of terpenes on the cardiovascular system: current advances and future perspectives. *Current medicinal chemistry, 23:* 4559-4600.

Andersen, M. L., Velasco, J., Skibsted, L. H. 2005. Analysis of lipid oxida¬tion by ESR spectroscopy. In Kamal-Eldin A, Pokorny J (eds) Analysis of lipid oxida¬tion. American Oil Chemists' Society Press, Illinois 2005, p127-151.

Aguirrezábal, M. M., Mateo, J., Domínguez, M. C., Zumalacárregui, J. M. 2000. The effect of paprika, garlic and salt on rancidity in dry sausages. Meat Sci. 54(1): 77-81.

Aruoma, O. I., Halliwell, B., Williamsom, G. (1997). *In vitro* methods for characterizing potential prooxidant and antioxidant actions of nonnutritive substances in plant foods. In *Antioxidant Methodology*; Aruoma, O. I., Cuppett, S. I., Eds.; AOCS Press: Champaign, IL.173-204.

Asensio, C. M., Grosso, N. R., Juliani, H. R. (2015). Quality characters, chemical composition and biological activities of oregano (Origanum spp.) essential oils from central and southern Argentina. Industrial crops and products, 63: 203-213.

Balusamy, S. R., Perumalsamy, H., Huq, Md. A., Balasubramanian, B. (2018). Anti-proliferative activity of *Origanum vulgare* inhibited lipogenesis and induced mitocondrial mediated apoptosis in human stomach cancer cell lines. *Biomedicine & pharmacotherapy, 108:* 1835-1844.

Bhargava, K., Conti, D. S., da Rocha, S. R., & Zhang, Y. (2015). Application of an oregano oil nanoemulsion to the control of foodborne bacteria on fresh lettuce. Food Microbiology, 47, 69–73.

Begnini, K. R., Nedel, F., Lund, R. G., Carvalho, P. H. D., Rodrigues, M. R. A., Beira, F. T. A., Del Pino, F. A. B. (2014). Composition and antiproliferative effect of essential oil of *Origanum vulgare* against tumor cell lines. *Journal of medicinal food, 17:* 1129-1133.

Bolumar, T., Anedersen, M. L., Orlien, V. (2011). Antioxidant active packaging for chicken meat processed by high pressure treatment. Food Chemistry, 129: 1406-1412.

Catarino, M. D., Alves-Silva, J. M., Fernandes, R. P., Gonçalves, M. J., Salgueiro, L. R., Henriques, M. F., Cardoso, S. M. (2017). Development and performance of whey protein active coatings with *Origanum virens* essential oils in the quality and shelf life improvement of processed meat products. *Food control, 80:* 273-280.

Carlsen, C. U., Rasmussen, K. T., Kjeldsen, K. K., Westergaard, P., Skibsted, L. H. (2003). *European Food Research Technology*. 217: 195-200.

Chang, T. W. & Pan, A. Y. (2008). Chapter 2: Cumulative Environmental Changes, Skewed Antigen Exposure and the Increase of Allergy. In: *Advances in Inmunology*, 98, 39-83.

Chang, Y., McLandsborough, L., & McClements, D. J. (2012). Physical properties and antimicrobial efficacy of thyme oil nanoemulsions: Influence of ripening inhibitors. *Journal of Agricultural and Food Chemistry*, 60(48), 12056–12063.

Chouliara, E., Karatapanis, A., Savaidis, I. N., Kontominas, M. G. (2007). Combined effect of oregano essential oil and modified atmosphere packaging on shelf life extensión of fresh chicken breast meat, stored at 4ºC. *Food microbiology, 24:* 607-617.

Clough, S. R. (2014). Sodium Sulfite. Reference Module in Biomedical Sciences. In: Encyclopedia of Toxicology (3ª Edition), 341-343.

Costa-Menezes, N. M., Figueiredo-Martins, W., Angelo-Longui, D., Falcão-de Aragão, G. M. (2018). Modeling the effect of oregano essential oil on shelf-life extensión of vacuum-packed cooked sliced ham. *Meat science, 139:* 113-119.

Croteau, R., Kutchan, I. M., Lewis, N. G. (2015). Natural products (secondary metabolites). In: Buchanan, B., Gruissem, W., Jones, R. (2015). *Biochemistry & Molecular Biology of Plants*. Eds: American Society of Plants, Rockville, MD, USA: 1250-1318.

Dantas, B. P. V., Alves, Q. L., de Assis, K. S., Ribeiro, T. P., de Almeida, M. M., de Vasconcelos, A. P., de Araújo, D. A. M., de Andrade Braga, V., de Medeiros, I. A., Alencar, J. L. et al., (2015). Participation of the trp channel in the cardiovascular effects induced by carvacrol in normotensive rat. *Vascular pharmacology, 67-69:* 48-58.

Desvasagayam, T. P. A., Tilka, J. C., Boloor, K. K., Sane, K. S., Ghaskadb, I., Lele, R. D. (2004). Free radicals and antioxidants in human health: current status and future prospects. *Journal of the Association of Physicians of India, 52:* 794-804.

Dorman, H. J.; Deans, S. G. Antimicrobial agents from plants: Antibacterial activity of plant volatile oils. *J. Appl. Microbiol.* 2000, 88, 308–316.

Dutra, T. V., Castro, J. C., Menezes, J. L., Ramos, T. R., do Prado, I. N., Junior, M. M., Mikcha, J. M. G., de Abreu Filho, B. A. (2019). Bioactivity of oregano (*Origanum vulgare*) essential oil against *Alicyclobacillus* spp. *Industrial crops & products, 129:* 345-349.

Emiroğlu, Z. K., Yemiş, G. P., Coşkun, B. K, Candoğan, K. (2010). Antimicrobial activity of soy edible films incorporated with thyme and oregano essential oils on fresh ground beef patties. *Meat science, 86:* 283-288.

Estévez, M. (2011). Protein carbonyls in meat systems: a review. *Meat Science, 89(3),* 259-279. DOI: 10.1016/j.meatsci.2011.04.025.

Farag RS, Daw ZY, Hewedi FM, El-Baroty GSA (1989) Antimicrobial activity of some Egyptian spice essential oils. *Journal of Food Protect* 52 (9): 665–667.

Fernandes, R. P. P., Trindade, M. A., Lorenzo, J. M., de Melo, M. P. (2018). Assessment of the stability of sheep sausages with the addition of different concentrations of *Origanum vulgare* extract during storage. *Meat science, 137:* 244-257.

Fernandes, R. P. P., Trindade, M. A., Tonin, F. G., Pugine, S. M. P., Lima, C. G., Lorenzo, J. M., de Melo, M. P. (2017). Evaluation of oxidative stability of lamb burger with *Origanum vulgare* extract. *Food chemistry, 233:* 101-109.

Fasseas, M. K., Mountzouris, K. C., Tarantilis, P. A., Polissiou, M., Zervas, G. (2007). Antioxidant activity in meat treated with oregano and sage essential oils. *Food Chemistry, 106:* 1188-1194.

Fernandes, R. P. P., Trindade, M. A., Lorenzo, J. M., de Melo, M. P. (2018). Assessment of the stability of sheep sausages with the addition of different concentrations of *Origanum vulgare* extract during storage. *Meat science, 137:* 244-257.

Fernandes, R. P. P., Trindade, M. A., Tonin, F. G., Pugine, S. M. P., Lima, C. G., Lorenzo, J. M., de Melo, M. P. (2017). Evaluation of oxidative stability of lamb burger with *Origanum vulgare* extract. *Food chemistry, 233:* 101-109.

Fernández-Pachón, M. S., Villano, D., Troncoso, A. M., García-Parrilla, M. C. (2008). Antioxidant activity of phenolic compounds: from in vitro results to in vivo evidence. *Critical Reviews in Food Science and Nutrition, 48(7):* 649-671.

Fernández-Pan, I., Mendoza, M., Maté, J. I. (2013). Whey protein isolate edible films with essential oils incorporated to improve the microbial quality of poultry. *Journal of the science of food and agriculture, 93(12):* 2986-2994.

Ferreira, J., Alves, D., Neves, O., Silva, J., Gibbs, P., & Teixeira, P. (2010). Effects of the components of two antimicrobial emulsions on food-borne pathogens. *Food Control,* 21(3), 227–230.

Giatrakou, V., Ntzimani, A., & Savvaidis, I. (2010). Effect of chitosan and thyme oil on a ready to cook chicken product. *Food Microbiology*, 27(1), 132–136.

Gonçalves, S., Moreira, E., Grosso, C., Andrade, P. B., Valentão, P., Romano, A. (2017). Phenolic profile, antioxidant activity and enzyme inhibitory activities of extracts from aromatic plants used in mediterranean diet. *Journal of Food Science and Technology, 54:* 219–227.

Govaris, A., Solomakos, N., Pexara, A., Charzopoulou, P. S. (2010) The antimicrobial effect of oregano essential oil, nisin and their combination against *Salmonella enteritidis* in minced sheep meat during refrigerated storage. *International journal of food microbiology, 137:* 175-180.

Gutiérrez-Grijalva, E. P., Antunes-Ricardo, M., Acosta-Estrada, B. A., Gutiérrez-Uribe, J. A., Heredia, J. B. (2019). Cellular antioxidant activity and *in vitro* inhibition of α-glucosidase, αamylase and pancreatic lipase of oregano polyphenols under simulated gastrointestinal digestion. *Food research international, 116:* 676-686.

Gutiérrez-Grijalva, E. P., Picos-Salas, M. A., Leyva-López, N., Criollo-Mendoza, M. S., Vazquez-Olivo, G., Heredia, J. B. (2017). Flavonoids and phenolic acids from oregano: occurrence, biological activity and health benefits. Review. Plants, 7(2). doi: 10.3390/plants7010002.

Ghosh, V., Mukherjee, A., & Chandrasekaran, N. (2013). Formulation and characterization of plant essential oil based nanoemulsion: Evaluation of its larvicidal activity against Aedes aegypti. Asian Journal of Chemistry, 25(Supplementary Issue), S321.

Hammer, K. A.; Carson, C. F.; Riley, T. V. Antimicrobial activity of essential oils and other plant extracts. *J. Appl. Microbiol.* 1999, 86, 985–990.

Haytowitz, D. B. & Bhagwat, S. (2010). USDA Database for the Oxygen Radical Absorbance Capacity (ORAC) of Selected Foods, Release 2. U.S. Department of Agriculture (USDA), Maryland, USA.

Hulankova, R., Borilova, G., Steinhauserova, I. (2013). Combined antimicrobial effect of oregano essential oil and caprylic acid in miced beef. *Meat science, 95:* 190-194.

Jongberg, S., Lund, M. N., Østdal, H., & Skibsted, L. H. (2012). Phenolic antioxidant scavengingof myosin radicals generated by hypervalent myoglobin. *Journal of Agricultural and Food Chemistry*, 60, 12020–12028.

Koutsoumanis, K., Lambropoulou, K., & Nychas, G. J. F. (1999). A predictive model for the non-thermal inactivation of Salmonella Enteritidis in a food model system supplemented with a natural antimicrobial. *International Journal of Food Microbiology*, 49, 63–74.

Leyva-López, N., Nair, V., Bang, W. Y., Cisneros-Zevallos, L., Heredia, J. B. (2016). Protective role of terpenes and polyphenols from three species of oregano (Lippia graveolens, Lippia palmeri and Hedeoma patens) on the suppression of lipopolysaccharide-induced inflammation in RAW 264.7 macrophage cells. *Journal of Ethnopharmacology*, 187: 302–312.

Liang, R., Xu, S., Shoemaker, C. F., Li, Y., Zhong, F., & Huang, Q. (2012). Physical and antimicrobial properties of peppermint oil nanoemulsions. *Journal of Agricultural and Food Chemistry*, 60(30), 7548–7555.

Mariutti, L. R. R., Orlien, V., Bragagnolo, N., Skibsted, L. H. (2008). Effect of sage and garlic on lipid oxidation in high-pressure processed chicken meat. *European Food Research and Technology*. 227: 337-344.

Monahan, FJ., Grat, JI., Asghar, A., Haug, A., Shi, B., Buckley, DJ. (1993). Effect of dietary lipid and vitamin E supplementation on free radical production and lipid oxidation in porcine muscle microsomal fractions. *Food Chem*. 46:1-6.

Nieto, G., Jongberg, S., Andersen, M. L., Skibsted, L. H. (2013). Thiol oxidation and protein cross-link formation during chill storage of pork patties added essential oil of oregano, rosemary, or garlic. *Meat Science*, 95(2), 177-18.

Nieto, G., Huvaere, K., Skibsted, L. H. 2011. Antioxidant activity of rosemary and thyme by-products and synergism with added antioxidant in a liposome system. *European Food Research and Technology*. 233: 11-18.

Nieto, G., Díaz, P., Bañón, S., Garrido, M. D. (2010). Dietary administration of ewe diets with a distillate from rosemary leaves (Rosmarinus o_cinalis L.): Influence on lamb meat quality. *Meat Science*, 84, 23–29.

Nieto, G., Bañon, S., Garrido, M. D. (2011). Effect of supplementing ewes'diet with thyme (Thymus zygis ssp. Gracilis) leaves on the lipid oxidation of cooked lamb meat. *Food Chemistry*, 125, 1147–1152.

Oussalah, M., Caillet, S., Salmiéri, S., Saucier, L., Lacroix, M. (2004). Antimicrobial and antioxidant effects of milk protein-based film containing essential oils for the preservation of whole beef muscle. *Journal of agricultural and food chemistry*, 52(18): 5598-5605.

Paparella, A., Mazzarino, G., Chaves-López, C., Rossi, C., Sacchetti, G., Guerrieri, O., Serio, A. (2016). Chitosan boosts the antimicrobial activity of Origanum vulgare essential oil modified atmosphere packaged pork. *Food microbiology*, 59: 23-31.

Peñalver P, Huerta B, Borge C, Astorga R, Romero R, Perea A. (2005) Antimicrobial activity of five essential oils against origin strains of the Enterobacteriaceae family. *Acta Pathol Microbiol Immunol Scand* 113: 1–6.

Pattnaik S, Subramanyam VR, Bapaji M, Kole CR. (1997) Antibacterial and antifungal activity of aromatic constituents of essentials oils. *Microbios* 89: 39–46.

Rahn K, Grandis SA, Clarke RC, McEwen SA, Galan JE, Ginocchio C, Curtiss R, Gyles CL. (1992) Amplification of an invA gene sequence of Salmonella typhimurium by polymerase chain reaction as a specific method of detection of Salmonella. *Mol Cell Probes* 6: 271– 279.

Rødtjer, A., Skibsted, L. H., Anderesen, M. L. 2006. Antioxidative and prooxidative effects of extracts made from cherry liqueur pomace. *Food Chemistry*, 99: 6-14.

Seydim AC, Sarikus G. (2006) Antimicrobial activity of whey protein based edible films incorporated with oregano, rosemary and garlic essential oils. *Food Research International*, 39:639–644.

Shange, N., Makasi, T., Gouws, P., Hoffman, L. C. (2019). Preeservation of previously frozen black wildebeest meat (Connochaetes gnou) using oregano (Oreganum vulgare) essential oil. *Meat science*, 148: 88-95.

Skendi, A., Irakli, M., Chatzopoulou, P. (2017). Analysis of phenolic compounds in Greek plants of Lamiaceae family by HPLC. *Journal of applied research on medicinal and aromatic plants*, 6: 62-69.

Thomsen, MK., Jacobsen, C., Skibsted, L. H. (2000). Mechanism of initiation of oxidation in mayonnaise enriched with fish oil as studied by electron spin resonance spectroscopy. *European Food Research and Technology*. 211: 381-386.

Ultee A, Bennink MHJ, Moezelaar R. (2002). The phenolic hydroxyl group of carvacrol is essential for action against the foodborne pathogen Bacillus cereus. *Appl Environ Microbiol* 68 (4): 1561–1568.

Viuda-Martos M, Ruíz-Navajas Y, Fernández-López J, Pérez-Álvarez JA. (2007) Chemical composition of the essential oil obtained from some spices widely used in Mediterranean region. *Acta Chim. Slov* 54:921–926.

Velasco, J., Andersen, ML., Skibsted, L. H. (2004). Evaluation of oxidative stability of vegetable oils by monitoring the tendency to radical formation. A comparison of electron spin resonance spectroscopy with the rancimat method and differential scanning calorimetry. *Food Chemistry*. 85: 623-632.

Yang, G. C., Yasaei, P. M., Page, S. W. 1993. Garlic as antioxidants and free radical scavengers. *J Food Drug Anal*. 1(4): 357-364.

EDITOR'S CONTACT INFORMATION

Gema Nieto
Department of Food Technology, Food Science and Nutrition,
Faculty of Veterinary Sciences, Regional
Campus of International Excellence "Campus Mare Nostrum",
Espinardo, Murcia, Spain
gnieto@um.es

INDEX

I

L

M

N

O

P

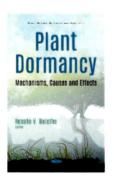

Related Nova Publications

Micropropagation: Methods and Effects

Editor: Valdir M. Stefenon, Ph.D.

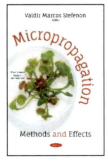

Series: Plant Science Research and Practices

Book Description: In *Micropropagation: Methods and Effects,* the authors aimed to shortly present some of these advances, as well as practical results of using this biotechnology towards the conservation of plant genetic resources.

Softcover ISBN: 978-1-53614-968-5
Retail Price: $82

Germination: Types, Process and Effects

Editors: Rosalva Mora-Escobedo, PhD, Cristina Martinez, and Rosalía Reynoso

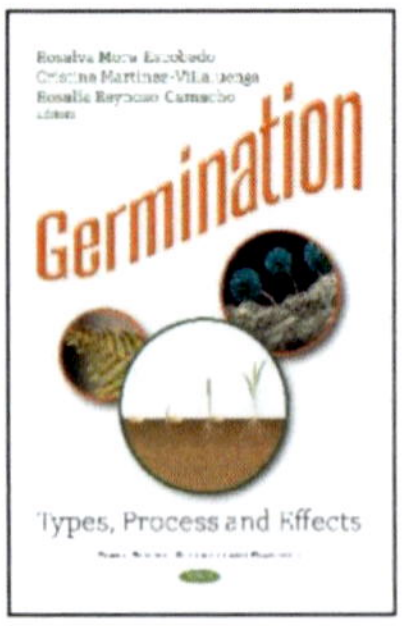

Series: Plant Science Research and Practices

Book Description: *Germination: Types, Process and Effects* is a book that brings together the contribution of new and relevant information from many experts in the fields of food and biological sciences, nutrition, and food engineering, to provide the reader with the latest information of fundamental and applied research in the role of edible seeds and discuss the benefits of consuming them.

Hardcover ISBN: 978-1-53615-973-8
Retail Price: $230

To see a complete list of Nova publications, please visit our website at www.novapublishers.com